EATING DISORDERS IN ADULT WOMEN

EATING DISORDERS IN ADULT WOMEN

JULIAN N. FUCHS
EDITOR

Nova Science Publishers, Inc.
New York

For permission to use material from this book please contact us:
Telephone 631-231-7269; Fax 631-231-8175
Web Site: http://www.novapublishers.com

Library of Congress Cataloging-in-Publication Data

Eating disorders in adult women / Julian N. Fuchs (editor).

p. ; cm.

Includes bibliographical references and index.

ISBN 978-1-60456-673-4 (hardcover)

1. Eating disorders in women. I. Fuchs, Julian N.

[DNLM: 1. Eating Disorders--psychology. 2. Adult. 3. Women. WM 175 E14735 2008]

RC552.E18 E2821145

616.85'260082--dc22 2008014995

Published by Nova Science Publishers, Inc. ≈ New York

CONTENTS

PREFACE

Recent decades have seen a rise in the prevalence of eating disorders, especially among adult women. The etiology and development of these disorders involve numerous biological, psychological, and familial factors that extend beyond adolescence into emerging adulthood. This new book provides leading research in this field.

Chapter 1 - Recent decades have seen a rise in the prevalence of eating disorders, especially among emerging adult women. The etiology and development of these disorders involve numerous biological, psychological, and familial factors that extend beyond adolescence into emerging adulthood. More recently, scholarship by communication researchers adds to existing research to reveal knowledge linking psychological factors, parent-child communication, and disordered eating behaviors. In this chapter the authors review scholarship on parent-child communication and disordered eating and provide empirical data from a study of 273 emerging adults revealing a significant relationship between parent-emerging adult child communication and disordered eating. Highlights of the chapter include a review of relevant communication research as it relates to health behaviors and a presentation of findings from an empirical study examining connections amongst parent-emerging adult child communication, psychological and interpersonal dimensions of self differentiation, and disordered eating. This chapter argues for the importance of studying communication processes when trying to understand the etiology of disordered eating. Information about how parent-child communication patterns affect offspring's eating behavior may allow for earlier detection of disorders and enhance prevention efforts.

Chapter 2 - Objective: Study aims were to develop an instrument to assess a proposed construct, "dysregulated eating," and investigate its association with potential risk factors. Method: A scale measuring dysregulated eating was developed and validated in a convenience sample of graduate students (n=186). Covariates hypothesized to be associated with dysregulated eating were investigated with multiple linear regression. Results: Factor analysis supported two latent constructs underlying dysregulated eating, which were glossed as schedule-constrained eating and distraction-related eating. Cronbach's coefficient alphas were >.7 for the overall scale and two subscales. In a fully adjusted multivariable linear regression model, female gender, frequent caffeine consumption, higher perceived stress, inadequate sleep, and high fast food consumption were significant predictors of a higher mean scale score. The model adjusted R2 was 0.48. Discussion: This scale appears to have acceptable internal consistency reliability and construct validity in a graduate student population. A multivariable linear regression model suggests modifiable risk factors for dysregulated eating.

Chapter 3 - In the last twenty years a lot has been written about eating disorders (EDs). The spreading of these disorders, which grew remarkably until ten years ago, seems to have become steady today, with percentages ranging between 0.2-1% for anorexia nervosa (AN) and 1-3% for bulimia nervosa (BN) in samples of adolescent women in western countries.

The stabilisation of complete clinical syndromes was associated with an increase in subthreshold diagnoses, called partial or subclinical EDs, that is conditions which, while displaying the psycho-pathological aspects typical of eating disorders (intense fear of gaining weight, self-esteem entirely dependent on physical appearance and body weight), do not reach such levels of clinical severity as to meet all the criteria established by the DSM-IV for an ED to be diagnosed. A research carried out on a sample of 788 adolescents aged between 12 and 14 showed that 9.4% of the subjects met the criteria for a partial diagnosis of ED. In the study carried out by Cotrufo et al. (1998) the subthreshold ED diagnosis concerned 10.7% of the female students aged between 14 and 19. Largely consistent results have been obtained by several authors who have studied partial syndromes. In 2005 the authors suggested some diagnostic criteria based on those of the DSM-IV (APA, 1994) to diagnose subtrheshold EDs.

Although there are no formal epidemiological studies available, in the last few years several authors have suggested an increasing prevalence of eating disorders and the adoption of abnormal eating behaviours also in developing countries.

Chapter 4 - The construction of Western social structures has been highly influenced by religious ideals, especially those related to Christianity. Ascetics are among the most remarkable ones, and have an important role by stimulating simplicity and self-discipline in the detriment of physical pleasures. Such features can be easily identified in the life story of Middle Age anorexic saints, such as Catherine of Siena and Mary Magdalene of Pazzi. Their search for sin redemption, spiritual purification and reconnecting with God was made through a system of moral values and practices where penitence and suffering prevailed. Nowadays, thinness has been, especially among women, overvalued as a basic attribute of beauty and success. This has been widely spread by the media, which use ascetic precepts as a tool to build and keep the "ideal woman" image in modern society. Therefore, the current study aimed to recognize and analyze ascetic and religious messages that are used in advertising directed to adult women. The authors found that many beauty rites that have been socially scattered and accepted reproduce forbidden rules. The ancient chastity dedicated to a religious god is now replaced by the oral chastity for the god of beauty, aiming to reach self-control. By transferring the feminine guilt from sex to eating, food consumption is not experienced by women as a pleasure, but merely as a way to satisfy nutritional needs. The dilemma between food production and consumption is reflected on advertising, which are conflicting, since they deliver concomitantly the ideas of controlling, dieting and overeating. Therefore, there is a conflict between redemption and sin, salvation and temptation, where eating appears as a desire that does not comply with good manners nor is socially accepted, though inevitable. Finally, the widely spread image of the ideal woman as well as this feeling of guilt may lead to the lack of acceptance of body shape and size. This generates the adoption of restrictive practices in order to fulfill current patterns and also creates a cycle that frequently leads to eating disorders.

Chapter 5 - Typically anorexia nervosa is diagnosed as a condition of teenage girls where the rates of mortality and morbidity are very high and recovery rates very low. This chapter discusses the condition as experienced by older women who have either lived with anorexia during adolescence and as young women or who have been diagnosed later in life. The discussion will traverse issues of consent to treatment or its refusal, capacity to provide consent, and the application of human right protections arising from various human rights instruments.

Chapter 6 - Although there is no psychological existence without the body, there are times when psychological motivations and defensive maneuvers take over basic bodily functions. Dissociation is considered as a psychological mechanism that enables such taking over or enables distance from one's troubling experience. An extreme use of dissociation can lead to complete disregard of painful memories and emotions, neglecting elementary bodily functions, and to full ignorance of painful sensations. Then, a vicious cycle may ensue, in which less attention is ascribed to basic bodily needs, more importance is tied to psychological motivations, and then again, less consideration is paid to bodily needs, and so on. This mechanism is suggested to play a major role in the etiology of eating disorders. By dissociating one's thoughts from the physical discomfort caused by endless dieting and intensive exercising, patients with eating disorders manage to eat less and exercise more. In this chapter, the authors will present an integrative perspective on the relationship between dissociation and eating disorders in women. They will commence with a short description of eating disorders. Then, they will review studies that evaluated dissociation in patients with eating disorders. Subsequently, the physiological processes in women will be discussed, that may teach them to dissociate themselves from physical discomfort and pain. Following that, the authors will describe several psychological characteristics of women regarding eating disorders that differentiate them from men. They will explain the impact of these psychological tendencies on the ability of women with eating disorders to dissociate themselves from their bodily needs. Finally, they will discuss the clinical implications of their integrative perspective on the treatment of women with eating disorders. Specifically, they will discuss preventive efforts of eating disorders in women: namely educational efforts, identification of high risk individuals, and hypnotherapy of women with eating disorders.

Chapter 7 - This chapter reviewed the gender perspective approach to eating disorders and analyzed certain socio-cultural and psychological aspects related to the development of the latter, such as the relationship of food and emotions, control and identity, the acceptance of the feminine body and, the mother-daughter relationship. The study belongs within the field of the study of clinical psychology and uses a qualitative approach. In-depth interviews were conducted with patients with eating disorders currently receiving specialized treatment at the Ramón de la Fuente Muñiz National Institute of Psychiatry. The testimonies were audiotaped, transcribed and subsequently analyzed using meaning condensation and categorization. Certain themes were selected to be discussed in light of the gender perspective and were illustrated using the interviewees' testimonies. The chapter ends with a discussion of the importance of a qualitative approach in the study of these pathologies.

Chapter 8 - While global prevalence rates of eating disorders have been increasing, there still exists a wide disparity in rates between westernized countries and the rest of the world. In fact, eating disorders are often referred to as "culture bound" syndromes due to the near exclusivity of the disorders in westernized countries. One explanation for this disparity is the "thin ideal" represented in the media in countries with elevated rates of eating disorders. This proposed book chapter will explore the research on the relationship between eating disorders and media exposure. In particular the specific images and messages that are disseminated in the media and the influence that may have on body image, and in turn risk factor for eating disorders. Topics to be discussed include current research on media influences on body image, the relationship between media exposure and eating disorder symptomatology and intervention and prevention programs that have been developed to minimize the risk of such exposure.

Chapter 9 - The purpose of this investigation was to review the empirical evidence specific to the relationship between physical activity contexts and social physique anxiety (SPA). English language studies were located from computer and manual literature searches. Studies included in the meta-analysis presented at least one empirical effect for SPA between physical activity participants (i.e., athletes or exercisers) and non-physical activity participants. The final sample included sixteen studies with a total sample size of 3595. Studies were coded for mean SPA between physical activity participants and non-physical activity participants with type of physical activity participation serving as a moderator variable. Using Hunter and Schmidt's (2004) protocol, statistical artifacts were corrected. Results indicated that, practically speaking, those who were physically active reported lower levels of SPA than the comparison group (dcorr = -0.15; SDcorr. = 0.21). Moderator analysis generally reiterated this trend, although concerns over generalizability were noted. Results offer support for the potential bi-directionality of the relationship between physical activity and SPA; however, the direction of causality warrants additional investigation. Future consideration of the dose-response effects of physical activity on SPA, as well as the nature of exercise behavior and sport classification may help elucidate the role of physical activity contexts on SPA.

Chapter 10 - This article aims to explore the associations between four attitudinal dimensions of the EAT-26 and selected mental health measures among women aged 15 or older concerned about their weight. The dimensions it studies are food and body weight preoccupation, self-imposed dieting and external pressure to eat. The mental health measures selected are self-perceived mental health, having experienced a depressive episode in the last year and a diagnosis of an eating disorder.

The analyses are based on a sub-sample of women who are classified as concerned about their weight and who are surveyed as part of a national representative sample of the Canadian population in 2002. Weighted cross-tabulations were used to describe the characteristics of weight-concerned women. Logistic regression models were constructed to examine the associations between eating attitudes and mental h*ealth measures when selected confounders were controlled.*

Women preoccupied with food are more likely to rate their mental health negatively, to have experienced a depressive episode in the last year and to report having received a diagnosis of an eating disorder. Body image preoccupation was associated with depression and an eating disorder while external pressure to eat was related to a diagnosed eating disorder. Self-imposed dieting is not associated with the mental health indicators studied.

The findings presented are based on a national representative sample and are generally consistent with those obtained with smaller communities or clinical samples that have used the EAT-26. Thus, they are more generalizable. Moreover, significant associations between specific dimensions of eating attitudes and mental health indicators were revealed.

Chapter 11 - *Aim:* It is not easy for overweight women to participate in professional life. They are often considered less efficient. If you think about a ′typical businesswoman`, you expect her to be a slim and attractive person. But is that true? Are women executives slimmer than other women? If yes, how do they achieve this goal?

Method: The authors wanted to find out the answers to these questions through a questionnaire they sent out by e-mail in 2006 to 300 women in leading positions (top and middle management) in Germany. The questionnaire contained a mix of open- and closed-ended questions. The subject of eight of the 50 questions was nutrition and health.

Results: The authors found an average body mass index in the low to normal range. The group of underweight women was nearly twice as large as it is in the average German female population. Additional questions showed that many of these female executives achieve this goal of staying slim through restrained eating.

Conclusion: A slim and well-styled body shows, "I am successful, I am perfect. I am managing my life as successfully as my career." In order to keep such a slim body in our affluent society over a long period of time, one's eating behavior must permanently be geared to loose weight or avoid weight gain. In this context, cognitive control of eating behavior is of prime importance. Ignoring physiological hunger signals and psychological appetence signals are important as well. However, such kind of eating behavior may lead to impaired eating, which is a risk factor for developing an eating disorder.

Chapter 12 - It was hypothesized that higher levels of actual-desired BMI discrepency (ADBD) would be associated with higher binge eating symptoms, lower self concept, and higher body dissatisfaction for a clinical sample of women with Bulimia Nervosa (BN) and Binge Eating Disorder (BED). A theoretical frame for ADBD was put forward based on self discrepancy theory. Also hypothesized was that women with BN would have greater eating and self related pathology than those with BED. Fifty-one participants diagnosed with BN and 41 with BED drawn from a clinical sample completed questionnaires assessing eating disorder and general psychopathology. Greater ADBD was related to greater body dissatisfactionfor the BN and BED groups, and lower self concept for the BN group. Those with BN had more self-related pathology. ADBD can be easily assessed by clinicians and may be used as an index of body dissatisfaction and overall self concept. ADBD may be a vulnerability factor for developing an eating disorder for women.

In: Eating Disorders in Adult Women
Editor: Julian N. Fuchs

ISBN 978-1-60456-673-4

Chapter 1

PARENT-EMERGING ADULT CHILD COMMUNICATION AND DISORDERED EATING PATTERNS

***Michelle A. Miller-Day**[*1] **and Carla L. Fisher**[2]*

1. The Pennsylvania State University, Department of Communication Arts and Sciences 234 Sparks Building, University Park, PA 16802-6207, USA
2. The Pennsylvania State University, Department of Communication Arts and Sciences 234 Sparks Building, University Park, PA 16802-6207, USA

ABSTRACT

Recent decades have seen a rise in the prevalence of eating disorders, especially among emerging adult women. The etiology and development of these disorders involve numerous biological, psychological, and familial factors that extend beyond adolescence into emerging adulthood. More recently, scholarship by communication researchers adds to existing research to reveal knowledge linking psychological factors, parent-child communication, and disordered eating behaviors. In this chapter we review scholarship on parent-child communication and disordered eating and provide empirical data from a study of 273 emerging adults revealing a significant relationship between parent-emerging adult child communication and disordered eating. Highlights of the chapter include a review of relevant communication research as it relates to health behaviors and a presentation of findings from an empirical study examining connections amongst parent-emerging adult child communication, psychological and interpersonal dimensions of self differentiation, and disordered eating. This chapter argues for the importance of studying communication processes when trying to understand the etiology of disordered eating. Information about how parent-child communication patterns affect offspring's eating behavior may allow for earlier detection of disorders and enhance prevention efforts.

---

[*] mam32@psu.edu.

Keywords: *eating disorders, parent-child relationships, communication, autonomy, control, differentiation, convergence, emerging adulthood*

INTRODUCTION

Eating disorders are an important public health issue in the United States. Each of these disorders involves a serious disturbance in eating behavior and is characterized by over evaluation of and possible distress about shape and weight, as well as judgment of self-worth largely in terms of shape, weight, and the ability to control them (Fairburn and Harrison, 2003; National Institute on Mental Health [NIMH], 2007). Scholars and clinicians recognize that the development of eating disorders involves numerous biological, psychological, social, and familial factors and one such familial factor—family environment—has been particularly useful in better understanding how an individual's family context contributes to the development of this negative health outcome.

Etiological research in the past 30 years (much of which has focused on a specific kind of disordered eating, anorexia nervosa, Fairburn and Harrison, 2003) has pointed to specific family patterns that contribute to the development, maintenance, and continuation of disordered eating (McGrane and Carr, 2002). For instance, a plethora of clinical research (Levitt, Sansone, and Cohn, 2004; Minuchin, Rosman, and Baker, 1978; Steiger, Liquornik, Chapman, and Hussain, 1991; Stierlin and Weber, 1989) has depicted the families of adolescent females with anorexia as enmeshed and rigid with blurred personal boundaries. Although this research is abundant and establishes the connection between family environment and disordered eating development, it is also deficient. For instance, scholars and practitioners still lack a complex understanding of which family behaviors cultivate such environments and, hence, how family communication facilitates the development of disordered eating. As eating disorders are currently considered a national public health concern, further exploration is needed.

In this chapter we review recent research in communication scholarship to provide scholars and health professionals with insight on how communication behavior can promote the development of disordered eating and, simultaneously, highlight the importance of interdisciplinary research to better understand how and why eating disorders have become a pressing public health concern. We also present empirical evidence of an association between parent-child communication and disordered eating behaviors in a sample of emerging adults[†]

LITERATURE REVIEW

Conceptualizing Disordered Eating

There are several types of disordered eating categories in the clinical literature. The main types of eating disorders are anorexia nervosa (AN), which an estimated 0.5% - 3.7% of

[†] Arnett (2000) referred to the transitional period from high school lto young adulthood as emerging adulthood. Thisstage of lifeis defined as the period from the end of secondary school through the attainment of adult status (Arnett, 2005).

females will develop in their lifetime, and bulimia nervosa (BN), which an estimated 1.1% - 4.2% of females will develop in their lifetime (NIMH, 2007). Binge eating disorder (BED) has only recently garnered scientific attention in the medical community (Devlin and Goldfein, 2003; Hudson, Lalonde, Berry, et al., 2006) and is estimated to affect 2%-5% of Americans. Although males also develop disordered eating, it is much less prevalent than in females. Males comprise only 5% - 15% of those with AN or BN and around 35% of those with BED (NIMH). And finally, a more common form of disorder is referred to as eating disorders not otherwise specified (EDNOS). This disorder is a significant predictor for the development of both AN and BN (Fairburn and Harrison, 2003).

Anorexia nervosa. Individuals with AN resist maintaining normal body weight, have an intense fear of gaining weight, a significant disturbance in body image and evaluation, and often involves a cessation of menstruation in women who have reached puberty (NIMH, 2007). AN is often accompanied by other strategies to control weight such as over-exercising, laxative use, or self-induced vomiting. The disorder is most prevalent in women ages 15-24 and is often accompanied by depression, irritability, and obsessional features (Fairburn and Harrison, 2003; NIMH). Anorexics are more likely than bulimics to view weight control as an accomplishment rather than a disorder and, therefore, may have limited motivation to seek or follow through with treatment (Fairburn and Harrison).

Bulimia nervosa. BN is characterized by a pattern of eating involving episodes of binge eating followed by purging (Fairburn and Harrison, 2003; NIMH, 2007). BN symptoms include feelings of low control over the binge and purge episode (which occur an average of twice a week for at least 3 months), a self-evaluation extremely influenced by body shape and weight, and frequent inappropriate compensation to prevent weight gain including vomiting, laxative misuse, fasting and excessive exercise (NIMH). Unlike AN, BN is not usually associated with abnormal body weight due to the binge and purge cycle (Fairburn and Harrison; NIMH). Bulimics usually characterize their binge and purge episodes as failures to control their eating and are likely to develop symptoms of depression and anxiety disorders (Fairburn and Harrison).

Eating disorders not otherwise specified. The two main types of eating disorders are anorexia nervosa and bulimia nervosa, but there is a third category of "eating disorders not otherwise specified (EDNOS)," which includes several variations of eating disorders. Most of these disorders are similar to anorexia or bulimia but with slightly different characteristics. Binge-eating disorder, which has received increasing research and media attention in recent years, is one type of EDNOS. Binge-eating disorder is characterized by recurrent binge-eating episodes during which a person feels a loss of control over his or her eating. Unlike bulimia, binge-eating episodes are not followed by purging, excessive exercise or fasting. As a result, people with binge-eating disorder often are overweight or obese (NIMH, 2007).

EDNOS is a diagnostic category of mental disorders that involve disordered eating patterns and is described in the DSM-IV-TR as a category of disorders of eating that do not meet the criteria for any specific eating disorder. EDNOS are sometimes referred to as atypical eating disorders (Fairburn and Harrison, 2003). In many cases, EDNOS are virtually identical to AN or BN but do not meet one of the precise criteria required for diagnosis. Still, all individuals with EDNOS exhibit maladaptive eating behaviors, and overevaluation of shape and weight is also present in most cases (Fairburn and Harrison).

EDNOS is a significant predictor of developing AN or BN and even though it is widely recognized as the most prevalent form of disordered eating, it is the least studied (Anderson,

Bowers, and Watson, 2001; APA, 2000; Fairburn and Harrison). Although researching AN and BN is important, it is not entirely clear whether the findings concerning these specific disorders generalize to a broader array of disordered eating behaviors, or whether the family relationships correlated with AN and BN behave the same way in EDNOS. Given that the most common form of disordered eating is EDNOS, this area of study merits further attention.

Family Factors and Disordered Eating

Given the seriousness of the risks associated with eating disorders, an increasing number of scholars are examining the potential causes and treatments of these disorders, especially those associated with AN and BN. A complex set of factors is thought to contribute to the development of AN and BN, including biological, psychological, sociological, and familial factors (Botta and Dumalo, 2002; Fairburn and Harrison, 2003; Keel, 2004; Kog and Vandereycken, 1985; NIMH, 2001; Prescott and Le Poire, 2002). In regards to the latter factor, disordered eating has been linked to family environments that stress conformity, discourage separation and autonomy, and are high in enmeshment (Dominy, Johnson, and Koch, 2000; Kent and Clopton, 1992; Kog and Vandereycken, 1985; Waller, Slade, and Calam, 1990). Some contemporary research does link family communication to psychological factors related to the development of eating disorders. For instance, familial environment characteristics may contribute to the development of low self-esteem, perfectionism, and the need for control – psychological factors related to disordered eating (Fairburn and Harrison, 2003; Kent and Clopton, 1992; Miller-Day and Marks, 2006). In addition, this research establishes that communication in all parent-child relationships (e.g., mother-daughter, mother-son, father-daughter, and father-son) must be considered to fully capture the influence of the family on eating disorder development.

Although much of the research examining disordered eating and family relationships has focused primarily on communication in mother-daughter relationships (Prescott and Le Poire, 2002), increasing evidence has shown that both mother-child and father-child bonds contribute to disordered eating and other risk outcomes. For example, research has demonstrated that adolescents' self-esteem is affected differently in each parent-child bond. Botta and Dumalo (2002) observed that communication patterns within each parent-child bond differ, and this difference necessitates looking at both parents when assessing disordered eating behavior. They found that in eating disordered adolescents, the father-daughter relationship was more strongly linked to the development of daughters' self-esteem than was the mother-daughter relationship. However, this same pattern may not hold for the parent-son relationship for sons. Barber and Thomas (1986) found that, whereas self-esteem in daughters was linked to general support from mothers and physical affection from fathers, it was companionship from mothers and sustained contact from fathers that were predictive of self-esteem in sons.

In addition, communication research shows that perfectionism and control may function differently in the development of disordered eating in different types of parent-child relationships. Whereas Miller-Day and Marks (2006) found that father-child conformity communication patterns and expectations of perfection were more predictive of disordered eating in a non-clinical sample, Prescott and Le Poire (2002) found that mothers who were controlling were more likely to reinforce daughters' disordered eating and this was linked to daughters' recidivism. Conformity orientation and expectations of perfection were also found to interact differently with different parents in the context of other risk behaviors, with female suicidal ideation linked to a conformity communication orientation in fathers and high expectations of perfection from mothers (Miller-Day and Lee, 2001).

The research reviewed above not only demonstrates the importance of examining communication in multiple parent-child bonds to fully understand how eating disorders develop, but establishes connections between family environment (in particular communication), disordered eating, and psychological factors like self-esteem, control, and perfectionism. Still, the following two additional phenomena may further explain connections amongst family environment, psychological factors, and disordered eating and also help illuminate how parent-child communication contributes to disordered eating: 1) differentiation-of-self—a psychological and interpersonal factor cultivated in family environments; and 2) necessary convergence communication—a parent-child communication pattern.

Differentiation-of-Self

Differentiation-of-self is a multidimensional construct that relates to emotional functioning, intimacy, and autonomy in interpersonal relationships (Skowron and Schmitt, 2003). Differentiation-of-self is the ability to maintain autonomy and a sense of self within the context of close personal relationships. It can be conceptualized as both a process and as an individual trait. The process of differentiating usually occurs during adolescence and emerging adulthood and involves the creation and maintenance of an individual identity separate from family, while simultaneously maintaining ties with family members (Jenkins, Buboltz, Schwartz, and Johnson, 2005).

Differentiation-of-self as a personality trait involves both intrapsychic and interpersonal dimensions. The intrapsychic dimension describes the ability to distinguish between thinking and feeling, as well as the ability to achieve a firm sense of self, to think independently, and to take what is referred to as an "I" position (Skowron and Schmitt, 2003). Individuals low in differentiation are likely to be overwhelmed by emotions and highly emotionally reactive (Skowron and Friedlander, 1998). Individuals highly differentiated are characterized by comfort with intimacy, autonomy in close personal relationships, as well as the ability to maintain connections with others while retaining a sense of self (Skowron, Holmes, and Sabatelli, 2003). A lack of a differentiation may manifest itself as either interpersonal fusion (i.e., a blurring of boundaries between individuals or family members characterized by few firmly held beliefs and seeking acceptance and approval above all else) or as emotional cutoff (i.e., experiencing intimacy as profoundly threatening and engaging in distancing behavior that often is characterized by a façade of extreme independence and isolation) (Skowron and Friedlander; Skowron and Schmitt). Difficulties with differentiation-of-self are related to different outcomes in men and women; men report more problems with emotional cutoff whereas women exhibit more emotional reactivity (Skowron et al.). Interestingly, these same issues linked to an undifferentiated self are also described as risk factors for disordered eating (see Green, Scott, DeVilder, Zeiger; Darr, 2006; and Tantillo, 2006). Yet, little research has systematically examined the relationship of differentiation-of-self to disordered eating.

Differentiation and disordered eating. Research has linked a lack of differentiation-of-self to a variety of negative outcomes including a higher likelihood of irresponsible attitudes toward alcohol, high levels of internalized distress, chronic anxiety, and difficulty coping with stress (Bartle and Sabatelli, 1989; Cohen, Vasey, and Gavazzi, 2003; Jenkins et al., 2005; Murdock and Gore, 2004; Skowron, Wester, and Azen, 2004). Additionally, other research suggests a possible connection between family communication patterns, low levels of differentiation, and anorexia nervosa (Kog and Vandereycken, 1985).

Individuals with disordered eating behaviors live in families generally characterized by the presence of both enmeshment and a strict rule structure, involving a pattern of control and interdependence (Kog and Vandereycken, 1985) and families of eating disordered patients often exhibit unusual degrees of blurring generational boundaries (Waller, Slade, and Calam, 1990). Interestingly, these findings describe patterns associated with a state of emotional fusion linked to poor differentiation-of-self. Families of those with BN and BED often discourage separation and autonomy, engage in conflict, are controlling, lack expressed affection, and exhibit a high pressure to conform (Botta and Dumalo, 2002; Dominy et al., 2000; Kog and Vandereycken, 1985). These enmeshed and overly interdependent family patterns show a low tolerance for independence and suggest a family environment that discourages differentiation-of-self. Although less research has focused on EDNOS, it is likely that individuals diagnosed with AN, BN, and BED may also have a low or undifferentiated self.

Necessary Convergence Communication

Exploratory research by Miller (1995; Miller-Day, 2004) suggests that in addition to differentiation-of-self, a specific communication pattern may play a role in predicting disordered eating. Necessary Convergence Theory is a grounded theory that grew out of Miller-Day's (2004) research with grandmothers, mothers, and adult daughters and her earlier work with four generations of maternal relationships in one family (Miller, 1995). Miller-Day has since adapted the theory to apply not only to maternal relationships but as a general relational influence theory accounting for dominant-submissive communication. The theory explains how chronic participation in a specific interaction routine (or script) called *necessary convergence communication* (NCC) may lead to negative outcomes for submissive relational partners, specifically resulting in poor mental health outcomes such as disordered eating or depression (Miller-Day, 2004; Miller, 1995). NCC has been defined as, "an interaction routine where submissive partners feel compelled to interpret the world around them in ways consistent with the dominant partner" (Miller-Day, 2006, p. 13). According to the theory, deference to a dominant partner's relational power leads to convergence of meaning where a submissive partner replaces his or her own opinions, beliefs, or attitudes with those of the dominant partner. Miller-Day (2004) characterizes this as interpersonal "hijacking of meaning."

Miller-Day reported links among women with disordered eating patterns, undifferentiated maternal relationships, and NCC patterns. For instance, she observed that "adult daughters and granddaughters would defer to the higher-status woman in the family, overaccomodate the higher-status woman's interpretation of events, and ultimately converge toward her interpretive frame for relational maintenance purposes" (Miller-Day, 2004, p. 201).

Coinciding with this pattern of relational influence was a high incidence of risk-behaviors including attempted suicide, alcohol and drug abuse, and disordered eating.

NCC and disordered eating. Necessary convergence theory posits that increased degree and chronicity of NCC will increase the probability of negative outcomes—such as disordered eating—for submissive relational partners (Miller-Day, 2004). Adding to the literature that reports associations between parental control efforts that discourage offspring's separation from family and personal autonomy (Botta and Dumalo, 2002; Kog and Vandereycken, 1985; Miller-Day and Marks, 2006; Prescott and Le Poire, 2002), Miller-Day's (2004) findings suggest that both parental control efforts and differentiation have been linked to NCC patterns (Miller-Day, 2004). Disordered eating often occurs when a person, unable to control other aspects of his or her life displaces this need for control into a preoccupation with food and weight (Fairburn and Harrison, 2003). It seems plausible that individuals who are in the habit of deferring to more powerful others in an interpersonal context, as in NCC, might develop disordered eating in an effort to exert personal control over one aspect of his or her life.

Sex and Parent-Child Relational Differences

Linking NCC to disordered eating in a non-clinical population extends the usefulness and descriptive power of the theory. Moreover, to refine knowledge about family communication patterns associated with disordered eating, we examine NCC in the specific context of parent-offspring communication.

NCC, disordered eating, differentiation, and sex differences. Given the abundance of research demonstrating that family interaction patterns may lead to different outcomes with respect to sex differences, it is important to consider mother-son, father-son, mother-daughter, and father-daughter interactions. Attention to sex differences in this area of research is important for several reasons: (1) disordered eating is rarely examined with respect to male populations, and (2) family communication patterns associated with women may not hold for men. It is possible that aspects of NCC and differentiation-of-self may be salient for the mother-daughter relationship but not the father-daughter or mother-son relationship, with respect to eating disorders. Nevertheless, these differences have yet to be determined. To further explore the potential link between disordered eating, differentiation-of-self, and convergence communication an original study was conducted.

Although associations among convergence communication, differentiation of self, and disordered eating were observed in previous observational research (see Miller-Day, 2004), these relationships remain untested. To build on this previous research and further examine the associations between disordered eating, differentiation of self and NCC, the following hypotheses and research question were proposed:

H1: Disordered eating is positively associated with a low differentiated self.
H2: Disordered eating is positively associated with necessary convergence communication.
H3: A low differentiated self is positively associated with necessary convergence communication.
RQ1: Are there significant sex (son/daughter) or parental (mother/father) differences in the associations among the study variables?

STUDY METHODS

Participants and Procedures

Scholars have shown that emerging adulthood is an impressionable developmental period—a time in which individuals reassess their beliefs, worldview, and identity (Perry, 1999). As adolescents transition into adulthood their thinking patterns change (Schaie, 1977), their relationships with their parents evolve (Arnett, 2000, 2001), as does their ability to think independently (Arnett, 1998, 2000; Greene, Wheatley, and Aldava, 1992). Since this study was intended to assess differentiation-- maintenance of an individual identity separate from family—an emerging adult sample was utilized.

A confidential, self-report, online questionnaire was administered to 270 introductory speech communication students at a large northeastern U.S. university. Students received course credit for their participation, and another option for equal credit was made available. Of the 270 participants, 49.3 % (n = 133) were men and 50.7% (n = 137) were women. The majority of participants (96.3%) were within the 18 - 23 age range with a mean age of 20.07 years.

This study was part of a larger study to examine family communication variables. The items discussed here were embedded in a larger survey that examined emerging adults' perceptions of parent-child communication variables for each parent as well as several individual risk behaviors such as disordered eating and depression.

After completing the short demographic section of the survey, participants were instructed to answer a series of questions about their interactions with their parents. They were asked to answer questions as honestly as possible and were reminded that their answers would remain confidential. The entire survey took approximately 40 minutes to complete and included 242 closed-ended items.

Measures

Disordered eating: The SCOFF questionnaire. Disordered eating was operationalized with the SCOFF instrument (Morgan, Reid, and Lacey, 1999) designed to measure the likelihood of maladaptive eating patterns. This measure consists of a set of five yes or no questions about body and food attitudes and was initially developed to be used as a short, simple assessment for use in clinical settings. A threshold of two or more positive answers out of five items on the SCOFF instrument indicates a possibility that the participant has some type of disordered eating though it does not specifically diagnose AN, BN, or BED (Morgan et al., 1999). SCOFF has been found to be very effective in ruling in the possibility of disordered eating such as a "mixed eating disorder" or EDNOS (Cotton, Ball, and Robinson, 2003). This study utilized the U.S. version of the SCOFF questionnaire. In this version SCOFF stands for **S**ick ("Do you make yourself sick because you feel uncomfortably full?), **C**ontrol ("Do you worry you have lost control over how much you eat?"), Others ("Do you believe yourself to be fat when others say you are too thin?"), Fourteen ("Have you recently lost more than fourteen pounds in a three month period?"), and Food ("Would you say that food dominates your life?") (Perry et al., 2002). In tests of the SCOFF instrument, sensitivity (percentage of those with an eating disorder positively identified by the instrument) has ranged from 78% to 100% (Cotton et al. 2003; Luck et al., 2002; Morgan et al.) and specificity (percentage of those identified by the instrument who are actually eating disordered) has ranged from 87% to 89.6% (Cotton et al.; Jacobi, Abascal, and Taylor, 2004; Luck et al., 2002; Morgan et al.).

Differentiation-of-self. The Differentiation-of-self Inventory (DSI) is a multidimensional measure of differentiation focusing on adults and their current significant relationships, including those with their family of origin, and was designed to measure the differentiation-of-self construct from Bowen theory (Skowron and Friedlander, 1998). This 43-item Likert-type scale ranging from 1 (*not at all true of me*) to 6 (*very true of me*) has four subscales: (1) Emotional Reactivity (ER) – 11 items assessing the degree to which a person responds to events with emotional flooding and hypersensitivity; (2) I Position (IP) – 11 items reflecting a clearly defined sense of self and the ability not to be swayed from one's convictions by others; (3) Emotional Cutoff (EC) – 13 items assessing feeling threatened by intimacy, fears of engulfment and utilization of defensive behaviors such as distancing; and (4) Fusion With Others (FO) – 9 items assessing emotional over-involvement with others including parents (Johnson et al., 2003).

Although Cronbach's alpha has been generally high for the DSI scale and the majority of its subscales (DSI, $\alpha = .74 - .88$; ER, $\alpha = .84 - .88$; IP $\alpha = .76 - .85$; EC $\alpha = .79 - .83$), the FO subscale was notably less reliable with alphas ranging from .59 - .74 (Johnson et al.; Murdock and Gore, 2004; Skowron and Friedlander, 1998; Skowron et al., 2003; Skowron et al., 2004). To address the low reliability in the FO subscale, the items in this subscale were reworked, and the new items were added to form the 46-item Revised Differentiation-of-self Inventory (DSI-R) that was used in this present study. The new FO subscale consists of 11 items and measures emotional over-involvement with others, including parents, as in the DSI, and also measures heavy reliance on others in decision making (Skowron and Schmitt, 2003). Cronbach's alpha for the DSI-R is improved over the DSI, with DSI-R, $\alpha = .92$; ER $\alpha = .84$; IP $\alpha = .81$; EC $\alpha = .84$; FO $\alpha = .86$ (Skowron and Schmitt,).

Sample items from the DSI-R include "At times my feelings get the best of me and I have trouble thinking clearly" (ER), "I am able to say 'no' to others even when I feel pressured by them" (IP), "I'm often uncomfortable when people get too close to me" (EC), and "I feel a need for approval from virtually everyone in my life" (FO). The ER, EC, and FO subscales are reverse-scored, so that higher scores indicate lower differentiation-of-self, more emotional reactivity, a lack of ability to take an "I" position, more emotional cutoff, and more fusion with others. For the present study, Cronbach's alpha was .91 for this measure.

Necessary convergence communication. The Necessary Convergence Communication Scale (NCC, Miller-Day, 2007) is a 38-item instrument designed to measure the perception of convergent communicative interaction. Participants were asked to fill out this questionnaire assessing their perception of their communication with their mother and also their father. With the prompt, "Generally, when I interact with this person (in person or on the telephone)…" respondents were asked to answer items assessing the level of convergence, motivation for convergence, and amount of equal participation in typical interactions with his or her mother and father. The NCC is assessed using a 5-point Likert-type scale ranging from 1 (*Not at all*) to 5 (*Very Much*) and has four subscales: Motivation (9 items), Convergence (8 items), Equilibrium-Participation (4 items), and Equilibrium-Consideration (4 items). Sample items include "I run the risk of losing my mother's affection if I do not defer to her,"

(Motivation); "I generally embrace my mother's point of view as my own" (Convergence); "Both of us share our individual attitudes and beliefs with each other" (Equilibrium-Participation); and "Both of us respect each other's opinions, even if we disagree" (Equilibrium-Consideration). Equilibrium items are reverse-scored, resulting in a scale where higher scores indicate a greater perceived need for convergence. Internal consistency estimates demonstrated high reliability for the NCC-parent instrument with a Cronbach's alpha of .91.

STUDY RESULTS

Descriptive Statistics

Disordered eating. Responses to the SCOFF questionnaire were coded into two dichotomous categories: "Disordered eating" and "Not disordered eating." An affirmative response to 0-1 of the items classified the individual as falling into the "not disordered eating" category and an affirmative response to less than two items classified the individual as "disordered eating." Results showed that 18.4% (N = 48) of the 261 respondents who completed this scale answered two or more questions affirmatively, indicating disordered eating behaviors among these respondents. Ten men and 38 women were classified as reporting disordered eating behaviors. This translates to a disordered eating classification for 7.5% of the men in the sample and 28% of the women.

Differentiation-of-self. The necessary items of the DSI-R were reverse-scored so that higher scores reflect a lower degree of differentiation-of-self. Among the entire sample, the mean score for differentiation was 3.0 (SD = .59). Women (M = 3.09, SD = .58) had a lower mean score for differentiation-of-self than men (M = 2.91, SD = .59).

Necessary convergence communication. The necessary items of the NCC scale were reverse-scored so that higher scores reflect a higher degree of NCC. NCC was initially calculated separately for communication with mother (NCC-mom) (M = 2.04, SD = .55) and for communication with father (NCC-dad) (M = 2.19, SD = .56) and then items combined for a parental average score (NCC-parent) (M = 2.12, SD = .50).

Inquiries

To examine our inquiries, we computed correlation coefficients (see Table 1) for all study variables. A positive correlation was discovered between disordered eating and differentiation-of-self (r = .30, p < .01), suggesting an association between a low differentiated self and disordered eating behaviors (H1). A significant positive relationship was also found between parental NCC and a low differentiated self (r = .29, p < .01) (H2) and a weaker, but significant, positive relationship was discovered between disordered eating and parental NCC (r = .07, p < .05) (H3).

Table 1. Correlations for total sample

	1	2	3
1. Differentiation-of-self	---	.30**	.32**
2. Disordered Eating		---	.07*
3. NCC –parents			---

** Correlation is significant at the 0.01 level (two-tailed).
* Correlation is significant at the 0.05 level (two-tailed).

Table 2. Correlations for Females Only

	1	2	3	4
Differentiation-of-self	---	.29**	.32**	.35**
Disordered Eating		---	.14	.18*
NCC-mom			---	.58**
NCC-dad				---

** Correlation is significant at the 0.01 level (two-tailed).
* Correlation is significant at the 0.05 level (two-tailed).

Table 3. Correlations for Males Only

	1	2	3	4
Differentiation-of-self	---	.27**	.36**	.28**
Disordered Eating		---	-.07	.01
NCC-mom			---	.68**
NCC-dad				---

** Correlation is significant at the 0.01 level (two-tailed).

In order to determine whether sex (son/daughter) or parental (mother/father) differences existed (RQ1), separate correlation coefficient analyses were computed for mothers and fathers across females only and males only. Additionally, we then conducted t-test sex comparisons of the study variables.

Correlation coefficients revealed the following significant relationships for females only (see Table 2) and males only (see Table 3). For females, disordered eating was positively correlated with a low differentiated self (r = .29, p < .01), and an increased degree of convergent communication with fathers only (NCC_{mom}, p = ns; NCC_{dad}, r = .18, p < .05). Additionally, for females NCC with both mothers and fathers was positively associated with a low differentiated self (NCC_{mom}, r = .32, p < .01; NCC_{dad}, r = .35, p < .01). For males, disordered eating was also positively correlated with a low differentiated self (r = .27, p < .01), but parental NCC appeared to not be associated with disordered eating (NCC_{mom}, p = ns; NCC_{dad}, p = *ns*). Additionally, similar to the pattern for females, NCC with both mothers and fathers was positively associated with a low differentiated self (NCC_{mom}, r = .36, p < .01; NCC_{dad}, r = .28, p < .01).

T-test and Chi-square comparisons revealed several significant sex differences. A Pearson chi-square analysis revealed that females reported more disordered eating behaviors than males (χ^2 (1) = 19.21, p < .001).

Table 4. Levels of study variables by sex

	N	*M*	*SD*	*t-value*	*sig*	
Diff of self						
male		131	2.90	.59	-2.46	.01
female	136	3.08	.57			
NCC parents					3.13	.002
Male	133	2.21	.49			
Female	137	2.02	.49			

Higher scores in Differentiation of self indicate less differentiated self
Higher scores in NCC indicate more convergence

Table 5. Levels of variables by disordered and nondisordered eating for females only

		N	*M*	*SD*	*t-value*	*sig*
Diff of self						
Disordered		48	3.37	.54	–5.05	.000
Nondisord	215	2.99	.56			
NCC parents						
Disordered		48	2.15	.50	ns	ns
Nondisord	215	2.09	.49			

Higher scores in Differentiation of self indicate less differentiated self.
Higher scores in NCC indicate more convergence.

Further t-test analyses also revealed significant sex differences regarding differentiation-of-self, with females reporting less differentiated selves than males (t = -2.46, df = 268, p < .01) and significant gender differences regarding convergent communication with parents, with males reporting more convergence communication than females (t = 3.13, df = 268, p < .01) (see Table 4). It is interesting to note that when post-hoc t-tests were run for individual subscales in both the differentiation-of-self and the parental NCC measures, additional sex differences significant at least at the .05 level included females reporting more fusion with others (t = -3.13, df = 265, p < .01), more equal participation in conversations with mother (t = 5.38, df = 268, p < .01), more equal consideration of ideas by mother (t = 4.71, df = 268, p < .001), and slightly more equal participation in conversations with father (t = 2.03, df = 269, p < .05) than males.

T-test analyses also revealed significant differences between participants with and without disordered eating behaviors (see Table 5). These analyses indicated that participants with disordered eating behaviors reported significantly less differentiation-of-self; that is, they tended to be more fused and undifferentiated than the non-disordered participants (t = -5.05, df = 261, p < .001). There were, however, no significant differences in parental convergent communication for those with or without disordered eating behaviors (t = -.772, df = 261, p = ns).

Conclusion

This chapter provides a review of scholarship focusing on parent-child communication and disordered eating and provides empirical evidence of a significant relationship between parent-emerging adult child communication and disordered eating. The study reported here examined the relationships among disordered eating, communication characterized by necessary convergence, and differentiation-of-self in a sample of emerging adults. Sex (male/female) and parental differences (mother/father) were also examined.

Sex Differences and Concerns

The results from this study revealed more than three times as many females than males who reported disordered eating behaviors. This is not surprising as this finding is reflected in previous prevalence data (NIMH, 2007). However, this sample did represent a greater overall percentage of both females (28%) and males (7.5%) reporting disordered eating behavior than in comparable populations (for example see Einar Kjelsa°s, E., Bjørnstrøm, C., and Go¨testam, K. G., 2004).

Across both males and females, disordered eating was significantly associated with low levels of differentiation. Nonetheless, the present study makes clear that an examination of sex differences is warranted when studying disordered eating—even at subclinical levels. Females were less differentiated as autonomous, emotionally independent individuals than males in this study. This finding has implications for those who work with emerging adult populations. As females are reportedly more likely to be at risk for disordered eating (and low levels of differentiation are associated with disordered eating), it seems particularly important that clinicians attend to emerging adult women's sense of self and individuation.

In this study, convergence communication with both mothers and fathers was related to less differentiated selves for both males and females, but—for females specifically—convergence communication with fathers is linked to disordered eating. In addition, for females, the results indicate that one particular dimension of a low differentiated self—fusion with others—appeared to be significant when examining differentiation and disordered eating. As fusion refers to a blurring of interpersonal boundaries and desire for approval above all else, this finding suggests that an under-developed autonomous identity may be a critical predictor of disordered eating, especially when combined with dominant paternal communication.

There is concern that emerging female adults, whose parents discourage autonomy by inhibiting their daughter's expression of opinions, beliefs, or attitudes, may also be increasing her risk of negative health outcomes—such as eating disorders. Still, emerging male adults should not be ignored, particularly because our findings suggest that sons seem to perceive more convergence communication with their mothers in comparison to daughters' perceptions. In other words, males reported particularly less participation in and consideration during conversations with their mothers.

Family Communication, Differentiation, and Eating Disorders

Upon closer inspection, whereas convergence communication and low levels of differentiation are both associated with disordered eating, convergence communication is most strongly correlated with differentiation. The direction and strength of the association between convergence communication and disordered eating suggests a possible interaction effect. Moreover, given the expected low rates of reported disordered eating within the entire sample, the associations reported in this study reveal impressive effect sizes—especially among differentiation-of-self and disordered eating. The present results also suggest that the link between differentiation-of-self and disordered eating is one that deserves additional study. With post-hoc analyses indicating that fusion is a particularly strong correlate with disordered eating behavior, it would be worthwhile in future research to test whether this or other subscales of the DSI-R adequately predict disordered eating in general.

The study reported in this chapter clearly demonstrated connections amongst differentiation-of-self, disordered eating, and NCC in an emerging adult population. The developmental literature on adolescence and emerging adulthood may not only help to explain these linkages but highlight areas practitioners and therapists can focus on in their intervention and counseling efforts.

Emerging adults' developmental needs and health. The study's results suggest that individuals who do not have a strong differentiation-of-self are also more likely to exhibit disordered eating. In light of this finding, it is important to recall that differentiation-of-self has been theoretically (Bray and Harvey, 1992; Carter and McGoldrick, 1999) and empirically (Johnson et al., 2003) tied to identity formation, and that identity formation is a developmental task for psychosocial adjustment in both adolescence and emerging adulthood (Flanagan, 2004). This connection between identity formation and psychosocial development has been thoroughly researched. Although linkages between differentiation-of-self and psychosocial development are less explored, in one of the only studies that examined this relationship, Jenkins et al. (2005) found that emerging adults' level of differentiation-of-self predicts adjustment in all of Erikson's (1950/1963) eight psychosocial stages, including identity formation. Hence, like identity formation, differentiation-of-self is critical to an emerging adult's psychosocial development. It is likely that because identity formation and, thus differentiation-of-self, are critical to an emerging adult's development, failure to do so can result in negative health implications. This negative result is in accord with Erikson's widely cited developmental literature in which he asserts that "health is achieved by successful resolution of a series of eight psychosocial stages throughout the life span" (Jenkins et al., 2005 p. 253). Moreover, as was noted in our review of prior research, it is not surprising then that poor differentiation has been linked with outcomes that can negatively impact health (Bartle and Sabatelli, 1989; Cohen et al., 2003; Jenkins et al., 2005; Murdock and Gore, 2004; Skowron et al., 2004).

Family communication and disordered eating. The present study reveals insight on the role of family communicative behavior in this negative health outcome that practitioners can use to ensure emerging adults are in an environment that allows them to cultivate an autonomous self (and, hopefully at the same time, reduce the prevalence of eating disorder development amongst emerging adults). Our results bring to light an important parent-child communication factor—NCC—that can inhibit emerging adults' ability to develop an autonomous sense of self (recall that NCC was most strongly correlated with differentiation-of-self). In previous research, Miller-Day (2004) established that NCC is a script enacted in parent-child interactions wherein parents communicatively discourage children's autonomy, and prior evidence supports the notion that family-of-origin interaction patterns impact individual development in the area of identity development (Anderson and Fleming, 1986; Bartle and Sabatelli, 1989; Fleming and Anderson, 1986). Our study not only further supports this contention, but we also advance the literature by not focusing on interaction in a general manner. Instead we have illuminated the complexity of family communication behavior in the parent-child bond by demonstrating that specifically NCC can impede an emerging adult's ability to cultivate a sense of self separate from his/her family. Hence, it is important that practitioners ascertain whether emerging adults' parents engage in the NCC pattern of communication, as identity formation and differentiation-of-self are critical developmental tasks in emerging adulthood.

Implications for Practitioners and Scholars

Identity formation is undoubtedly present across the life span. Yet, because self-awareness and self-reflection notably increase during adolescence (Streigel-Moore, 1996), identity formation is likely particularly salient during adolescence and emerging adulthood. This should encourage practitioners and therapists to look more closely at how the presence of NCC in the family environment might contribute to an impeded differentiated self and, ultimately, the development of an eating disorder in emerging adulthood. Because no previous research formally tested the associations among NCC, disordered eating behavior, and differentiation-of-self, the results from this study provide an important contribution to existing knowledge on the etiology of disordered eating in relation to specific familial factors. The findings from this study reveal the importance of examining family communication patterns (such as convergence communication) when trying to understand disordered eating behaviors. These findings provoke interest in the role of convergence communication in the development of emerging adults, in particular in how it may affect differentiation-of-self and identity formation.

Professionals working with this population must consider the psychosocial and developmental importance of cultivating a sense of self and identity separate from one's family. When emerging adults are prevented from forming an independent identity, their psychosocial development is not fulfilled which then heightens their risk for negative health outcomes like disordered eating.

Further exploration of NCC as a mitigating factor in emerging adults' ability to form autonomous identities seems warranted and can help practitioners better understand their risk and potential development of eating disorders after adolescence. Moreover, future research efforts should utilize clinical samples to further examine the strength of convergence communication and differentiation-of-self as predictors for disordered eating at clinical levels. Given the preliminary findings linking parent-child communication patterns—specifically those patterns related to conformity and control--to eating behaviors (e.g., Miller-Day and Marks, 2006 and Prescott and Le Poire, 2002), future research might seek a broader context and more closely examine the *meanings* attached to interpersonal dominant-submissive interactions in the family, and not just those interactions surrounding food intake.

It may be fruitful for scholars to take a closer look at parenting differences and eating disorders—specifically, differences in how fathers and mothers communicate with their sons and daughters and the relationship between these parent-child communication patterns and disordered eating. Father-daughter communication, in particular, is increasingly being exposed as an important factor in daughters' disordered eating behaviors. As found in this study, father-daughter communication may indeed function differently than mother-daughter communication in its relationship to disordered eating (Botta and Dumalo, 2002; Kent and Clopton, 1992; Miller-Day and Marks, 2006). The current study builds on that previous research and highlights how communication among mothers and fathers and sons is often characterized by different patterns of communication than among mothers and fathers and daughters. In the present study, although women were more likely to develop disordered eating and have less self-differentiation, men reported higher levels of NCC with their mothers. Future scholars should examine both parents' and their child's perceptions (dyadic communication patterns) when assessing at-risk behaviors, especially with respect to disordered eating.

Given this review and the findings presented here, it seems imperative to honor the complexity of families when examining family factors contributing to eating disorders. This complexity includes family communication processes, such as interaction patterns and meanings attached to messages exchanged in family contexts, which occur across adolescence and into adulthood.

REFERENCES

American Psychiatric Association. (2000). *Diagnostic and statistical manual of mental disorders* (TR). Washington, DC: American Psychiatric Pub Group.

Anderson, A. E., Bowers, W. A., and Watson, T. (2001). A slimming program for eating disorders not otherwise specified. Reconceptualizing a confusing residual diagnostic category. *Psychiatric Clinics of North America, 24*, 271-280.

Anderson, S. A., and Fleming, W. M. (1986). Late adolescents identity formation: Individuation from the family of origin. *Adolescence, 21,* 786–796.

Arnett, J. J. (2005). The developmental context of substance use in emerging adulthood. *Journalof Drug Issues,* 35, 235–253.

Arnett, J. J. (2001). Conceptions of the transition to adulthood: Perspectives from adolescence through midlife. *Journal of Adult Development, 8*, 133-143.

Arnett, J. J. (2000). Emerging adulthood: A theory of development from the late teens through the twenties. *American Psychologist, 55*, 469-480.

Arnett, J. J. (1998). Learning to stand alone: The contemporary American transition to adulthood in cultural and historical context. *Human Development, 41*, 295-315.

Barber, B. K., and Thomas, D., L. (1986). Dimensions of fathers' and mothers' supportive behavior: The case for physical affection. *Journal of Marriage and the Family, 48*, 783-794.

Bartle, S. E., and Sabatelli, R. M. (1989). Family systems dynamics, identity development, and adolescent alcohol use: Implications for family treatment. *Family Relations, 38*, 258-265.

Botta, R., and Dumalo, R. (2002). How do conflict and communication patterns between fathers and daughters contribute to or offset eating disorders? *Health Communication, 14*, 199-219.

Bray, J. H., and Harvey, D. M. (1992). Intimacy and individuation in young adults: Development of the young adult version of the personal authority in the family system questionnaire. *Journal of Family Psychology, 6*, 152–163.

Carter B., and McGoldrick M. (1999). *The expanded family life-cycle: Individual, family, and social perspectives* (3rd ed.). Boston: Allyn and Bacon.

Caughlin, J. P. (2002). The Demand/Withdraw Pattern of Communication as a Predictor of Marital Satisfaction Over Time: unresolved issues and future directions. *Human Communication Research, 28*(1), 49-85.

Cohen, E. A., Vasey, M. W., and Gavazzi, S. M. (2003). The dimensionality of family differentiation and the prediction of adolescent internalized distress. *Journal of Family Issues, 24*, 99-123.

Cotton, M.-A., Ball, C., and Robinson, P. (2003). Four simple questions can help screen for eating disorders. *Journal of General Internal Medicine, 18*, 53-56.

Dominy, N. L., Johnson, B. W., and Koch, C. (2000). Perception of parental acceptance in women with binge eating disorder. *The Journal of Psychology, 134*, 23-36.

Eating Disorder Coalition for Research, Policy, and Action (2002). *Testimony of The EDCRPA: The Promoting Healthy Eating Behaviors in Youth Act of 2002.* Submitted to the Senate Health, Education, Labor and Pensions Committee, Subcommittee on Public Health April 25. Accessed on January 9, 2006 at http://help.senate. gov/Hearings/2002_04_25_a/EatingDisorders.pdf

Fairburn, C. G., and Harrison, P. J. (2003). Eating Disorders. *The Lancet, 361*, 407-416.

Flanagan, C. A. (2004). Volunteerism, leadership, political socialization, and civic engagement. In R. M. Lerner and L. Steinberg (Ed.) *Handbook of Adolescent Psychology,* (2nd ed.) (pp. 721-746). New York: John Wiley and Sons.

Fleming, W. M., and Anderson, S. A. (1986). Differentiation within the family of origin and personal adjustment in late adolescence. *Journal of Marital and Family Therapy, 12,* 311–315.

Green, M. A., Scott, N. A., DeVilder, E. L., Zeiger, A., and Darr, S. (2006).Relational-Interdependent self-construal as a function of bulimic symptomology. *Journal of Clinical Psychology, 62* (7), 943-951.

Greene, A. L., Wheatley, S. M., and Aldava, J. F., IV. (1992). Stages on life's way: Adolescents'implicit theories of the life course. *Journal of Adolescent Research, 7,* 364-381.

Jacobi, C., Abascal, L., and Taylor, C. B. (2004). Screening for eating disorders and high-risk behavior: Caution. *International Journal of Eating Disorders, 36*, 280-298.

Jenkins, S. M., Buboltz, W. C., Schwartz, J. P., and Johnson, P. (2005). Differentiation-of-self and psychosocial development. *Contemporary Family Therapy, 27*, 251-261.

Johnson, P., Buboltz, W. C., and Seemann, E. (2003). Ego identity status: A step in the differentiation process. *Journal of Counseling and Development, 81*, 191-195.

Keel, P. K. (2004). *Eating disorders.* Prentice Hall.

Kent, J. S., and Clopton, J. R. (1992). Bulimic women's perceptions of their family relationships. *Journal of Clinical Psychology, 48*, 281-292.

Kog, E., and Vandereycken, W. (1985). Family characteristics of anorexia nervosa and bulimia: A review of the research literature. *Clinical Psychology Review, 5*, 159-180.

Levitt, J.L., Sansone, R.A., and Cohn, L. (Ed.) (2004). *Self harm and eating disorders: Dynamics, assessment, and treatment.* New York: Brunner-Routledge.

Luck, A. J., Morgan, J. F., Reid, F., O'Brien, A., Brunton, J., Price, C., et al. (2002). The SCOFF questionnaire and clinical interview for eating disorders in general practice: comparative study. *British Medical Journal, 325*, 755-756, 1331.

McGrane, D., and Carr, A. (2002). Young women at risk for eating disorders: Perceived family dysfunction and parental psychological problems. *Contemporary Family Therapy, 24* (2), 385-395.

Miller-Day, M. (2005). *Necessary Convergence of Meaning in Interpersonal Relationships.* Paper presented at the International Communication Association, New York.

Miller-Day, M., and Lee, J. W. (2001). Communicating disappointment: The viewpoint of sons and daughters. *The Journal of Family Communication, 1*, 111-131.

Miller-Day, M., and Marks, J. D. (2006). Perceptions of parental communication orientation, perfectionism, and disordered eating behaviors of sons and daughters. *Health Communication, 19*, 153-163.

Miller-Day, M. A. (2004). *Communication among grandmothers, mothers, and adult daughters: A qualitative study of maternal relationships*. Mahwah, NJ: Lawrence Erlbaum Associates.

Miller, M. (1995). An intergenerational case study of suicidal tradition and mother-daughter communication. *Journal of Communication Research, 23*, 247-270.

Minuchin, S., Rosman, B. L., and Baker, L. (1978). *Psychosomatic families: Anorexia nervosa in context.* Oxford, England: Harvard University Press.

Morgan, J. F., Reid, F., and Lacey, J. H. (1999). The SCOFF questionnaire: Assessment of a new screening tool for eating disorders. *British Medical Journal, 319*, 1467-1468.

Murdock, N. L., and Gore, P. A. J. (2004). Stress, coping, and differentiation-of-self: A test of Bowen theory. *Contemporary Family Therapy, 26*, 319-335.

National Institute of Mental Health. (2007). *Eating disorders.*. Bethesda (MD): National Institute of Mental Health, National Institutes of Health, US Department of Health and Human Services (NIH Publication Number: 07-4901). 13 pages. Retrieved February 4, 2008 and available from: http://www.nimh.nih.gov/publicat/NIMHeatingdisorder.pdf

Nussbaum, J. F., and Coupland, J. (Eds.) (2004). *Handbook of communication and aging research. 2nd edition*. Mahwah, NJ: LEA Publishers.

Perry, W. G. (1999). *Forms of ethical and intellectual development in the college years: A scheme.* San Francisco: Jossey-Bass. (Original work published in 1970).

Perry, L., Morgan, J. F., Reid, F., Brunton, J., O'Brien, A., Luck, A. J., et al. (2002). Screening for symptoms of eating disorders: Reliability of the SCOFF screening tool with written compared to oral delivery. *International Journal of Eating Disorders, 32*, 466-472.

Prescott, M. E., and Le Poire, B. A. (2002). Eating disorders and mother-daughter communication: A test of inconsistent nurturing as control theory. *The Journal of Family Communication, 2*, 59-78.

Rogers, E. L. (2006). Relational communication theory: An interactional theory. In D. O. Braithwaite and L. A. Baxter (Eds.), *Engaging theories in family communication: multiple perspectives* (pp. 115-129). Thousand Oaks: Sage.

Schaie, K. W. (1977). Toward a stage of adult theory of adult cognitive development. *Journal of Aging and Human Development, 8,* 129-138.

Skowron, E. A., and Friedlander, M. L. (1998). The differentiation-of-self inventory: Development and initial validation. *Journal of Counseling Psychology, 45*, 235-246.

Skowron, E. A., Holmes, S. E., and Sabatelli, R. M. (2003). Deconstructing differentiation: Self regulation, interdependent relating, and well-being in adulthood. *Contemporary Family Therapy, 25*, 111-129.

Skowron, E. A., and Schmitt, T. A. (2003). Assessing interpersonal fusion: Reliability and validity of a new DSI fusion with others subscale. *Journal of Marital and Family Therapy, 2*, 209-222.

Skowron, E. A., Wester, S. R., and Azen, R. (2004). Differentiation-of-self mediates college stress and adjustment. *Journal of Counseling and Development, 82*, 69-78.

Steiger, H., Liquornik, K., Chapman, J., and Hussain, N. (1991) Personality and family disturbances in eating-disorder patients: Comparison of "restricters" and "bingers" to normal controls. *International Journal of Eating Disorders, 10*, 501-512.

Stierlin, H., and Weber, G. (1989). *Unlocking the family door: A systemic approach to the understanding and treatment of anorexia nervosa.* Philadelphia, PA: Brunner/Mazel.

Striegel-Moore, R. (1996). Psychological factors in the etiology of binge eating. *Addictive Behaviors, 20*, 713-723.

Tantillo, M. (2006). A relational approach to eating disorders multifaceted therapy group: moving from difference and disconnection to mutual connection. *Families, Systems, and Heath, 24* (1), 82-102.

Waller, G. M., Slade, P., and Calam, R. (1990). Family adaptability and cohesion: Relation to eating attitudes and disorders. *International Journal of Eating Disorders, 9*, 225-228.

In: Eating Disorders in Adult Women
Editor: Julian N. Fuchs

ISBN 978-1-60456-673-4

Chaprer 2

DYSREGULATED EATING PATTERNS AMONG GRADUATE STUDENTS: SCALE DEVELOPMENT AND PREDICTORS

Anne E. Becker,[1] Laura Ferguson,.[*2] ,Sharon Iron-Segev[3], Malinda Kennedy[3], Binta Beard [3], Laura Kozek[†4], Erin Scheick[4], and Steven L. Gortmaker [3]

1. Eating Disorders Clinical and Research Program, Department of Psychiatry, Massachusetts General Hospital, Boston, MA, Department of Social Medicine, Harvard Medical School, Boston, MA USA
2. Program on International Health and Human Rights, Harvard School of Public Health, Boston, MA, USA
3. Department of Society, Human Development, and Health, Harvard School of Public Health, Boston, MA,USA
4. Department of Population and International Health, Harvard School of Public Health, Boston, MA,USA

ABSTRACT

Objective: Study aims were to develop an instrument to assess a proposed construct, "dysregulated eating," and investigate its association with potential risk factors. Method: A scale measuring dysregulated eating was developed and validated in a convenience sample of graduate students (n=186). Covariates hypothesized to be associated with dysregulated eating were investigated with multiple linear regression. Results: Factor analysis supported two latent constructs underlying dysregulated eating, which were glossed as schedule-constrained eating and distraction-related eating. Cronbach's coefficient alphas were >.7 for the overall scale and two subscales. In a fully adjusted multivariable linear regression model, female gender, frequent caffeine consumption,

[*] Correspondence to: Laura Ferguson: lferguso@hsph.harvard.edu. Dr. Becker and Ms. Ferguson contributed equally to this study.

[†] Affiliation at the time the study was conducted.

higher perceived stress, inadequate sleep, and high fast food consumption were significant predictors of a higher mean scale score. The model adjusted R2 was 0.48. Discussion: This scale appears to have acceptable internal consistency reliability and construct validity in a graduate student population. A multivariable linear regression model suggests modifiable risk factors for dysregulated eating.

Keywords: *dysregulated eating, scheduled-constrained eating, distraction-related eating, graduate students, "Freshman 15"*

INTRODUCTION

The transition to college has been found to be associated with an elevated risk of weight gain. Indeed, the risk of unwanted weight gain associated with transition to college is implicit to the popular phrase "the freshman 15". Several studies have reported an increased risk of weight gain among college freshmen [1,2,3,4,5,6]. For instance, one recent study found students enrolled in their first semester of college had a significantly greater rate of weight gain than expected in the general population. Similarly, a comparative study of university freshman women with age-matched non-university women found significantly greater excess weight gain among the former group. Finally, Anderson and colleagues found a statistically significant — although modest — weight gain occurred for most of their respondents during their college freshman year. This led them to conclude that for some, the college freshman year is a "critical period for weight gain".

Transition to a college or other academic environment may also enhance risk for psychological symptoms among vulnerable individuals [7] Anecdotal clinical experience suggests that disordered eating behaviors often emerge or become exacerbated after a transition from a home to a school environment. For example, two studies suggest that medical students may be at elevated risk for an eating disorder [8,9]. College campuses have also been recognized as environments that may potentially increase perceived pressure to be slim [10]. Whereas one longitudinal study of incoming Dartmouth freshman did not support an increase in risk for eating disorder behaviors with this transition, investigators did find a highly significant decrease in body satisfaction during the freshman year of college as compared with the senior year of high school. Of particular relevance for this study, an increase in BMI was significantly associated with decreased body satisfaction over this transition period [11]. In addition, the concern about weight gain during the freshman year has been linked to both weight concern and poorer body image [12].

Although changes in eating patterns associated with transition to college and to graduate school may contribute to considerable distress, poor nutrition, overweight, and body dissatisfaction in a variety of ways, phenomenologic data on eating patterns in academic environments and their impact on health are lacking. Moreover, family and peer environment have been studied and linked to the development of eating pathology [13,14,15,16,17,18], yet other dimensions of environmental influences on unhealthful eating patterns have received comparatively less emphasis in theoretical models and in empirical research on eating disorders. Disordered eating and excessive calorie intake may emerge in a college environment for many plausible reasons (e.g. loss of parental supervision, cafeteria style eating, peer pressure to binge, purge or diet, or change in access to clinical resources). For this study, we considered the possibility that a graduate academic program might also have adverse impact on eating patterns because of academic and scheduling pressures relating to assignments and performance expectations. A variety of stressors have been found to be associated with overeating or overweight in vulnerable individuals [19,20,21,22] Moreover, we considered that the food environment that typifies university life, characterized by cafeteria style dining as well as the high availability of fast food and vending machine products may influence dietary routines and choices. Increasing obesity has also been attributed to changes in the social environment that have promoted overconsumption of calorie dense fast foods [23].

We hypothesized that eating patterns may frequently become "dysregulated"—that is, uncoupled from healthy eating routines that are conventionally guided by both nutritional needs as well as a social frame. Although these healthy eating routines vary considerably across individuals and social contexts and it is impossible to define an absolute or common standard, we suggest that scheduled mealtimes, meals with healthful and balanced nutritional content, eating accompanied by social interaction and culturally derived protocols represent key features of a healthy standard across diverse contexts.

Because there is no formal or consensual definition of "healthful eating" a construct defined by reference to it is as problematic as it is important. Healthful eating can be assessed unidimensionally by the nutritional content of the diet [24,25]. For example, the Healthy Eating Index (HEI) relates specifically to dietary quality [26]. In contrast, healthy eating has also been defined as the absence of disordered eating patterns such as restrictive eating, binge eating, and purging [27]. Several assessments have been developed to measure constructs relating to motivation for eating and eating patterns. For example, the Emotional Eating Scale (EES) was developed to assess how eating is used to cope with negative affect, including anger/frustration, depression, and anxiety [28]. Relatedly, the Dutch Eating Behaviour Questionnaire (DEBQ) assesses the eating styles characterized by restraint, 'external eating' (eating motivated by external cues), and emotional eating [29]. Similarly, the Three-Factor Eating Questionnaire (TFEQ) assesses dietary restraint and disinhibition as well as hunger [30,31]. Next, the Motivations to Eat scale measures four psychological motivations to eat: coping (overlapping with the EES and DEBQ), social, 'compliance' and pleasure.

Although these assessments are useful tools in understanding how eating patterns and triggers contribute to overweight and disordered eating, they have not exhausted all of the dimensions of departures from healthy eating. In particular, we note that the social frame for eating often differs in a university environment in which there is less time for preparing food, setting a table, sitting down for a scheduled meal, washing dishes, and so forth. Moreover, eating is also potentially used for distraction from and reward for work done in student culture. Thus in this study, we sought to add another perspective in developing a complementary construct, "dysregulated eating".

This proposed new construct of "dysregulated eating" represents both behavioral and motivational dimensions of a departure from healthful eating. That is, this construct encompasses a variety of eating behaviors (e.g. eating meals while standing up or walking to class, or while studying, or on a schedule) and motivations (e.g. eating for reward, relaxation, comfort, or distraction) that may contrast with healthy eating in some dimensions. Whereas this construct partially overlaps with those in the above mentioned assessments of emotional eating and psychological motivations to eat, it assesses additional behavioral and motivational dimensions that relate to the unique requirements of an academic environment. Study aims were: (1) to develop and validate an instrument to assess this proposed construct, "dysregulated eating"; and (2) to investigate the association of demographic and other possible risk factors with this construct in a survey among graduate students. Identification of eating patterns associated with an academic environment that may also contribute to an eating disorder or obesity may suggest opportunities to modify risk.

METHODS

Development of the Dysregulated Eating Pattern Scale (DEPS)

We hypothesized two chief domains underlying the proposed construct: (1) eating behaviors that relate to schedule and time constraints (e.g., eating outside of mealtimes; snacking while studying; eating while standing, eating while walking from one place to another; etc.); and (2) eating behaviors that are motivated by desire for distraction, reward, and/or comfort (e.g., eating as a break from or reward for studying; eating when feeling stressed).

A self-report questionnaire was developed with 17 items scored on a Likert scale to evaluate these domains. The hypothesized domains and corresponding items were generated, evaluated, and selected by consensus among the investigators, all but one of whom were graduate students at the time and included two with clinical expertise in eating disorders. The 6 point Likert Scale included response options of Never/Less than once a month, 1-3 times per month, once per week, 2-4 times per week, 5-6 times per week, and at least once a day. Additional items assessed demographic characteristics and other covariates of interest relating to weight and height, years spent in this particular graduate school, lifestyle, and perceived stress. All lifestyle and perceived stress questions (i.e., "I don't get enough sleep;" "I drink more caffeinated coffee/sodas than I should;" "I get enough time for leisure;" "I eat fast food;" and "I feel stressed") requested responses on this 6 point Likert scale. Questions regarding demographic data (i.e. gender, age, U.S. vs. non-U.S. nationality, and living arrangements) and weight and height requested categorical responses to preserve subject anonymity. Finally, two open-ended response items were included to elicit qualitative descriptions of change in and contentment with eating and to augment evaluation of construct validity.

The questionnaire was pilot-tested on a small group of graduate students to assess the time required to complete the questionnaire as well as whether the items were interpreted easily and as intended. Items were then revised as necessary to enhance comprehensibility and relevance.

Design and Study Participants

The study design was cross-sectional. A convenience sample of graduate students in a private school of public health in New England was recruited from two large classes. One hundred and eighty-six respondents returned questionnaires (response rate = 70%). The study was approved by this academic institution's Human Subjects Committee.

Data Analysis

Data were analyzed with SAS 9.1. Initially, data were examined for outliers, distribution, and missing values. Subjects missing 2 or more responses on the Dysregulated Eating Patterns Scale (DEPS) (n=5) were excluded from the statistical analyses. For subjects missing just one item, values for this item were imputed. Imputed values were based on the individual respondent's average response for the other scale items. Data from an additional 9 respondents were excluded from these analyses due to missing information on demographic and other covariates of interest.

Demographic covariates were analyzed as categorical variables as follows: age as 18 to 29 years or > 30 years; years at graduate school as ≤ one year or > one year; nationality as U.S. or non-U.S.; living arrangement as with or without family; weight and height as between 19 kg/m^2 and 25 kg/m^2 or either < 19 kg/m^2 or > 25 kg/m^2. Lifestyle and perceived stress covariates were analyzed as mean scores based on the numeric value of the single item response to the corresponding question (listed above); corresponding predictors were characterized as "inadequate sleep," "frequent caffeine consumption," "high fast food consumption," and "higher perceived stress." The item relating to leisure was reverse coded so that a relatively higher score reflected "inadequate leisure."

Factor Analysis

We hypothesized that the DEPS would have two subscales, one related to schedule-constrained eating, the other to distraction-related eating. We conducted our factor analysis with an oblique rotation, and selected factors based on an examination of the scree plot and of Eigenvalues. The criteria for including an item in a factor were a loading of at least 0.30 and no greater loading on another factor.

Reliability

Internal consistency reliability of the DEPS was assessed using Cronbach's coefficient alpha in the overall sample and among males and females. Internal consistency reliability for each subscale (factor) of the DEPS was also assessed.

Validity

The known groups validation method was used to assess construct validity on the overall scale and each of the subscales of the DEPS. Based on previous literature, we expected higher mean DEPS scores for women as compared with men [32, 33], among respondents reporting higher perceived stress levels [34,35], among respondents living alone or with roommates compared with those living with family due to less support for meal preparation [36], among respondents reporting a change in eating patterns since arriving at graduate school, and for first year students compared with more advanced students.

Descriptive Statistics

Descriptive statistical analyses of our sample were conducted within gender subgroups as well as the overall sample to assess demographics, mean DEPS scores, median subscale scores (and their ranges), as well as the frequencies and means of other covariates of interest.

Qualitative Data

Two open-ended questions ("If so [if you think your eating patterns have changed since you came to this school], how have they changed?" and "How content are you with your eating patterns?") were reviewed for thematic content. Responses were independently coded by two investigators to reflect either no change or a positive or negative change for the former question for use in quantitative analyses; discrepancies in assignment were resolved in discussion with a third investigator. All observations with responses to either of these questions were retained for analysis of these qualitative data.

The association between DEPS score and responses to the qualitative items were evaluated with an ANOVA. Finally, excerpts from both representative and richly detailed statements were culled from the data to illustrate their range and provide context for the quantitative data and to suggest hypotheses for future research.

Regression Analysis

A multiple linear regression model was developed in order to examine which demographic and other hypothesized risk factors were associated with overall DEPS score and each of the subscale scores.

RESULTS

Characteristics of the study population are summarized in Table 1. The majority of respondents were from the United States and lived without family. A slight majority were female and a sizeable minority were at least 30 years old. The majority of both men and women were in their first year of graduate school at this institution.

Factor Analysis

Factor analysis supported the presence of two sub-scales underlying the construct of dysregulated eating patterns. Eigenvalues were 2.8 for Schedule-Constrained Eating and 5.7 for Distraction-Related Eating; together these captured 90% of the information in the overall scale, supporting a two-factor solution. Two items were eliminated from the scale because they did not meet criteria for loading onto either scale ("I drink more caffeinated coffee/sodas than I should" and "I eat fast food") (Table 2).

Table 1. Sample characteristics

	Men	Women	Total
Age			
18-29	20 (36.4%)	71 (60.7%)	91 (52.9%)
30+	35 (63.6%)	46 (39.3)%	81 (47.1%)
Years at Graduate School			
One year	43 (78.2%)	76 (65.0%)	119 (69.2%)
Two + years	12 (21.8%)	41 (35.0%)	53 (30.8%)
Nationality			
US	21 (38.2%)	87 (74.4%)	108 (62.8%)
Other	34 (61.8%)	30 (25.6%)	64 (37.2%)
Living arrangement			
With family	26 (47.3%)	36 (30.8%)	62 (36.1%)
Without family	29 (52.7%)	81 (69.2%)	110 (63.9%)
BMI score			
BMI between 19 kg/m^2 and 25 kg/m^2	33 (60.0%)	88 (75.2%)	121 (70.4%)
BMI < 19 kg/m^2 or > 25 kg/m^2	22 (40.0%)	29 (24.79%)	51 (29.6%)
Mean DEPS score	43.1 (23-69)	46.6 (21-76)	45.4 (21-76)
Mean Stress score	3.5	4.1	3.9
Mean Sleep score	3.9	3.9	3.9
Mean Leisure score	4.1	4.2	4.2
Mean Caffeine consumption score	3.1	3.1	3.1
Mean Fast food consumption score	1.5	1.4	1.4
Total n	55 (32.0%)	117 (68.0%)	172

Reliability

Acceptable internal consistency reliability of the questionnaire and its subscales was demonstrated with Cronbach's alpha >0.7 for the overall scale, each sub-scale, and by gender (Table 3).

Table 2. Promax-rotated factor loadings for dysregulated eating items based on two-factor solution

Item	Factor 1	Factor 2
Factor 1: Schedule-constrained eating		
My schedule dictates my meals	.41	-.010
I take the time to prepare my meals from scratch (as opposed to ready-made meals)	.43	-.10

Table 2. (Continued)

Item	Factor 1	Factor 2
I eat meals while walking from one place to another	.66	.05
I eat/drink straight out of the original carton/container (e.g. milk, ice cream)	.37	.13
I eat my meals standing up	.60	.09
I skip meals	.53	-.10
I eat with the refrigerator door open	.34	.32
I eat according to a regular schedule	.55	-.08
I eat meals while I am studying	.45	.32
Factor 2: Distraction-related eating		
Eating helps me unwind at the end of the day	-.29	.56
I eat more when I am stressed	-.03	.68
I reward myself with food for finishing an assignment/getting a good grade	-.04	.56
I eat as an excuse to take a break from studying	-.04	.79
I eat more than I should in order to stay up late	.06	.62
I have snack food available when studying	.12	.46
Items not retained from factor analyses		
I drink more caffeinated coffee/sodas than I should	.24	.25
I eat fast food	.29	.04

Note: Primary factor loadings in bold. All items and respective anchors (see below) appear with original wording. Italicized items were reverse coded prior to calculating mean factor so that a a higher score would more likely reflect a departure from conventional or healthful eating patterns on each question.

Table 3. Cronbach's alpha (Standardized) in each subscale by gender

	Overall	Men	Women
Dysregulated eating patterns	0.79	0.80	0.78
Distraction-related eating	0.76	0.73	0.76
Schedule-constrained eating	0.75	0.80	0.72

Construct Validity

As hypothesized, higher perceived stress, not living with family, and a reported change in eating patterns were all associated with significantly higher mean scores on the overall DEPS and on the distraction-related eating sub-scale as compared with lower perceived stress, living with family, and no reported change in eating patterns, respectively. Women had higher mean scores than men at the level of a trend on the overall scale and had significantly higher mean subscale scores on the distraction subscale. First year graduate students' mean scores were higher than those of more advanced students as expected, but this difference was not statistically significant. Finally, all of these predictors were positively associated with higher schedule-constrained sub-scale mean scores, although only the association with perceived stress reached statistical significance and the association with not living with family and with reported change in eating patterns since graduate school were marginally significant (Tables 4 and 6).

Qualitative Data

Responses to two open-ended questions relating to how eating habits had changed since arrival at graduate school, and how respondents felt about this change were assessed. Seventy percent (n=131) of study participants responded to one or both of these questions. Themes identified from the qualitative responses included changes in schedule, venue, and quality of eating as well as time-constrained and somewhat disorganized qualities to eating. Whereas the majority of responses suggested the changes were perceived as negative, some respondents reported their eating habits had improved since arriving at graduate school. Excerpts that illustrate these themes are listed in Table 5.

Those reporting a positive change in eating behavior since arriving at graduate school (n=8) reported a significantly lower mean DEPS than those who reported a negative change (n=45; p=0.01). Similarly those reporting improved quality in their diet had a significantly lower DEPS than those reporting that the quality of their diet had deteriorated since arriving at graduate school (p=0.03).

Regression Analyses

Five of the eleven candidate predictor variables were found to have a statistically significant unadjusted association with a higher mean overall DEPS score: non-family living arrangement (p =0.0050), insufficient sleep (p <0.0001), higher perceived stress (p <0.0001), frequent caffeine consumption (p <0.0001), high fast food consumption (p <0.0011). The direction of association of each of these covariates with the outcome measure was consistent with initial hypotheses (Table 6). In addition, older age group and female gender were positively associated with higher mean DEPS scores at the level of a trend (p=0.053 and p=0.066, respectively). All covariates were retained in the multivariable regression model regardless of association with the DEPS score because they were deemed scientifically plausible predictors, potential confounders, or conventionally included in similar analyses.

Table 4. Associations between covariates and DEPS overall and subscale mean scores

Scale	Men	Women	Difference	P-value
DEPS	43.1	46.6	3.5	0.0684
Distraction-related eating	14.4	17.2	2.8	0.0031
Schedule-constrained eating	22.9	24.6	1.7	0.1676
	Living with Family	Not living with family		
DEPS	42.2	47.3	5.1	0.0046
Distraction-related eating	14.4	17.3	2.9	0.0007
Schedule-constrained eating	22.8	24.7	1.9	0.0965
	No changed eating	Changed eating		
DEPS	42.2	47.8	5.6	0.0013
Distraction-related eating	14.7	17.5	2.8	0.0014
Schedule-constrained eating	22.9	24.9	2.0	0.0650
	1st year at graduate school	At least 2nd year at graduate school		
DEPS	46.1	44.0	2.1	0.2703
Distraction-related eating	16.5	15.8	0.7	0.4707
Schedule-constrained eating	24.4	23.3	1.1	0.3636

Table 5. Qualitative themes in open-ended responses relating to dietary changes and levels of discontentment

Theme	Selected excerpted open-ended responses
Changes in Schedule	Eats later at night I skip more meals Meal times are less regular More irregular More regular More snack and eating late . . Not in an appropriate time Not enough time to prepare food [. . .] I'm busy, sometimes no time to eat leisurely Faster, quicker meals [. . .] I take less time to eat. I am very busy with assignments and classes. I do not have time to sleep, eat most of the time. . . . Less time to chew, savor, digest Worse [. . .] more@ odd hours I am busier, so I eat things that are easier or eat more than I did before due to stress
Changes in Place	I eat watching news on TV Eat during class I eat what is in the dining café by my building

Theme	Selected excerpted open-ended responses
	. . . More on-the-go . . .
Changes in Quality of the Diet	I cook fewer meals and buy more pre-made meals Less cooking, less vegetables due to less time I eat more junk food, drink more caffeine More fast-food based now Eating lots of snacks (reward); gained weight; drink lots of soda/coke Gone bad
Perception of positive changes	Improved, higher calorie intake [. . .] more vegetables, since everyone eats them [. . .] More time and accessibility to go home and cook [. . .] I eat healthier-lost a couple of pounds even though I have less time to workout Eating breakfast now
Sources of discontentment: Time constraints	I would like more time to prepare and enjoy meals Want to cook more [. . .] need time to shop for healthy foods
Sources of discontentment: Dietary quality is suboptimal	I'm not happy with it. I would like to eliminate the junk food and stick to eating healthier food on a regular basis Not content; trying to eat more fruits/vegetables I eat too many snacks. Not enough fruits/vegetables. [. . .] I want more variety in my diet. [. . .] Would like to be eating less of high energy foods. Too many calories/carbs [. . .] I'd rather not have breakfast Wish I at[e] a more healthy diet less fat (fewer jun[k] food calories) [. . .] Would like to be eating less of high energy foods. . . . I need [. . .] less sugar. Not happy, but could be worse, I could be starving myself Not happy; feel sloggy; don't have energy Feel like I need to take better care of myself but always on the go [. . .] I wish I stuck to more standard eating times but sometimes am busy
Sources of discontentment: Dietary patterns are disorganized	Above makes me feel disorganized Much better pattern now; last year was crazy (my first year here) Very discontent. I eat poorly but am too busy/stressed to address changing my habits Not content-I've lost weight Not really [content], binge, skip meals, eat when stressed

The final model to predict DEPS score included five significant predictor variables: female gender, inadequate sleep, higher perceived stress, frequent caffeine consumption, and high fast food consumption. In addition, being a first year graduate student (versus a more advanced student) was marginally significantly associated with a higher mean DEPS score (Table 7). The adjusted R^2 of the final model is 0.48.

Table 6. Unadjusted association of candidate predictor variables with overall DEPS score and each subscale

	DEPS		Schedule-constrained		Distraction-related	
Predictor Variable	Parameter Estimate	p-value	Parameter Estimate	p-value	Parameter Estimate	p-value
Younger age group	-3.40	0.0530	-1.51	0.1700	-1.98	0.0272
Female	3.47	0.0656	1.69	0.1509	2.74	0.0041
US nationality	0.53	0.7720	-0.42	0.7138	-0.92	0.3224
1st year in graduate school	2.16	0.2583	1.11	0.3517	0.68	0.4884
Non-family living arrangement	5.10	0.0050	1.95	0.0876	2.89	0.0018
Inadequate sleep	2.95	<0.0001	1.55	0.0022	1.50	0.0003
Higher perceived stress	3.21	<0.0001	1.62	<0.0001	1.24	<0.0001
Frequent caffeine consumption	3.46	<0.0001	1.08	0.0001	0.76	0.0010
Inadequate leisure time	-0.30	0.6918	0.16	0.7390	-0.51	0.1919
High fast food consumption	3.51	<0.0001	1.71	0.0002	0.49	0.2113
BMI < 19 kg/m^2 or > 25 kg/m^2	1.40	0.4679	1.06	0.3784	-0.12	0.9003

Table 7. Final models from regression analyses

DEPS

Predictor	Parameter Estimate	95% Confidence Interval	P-value
Younger age group	-1.58	(-4.7,1.5)	0.3178
Female	5.32	(2.2,8.4)	0.0009
US nationality	0.32	(-2.9,3.5)	0.8456
1st year at graduate school	2.50	(-0.3,5.3)	0.0803
Non-family living arrangement	2.41	(-0.7,5.6)	0.1360
Inadequate sleep	1.74	(0.5,3.0)	0.0063
Higher perceived stress	1.93	(0.9,3.0)	0.0004
Frequent caffeine consumption	2.01	(1.3,2.7)	<0.0001
Inadequate leisure time	-0.97	(-2.2,0.2)	0.1088

Predictor	Parameter Estimate	95% Confidence Interval	P-value
High fast food consumption	3.42	(2.1,4.7)	<0.0001
BMI < 19 kg/m^2 or > 25 kg/m^2	0.73	(-2.2,3.7)	0.6243

Adjusted R-Square: 0.4753

Schedule-Constrained Eating

Predictor	Parameter Estimate	95% Confidence Interval	P-value
Younger age group	-1.03	(-3.4,1.3)	0.3922
Female	2.61	(0.3,5.0)	0.0316
US nationality	-0.31	(-2.8,2.2)	0.8078
1st year at graduate school	1.49	(-0.6,3.6)	0.1708
Non-family living arrangement	0.66	(-1.8,3.1)	0.5943
Inadequate sleep	0.73	(-0.2,1.7)	0.1320
Higher perceived stress	1.06	(0.3,1.9)	0.0097
Frequent caffeine consumption	0.59	(0.1,1.1)	0.0280
Inadequate leisure time	-0.14	(-1.0,0.8)	0.7690
High fast food consumption	1.83	(0.8,2.8)	0.0004
BMI < 19 kg/m^2 or > 25 kg/m^2	0.72	(-1.5,2.9)	0.5292

Adjusted R-Square: 0.2113

Distraction-Related Eating

Predictor	Parameter Estimate	95% Confidence Interval	P-value
Younger age group	-0.54	(-2.5,1.4)	0.5814
Female	2.72	(0.8,4.7)	0.0067
US nationality	0.63	(-1.4,2.6)	0.5443
1st year at graduate school	1.01	(-0.7,2.8)	0.2601
Non-family living arrangement	1.76	(-0.2,3.7)	0.0840
Inadequate sleep	1.01	(0.2,1.8)	0.0112
Higher perceived stress	0.87	(0.2,1.5)	0.0102
Frequent caffeine consumption	0.41	(-0.02,0.8)	0.0620

Table 7. (Continued)

Predictor	Parameter Estimate	95% Confidence Interval	P-value
Inadequate leisure time	-0.84	(-1.6,-0.1)	0.0283
High fast food consumption	0.59	(-0.2,1.4)	0.1607
BMI < 19 kg/m^2 or > 25 kg/m^2	0.01	(-1.8,1.8)	0.9888

Adjusted R-Square: 0.2108

In the fully adjusted multivariable model for the schedule-constrained subscale, female gender, frequent caffeine consumption, high fast food consumption, and higher perceived stress were associated with significantly higher mean scores as compared with male gender, infrequent caffeine consumption, low fast food consumption, and lower perceived stress. The adjusted R^2 of the final model is 0.21.

In the next fully adjusted multivariable model describing the association between covariates of interest and the distraction-related eating subscale, female gender, inadequate sleep, and higher perceived stress time were significantly positively associated with higher mean scores. Inadequate leisure time was significantly inversely associated with higher subscale scores. Frequent caffeine consumption and a non-family living arrangement were each also positively and marginally significantly associated with a higher score on the distraction-related eating subscale (p=0.06 and p=0.08 respectively). The adjusted R^2 of the final model is 0.21.

CONCLUSION

In this chapter we propose a construct of "dysregulated eating" that references eating behaviors and motivation that depart from healthful eating and that develop in relation to achievement pressures and scheduling constraints inherent to many tertiary academic environments. An assessment measure of dysregulated eating was developed which had two subscales—schedule-constrained eating and distraction-related eating—with acceptable internal consistency reliability and construct validity in a graduate student study population. Our exploratory analysis found that, in a multivariable model, high mean scores on the overall scale were associated with female gender, inadequate sleep, higher perceived stress, frequent caffeine consumption, and high fast food consumption. In addition, being a first year graduate student as compared with a more advanced student was associated with a marginally significant higher mean score. These findings suggest that dysregulated eating may be more common among women and may be associated with lifestyle changes or patterns that may reflect academic and social pressures in many graduate academic environments. Moreover, qualitative data support the hypothesis that the perception of academic pressure is associated with perceived dysregulated eating patterns.

Analysis of the schedule-constrained subscale of DEPS found that, in a multivariable model, it was associated with female gender, frequent caffeine consumption, high fast food consumption, and higher perceived stress. The multivariable model for the distraction-related eating subscale demonstrated that female gender, inadequate sleep, higher perceived stress were significantly and positively associated with high mean scores on this subscale. In addition, both frequent caffeine consumption and a non-family living arrangement were marginally significantly associated with a higher mean score on this subscale. Unexpectedly, inadequate leisure was significantly inversely associated with a higher mean score on the distraction-related eating subscale.

Causal inference about antecedents to dysregulated eating is limited by the cross-sectional design of this study; using the DEPS in a longitudinal study could suggest whether dysregulated eating among students does arise in an academic environment and also whether it might have adverse health outcomes such as increasing risk for clinically significant disordered eating or weight gain. The term dysregulated eating may also be a misnomer insofar as it implies a departure from a normative standard for "healthful eating". Even if such a standard were defined, we are unable to establish that study participants have progressed from "healthy" to dysregulated eating. However, the significantly higher mean scores on the DEPS among those who perceived a negative change in eating patterns since entering graduate school may suggest a progression toward this pattern in graduate school. This study is also limited by convenience sampling, and self-selection for participation in the study, which may have biased the results in an unknown direction. As this study is based on a self-report questionnaire, many of the responses are based on the participants' subjective assessments of their behavior; these interpretations might differ among participants. Furthermore, it is possible that social desirability and recall bias may have had an effect on responses to the survey. Finally, generalizability to populations in non-academic environments or even in other academic environments may be limited by culturally unique attributes of the institution where the research data were collected. On the other hand, these results suggest potential avenues for promoting healthful eating for students who may be vulnerable to weight gain and disordered eating.

Whereas the construct of dysregulated eating proposed in this study does not necessarily reference a clinical phenomenon, we suggest it may illustrate a meaningful departure from healthful eating patterns that may contribute to risk for excessive calorie intake. Both predictors of dysregulated eating and its effects on weight gain, body dissatisfaction, and disordered eating behaviors warrant further investigation.

Acknowledgements

We thank Malavika Subramanyam for her contributions, and Keri Conron for helpful comments on earlier versions of this work. We thank Bryn Austin for her extremely thoughtful and useful comments as a peer reviewer of this chapter. This work was supported in part by a grant from the National Institute of Mental Health K23 MH068575 (AEB).

References

[1] Morrow, ML; Heesch, KC; Dinger, MK; Hull, HR; Kneehans, AW; Fields, DA. Freshman 15: fact or fiction?. *Obesity*, 2006 14, 1438-43.

[2] Hoffman, DJ; Policastro, P; Quick, V; Lee, SK. Changes in body weight and fat mass of men and women in the first year of college: A study of the "freshman 15". *Journal of American College Health,* 2006 55, 41-5.

[3] Levitsky, DA; Halbamaier, CA; Mrdjenovic, G. The freshman weight gain: a model for the study of the epidemic of obesity. *International Journal of Obesity and Related Metabolic Disorders: Journal of the International Association for the Study of Obesity*, 2003 28, 1435-42.

[4] Hovell, MF; Mewborn, CR; Randle, Y; Fowler-Johnson, S. Risk of excess weight gain in university women: A three-year community controlled analysis. *Addictive Behaviors*, 1985 10,15-28.

[5] Butler, SM; Black, DR; Blue, CL; Gretebeck, R.J. Change in diet, physical activity, and body weight in female college freshman. *American Journal of Health Behavior*, 2004 28, 24-32.

[6] Anderson, DA; Shapiro, JR; Lundgren, JD. The freshman year of college as a critical period for weight gain: An initial evaluation. *Eating Behaviors*, 2003 4, 363-67.

[7] Compas, BE; Wagner, BM; Slavin, LA; Vannatta, K. A prospective study of life events, social support, and psychological symptomatology during the transition from high school to college. *American Journal of Community Psychology*, 1986 14, 241-57.

[8] Herzog, DB; Borus, JF; Hamburg, P; Ott, IL; *Concus A. Substance use, eating behaviors, and social impairment of medical students. Journal of Medical Education*, 1987 62, 651-7.

[9] Futch, LS; Wingard, DL; *Felice, ME. Eating pattern disturbances among women medical and graduate students. Journal of Adolescent Health Care*, 1988 9, 378-83.

[10] Striegel-Moore, RH; Silberstein, LR; Rodin, J. Toward an understanding of risk factors for bulimia nervosa. *American Psychologist*, 1986 41, 246-63.

[11] Vohs, KD; Heatherton, TF; Herrin, M. Disordered eating and the transition to college: A prospective study. *International Journal of Eating Disorders*, 2001 29, 280-88.

[12] Graham, MA; Jones, AL. Freshman 15: valid theory or harmful myth?. *Journal of American College Health*, 2002 50, 171-3.

[13] Lin, LF; Kulik, JA. Social comparison and women's body satisfaction. *Basic and Applied Social Psychology*, 2002 24, 115-123.

[14] Presnell, K; Bearman, SK; Stice, E. Risk factors for body dissatisfaction in adolescent boys and girls: A prospective study. *International Journal of Eating Disorders*, 2004 36, 389-401.

[15] Neumark-Sztainer, D; Falkner, N; Story, M; Perry, C; Hannan, PJ; Mulert, S. Weight-based teasing among adolescents: Correlations with weight status and disordered eating behaviors. *International Journal of Obesity*, 2002 26, 123-131.

[16] Mora-Giral, M; Raich-Escursell, RM; Segues, CV; Torras-Claraso, J; Huon, G. Bulimia symptoms and risk factors in university students. *Eating andWeight Disorders: EWD*, 2004 9, 163-9.

[17] Wade, TD; Gillespie, N; Martin, NG. A comparison of early family life events amongst monozygotic twin women with lifetime anorexia nervosa, bulimia nervosa, or major depression. *International Journal of* Eating Disorders, 2007 40, 679-86.

[18] Fernandez-Aranda, F; Krug, I; Granero, R; Ramon, JM; Badia, A; Gimenez, L; Solano, R; Collier, D; Karwautz, A; Treasure, J. Individual and family eating patterns during

childhood and early adolescence: an analysis of associated eating disorder factors. *Appetite*, 2007 49, 476-85.

[19] Timmerman, GM; Acton, GJ. The relationship between basic need satisfaction and emotional eating. *Issues in Mental Health Nursing*, 2001 22, 691-701.

[20] Lowe, MR; Fisher, EB Jr. Emotional reactivity, emotional eating, and obesity: A naturalistic study. *Journal of Behavioral Medicine*, 1983 6, 135-49.

[21] Musante, GJ; Costanzo, PR; Friedman, KE. The comorbidity of depression and eating dysregulation processes in a diet-seeking obese population: A matter of gender specificity. *International Journal of Eating Disorders*, 1998 23, 65-75.

[22] Pinaquay, S; Charbrol, H; Simon, C; Louvet, JP; Barbe, P. Emotional eating, alexithymia, and binge-eating disorder in obese women. *Obesity Research*, 2003 11, 195-201.

[23] Wadden, TA; Brownell, KD; Foster, GD. Obesity: responding to the global epidemic. *Journal of Consulting and Clinical Psychology*, 2002 70, 510-25.

[24] Evans, AE; Wilson, DK; Buck, J; Torbett, H; Williams, J. Outcome expectations, barriers, and strategies for healthful eating: A perspective from adolescents from low income families. *Family and Community Health*, 2006 29, 17-27

[25] Prochaska, JD; Sharkey, JR; Ory, MG; Burdine, JN. Assessing healthful eating among community dwelling rural older adults using self-reported fruit and vegetable consumption via a community-wide mail-out health status assessment. *Journal of Nutrition for the Elderly*, 2005 25, 101-12.

[26] Kennedy, ET; Ohls, J; Carlson, S; Fleming, K. The Healthy Eating Index: Design and applications. *Journal of the American Dietetic Association*, 1995, 95, 1103-08.

[27] Jackson, B; Cooper, ML; Mintz, L; Albino A. Motivations to eat: Scale development and validation. *Journal of Research in Personality*, 2003 37, 297-318.

[28] Arnow, B; Kenardy, J, Agras, WS. The Emotional Eating Scale: The development of a measure to assess coping with negative affect by eating. *International Journal of Eating Disorders*, 1995; 18:79-90.

[29] Wardle, J. Eating style A validation of the Dutch Eating Behaviour Questionnaire in Normal Subjects and Women with Eating Disorders. *Journal of Psychosomatic Research*, 1987 31, 161-69.

[30] Stunkard, AJ; Messick, S. The Three-Factor Eating Questionnaire to measure dietary restraint, disinhibition, and hunger. *Journal of Psychosomatic Research*, 1985 29, 71-83.

[31] Bond, MJ; McDowell, AJ; Wilkinson, JY. The measurement of dietary restraint, disinhibition and hunger: An examination of the factor structure of the Three Factor Eating Questionnaire (TFEQ). *International Journal of Obesity*, 2001 25, 900-906.

[32] Wardle, J; Marsland, L; Sheikh, Y; Quinn, M; Federoff, I; Ogden, J. Eating style and eating behaviour in adolescents. *Appetite*, 1992 18, 167-83.

[33] Johnson, CS; Bedford, J. Eating attitudes across age and gender groups: a Canadian study. *Eating and Weight Disorders*, 2004 9, 16-23.

[34] Wallis, DJ; Hetherington, MM. Stress and eating: The effects of ego-threat and cognitive demand on food intake in restrained and emotional eaters. *Appetite*, 2004 43, 39-46.

[35] Laitinen, J; Ek, E; Sovio, U. Stress-related eating and drinking behavior and body mass index and predictors of this behavior. *Preventive Medicine*, 2002 34, 29-39.

[36] Devine, CM; Connors, MM; Sobal, J; Bisogni, CA. Sandwiching it in: Spillover of work onto food choices and family roles in low-and moderate-income urban households. *Social Science and Medicine*, 2003 56, 617-30.

In: Eating Disorders in Adult Women
Editor: Julian N. Fuchs

ISBN 978-1-60456-673-4

Chapter 3

THE POSSIBLE LINK BETWEEN THE FEMALE PUBERTY AND THE EATING DISORDERS ONSET

Paolo Cotrufo* and Stefania Cella
Observatory on Eating Disorders, Department of Psychology,
Second University of Naples, Italy

Keywords: *Anorexia, Bulimia, Puberty, Menarche, Eating Disorders*

In the last twenty years a lot has been written about eating disorders (EDs). The spreading of these disorders, which grew remarkably until ten years ago (Hoek and Van Hoeken, 2003), seems to have become steady today, with percentages ranging between 0.2-1% for anorexia nervosa (AN) and 1-3% for bulimia nervosa (BN) in samples of adolescent women in western countries (A.P.A., 1994; Cotrufo et al., 1998; Rosenvinge et al., 1999; Hoek and Van Hoeken, 2003).

The stabilisation of complete clinical syndromes was associated with an increase in subthreshold diagnoses, called partial or subclinical EDs, that is conditions which, while displaying the psycho-pathological aspects typical of eating disorders (intense fear of gaining weight, self-esteem entirely dependent on physical appearance and body weight), do not reach such levels of clinical severity as to meet all the criteria established by the DSM-IV for an ED to be diagnosed (Dancynger and Garfinkel, 1995; Eagles et al., 1995, Cotrufo et al., 1998; Cotrufo et al., 2005). A research carried out on a sample of 788 adolescents aged between 12 and 14 showed that 9.4% of the subjects met the criteria for a partial diagnosis of ED (Zini et al., 2007). In the study carried out by Cotrufo et al. (1998) the subthreshold ED diagnosis concerned 10.7% of the female students aged between 14 and 19. Largely consistent results have been obtained by several authors who have studied partial syndromes (Crow et al., 2002; Fairburn and Walsh, 2002). In 2005 we suggested some diagnostic criteria based on those of the DSM-IV (APA, 1994) to diagnose subtrheshold EDs (Table 1; Cotrufo et al., 2005).

* Address for correspondence: Prof. Paolo Cotrufo, Department of Psychology, Via Vivaldi, 43 – 81100, Caserta, Italy.e-mail: paolo.Cotrufo@unina2.it.

Table 1. Full-, Partial- and Subclinical Eating Disorders diagnostic criteria, based on DSM-IV (Cotrufo et al., 2005)

	Full-syndrome	Partial-syndrome	Subclinical ED
Anorexia	1.Body weight less than 85% of that expected. 2.Intense fear of gaining weight or becoming fat, even though underweight. 3.Disturbance in the way in which one's body weight or shape is experienced, undue influence of body weight or shape on self-evaluation, or denial of the seriousness of the current low body weight. 4.In postmenarcheal females, amenorrhea.	1.Intense fear of gaining weight or becoming fat, even though underweight. 2.Disturbance in the way in which one's body weight or shape is experienced, undue influence of body weight or shape on self-evaluation, or denial of the seriousness of the current low body weight. 3.Body weight less than 85% of that expected; OR 4.In postmenarcheal females, amenorrhea.	1.Intense fear of gaining weight or becoming fat, even though underweight. 2.Disturbance in the way in which one's body weight or shape is experienced, undue influence of body weight or shape on self-evaluation, or denial of the seriousness of the current low body weight.
Bulimia	1.Recurrent episodes of binge eating. 1.a.Sense of lack of control during the episodes. 2.recurrent inappropriate compensatory behaviour in order to prevent weight gain. 3.The binge eating and inappropriate compensatory behaviours both occur, on average, at least twice a week for 3 months. 4.Self-evaluation is unduly influenced by body shape and weight. 5.The disturbance does not occur exclusively during episodes of Anorexia Nervosa.	1.Recurrent episodes of binge eating. 2.recurrent inappropriate compensatory behaviour in order to prevent weight gain. 4.Self-evaluation is unduly influenced by body shape and weight. 5.The disturbance does not occur exclusively during episodes of Anorexia Nervosa. 1.a.Sense of lack of control during the episodes. OR 3.The binge eating and inappropriate compensatory behaviours both occur, on average, at least twice a week for 3 months.	1.Recurrent episodes of binge eating. 2.recurrent inappropriate compensatory behaviour in order to prevent weight gain. 4.Self-evaluation is unduly influenced by body shape and weight. 5.The disturbance does not occur exclusively during episodes of Anorexia Nervosa.
BED	1.Recurrent episodes of binge eating. 1.a.Sense of lack of control during the episodes. 2.The binge eating episodes are associated with three of the following: 2.a.eating much more rapidly then normal, 2.b.eating until feeling uncomfortably full, 2.c.eating large amount of food not feeling physically hungry, 2.d.eating alone because of being	1.Recurrent episodes of binge eating. 2.The binge eating episodes are associated with three of the following: 2.a.eating much more rapidly then normal, 2.b.eating until feeling uncomfortably full, 2.c.eating large amount of food not feeling physically hungry, 2.d.eating alone because of being embarrassed, 2.e.feeling disgusted, depressed, or guilty after overeating.	1.Recurrent episodes of binge eating. 2.The binge eating episodes are associated with three of the following: 2.a.eating much more rapidly then normal, 2.b.eating until feeling uncomfortably full, 2.c.eating large amount of food not feeling physically hungry, 2.d.eating alone because of being embarrassed, 2.e.feeling disgusted, depressed, or guilty after overeating. 3.Marked distress regarded binge eating is present. 5.The binge eating is not associated with use of compensatory

	Full-syndrome	Partial-syndrome	Subclinical ED
	embarrassed, 2.e.feeling disgusted, depressed, or guilty after overeating. 3.Marked distress regarded binge eating is present. 4.The binge eating occur at least two days a week for 6 months. 5.The binge eating is not associated with use of compensatory behaviours.	3.Marked distress regarded binge eating is present. 5.The binge eating is not associated with use of compensatory behaviours. 1.a.Sense of lack of control during the episodes. OR 4.The binge eating occur at least two days a week for 6 months.	behaviours.

Although there are no formal epidemiological studies available, in the last few years several authors have suggested an increasing prevalence of eating disorders and the adoption of abnormal eating behaviours also in developing countries (Ghazal et al., 2001; Shroff and Thompson, 2004; Gentile et al., 2007).

In Turkey, the scores obtained by 7.9% of university students on the Eating Attitude Test – 40 were such that a tendency towards anorexic-bulimic behaviours was supposed (Altug et al., 2000). A study conducted on a sample of 414 female college students revealed figures concerning eating disorders (with the exception of bulimia nervosa) comparable to those of western countries (Uzun et al., 2006). Researchers expect an increasing number of cases in the next few years (Elal et al., 2000; Kiziltan et al., 2006). In the Philippines, 15% of girls and 14.5% of boys presented a dysfunctional eating behaviour (Lorenzo et al., 2002), while abnormal eating habits have recently been 10 ten times as many as those recorded in the United States (Madanat et al., 2006). Similar values were recorded in a population of university students in Brazil (Nunes et al., 2003). In Saudi Arabia too, a prevalence of anorexia nervosa has been recorded (2.0%), in line with the rest of the world (Eapen et al., 2006). In Iran, anorexia and bulimia were at 0.9% and 3.2% respectively (Nobakht and Dezhkam, 2000), whereas in Pakistan, out of 111 subjects two met the requirements for a diagnosis of bulimia and two met the diagnostic criteria for an ED NOS (Suhail and Zaib-u-Nisa, 2002). The sharp increase in the prevalence of EDs which was recorded in western countries between the 1960s and 1970s seems to be affecting, thirty years later, also the so-called developing countries.

Another interesting element to look at is the onset of the disorders, which occurs at an increasingly younger age. In the last decade clinical cases of anorexia nervosa and other EDs have been recorded more and more often among girls of prepuberal age, before the menarche and the somatic changes brought about by puberty. More generally, several authors draw attention to the high levels of drive for thinness and body dissatisfaction in children as young as 5 to 11 (Williamson and Delin, 2001; Sancho et al., 2007) and the following adoption of dysfunctional eating behaviours aimed at controlling body weight (Sands et al., 1997; Davis and Lambert, 2000; Ricciardelli and McCabe, 2001; Hausenblas et al., 2002; Knez et al., 2006).

The study by Rolland et al. (1997) on a sample of 244 students aged between 8 and 12 showed that 50% of females and 33% of males wished to lose weight, and that 40% and 24% respectively adopted strategies to counter the increase in body fat. Largely similar results are reported by Sasson et al. (1995) and by Schur et al. (2000). Quite high percentages also appear in the study carried out by Shisslak et al. (1998) on a sample of 523 pupils attending the primary and junior high schools (aged between 6 and 13): 50% and 66% of the children respectively adopted unhealthy practices for body weight control. The clinical picture of eating disorders observed in female children and preadolescent girls is very similar to that of adolescent girls and young women (Lask and Bryant-Waugh, 1994).

Alongside the increase in early forms of EDs, child obesity has grown remarkably. Although estimates are difficult to compare, research carried out in Italy indicates that obesity is much more widespread, particularly in the regions of southern Italy, than in other European countries like France and the Netherlands, and even than the US, which was considered as the country where this pathology recorded its highest values (Esposito-Del Puente et al., 1996). Most of these children remain overweight also in their adult age and, as early as the age of development, obesity is associated to metabolic and organ morbidity (Dietz, 1998).

While extending the risk period for EDs to pre-adolescence, however, these data do not link the onset of such disorders directly to body changes. A study highlighted how the experience of the menarche increases concern for body weight (O'Dea and Abraham, 1999) and how the idea of diet itself changes depending on whether the subject has already menstruated or not (Abraham and O'Dea, 2001). Other authors have shown that the perception of being overweight (Ackard and Peterson, 2001) and weight increase linked to the beginning of puberty may have a role in the adoption of dysfunctional eating behaviours, and that an early development may entail a greater risk of developing an ED (Striegel-Moore et al., 2001).

In a study carried out on a sample of 2657 subjects (1345 males and 1312 females) aged between 11 and 13, attending the junior high school (age: 10-13) in different areas of southern Italy (Cotrufo et al., 2007), we have found that interest in fitness and body weight, and the following adoption of dysfunctional eating behaviours concern a high percentage of preadolescents. Even when considering a general population sample, more than half the subjects showed a weak acceptance of their own bodies, and an equally relevant number stated they adopted strategies aimed to counter weight gain (8.7%) or particular diets, such as restrictions (39.5%) or binge eating (30.9%), sometimes as often as twice a week (Table 2). The data become even more interesting if we consider that 14.0% of the students went beyond the cut-off score of 14 in the scale of the impulse for thinness (IT) of the Eating Disorders Inventory – 2 (EDI – 2; Garner, 1991), corresponding to the 98th percentile for the screening of EDs. In addition, if we consider the Body Mass Index (BMI), that is considered as one of the main risk factors for the onset of an eating disorder (Friedman et al., 1995; Vander and Thelen, 2000), also in consideration the high percentage of obese and overweight subjects (22.0% and 24.3% respectively) found in the sample seems worth of note.

The original aim of our research project was to investigate the influence of body changes on the adoption of abnormal eating behaviours and on the concerns typically associated to an ED. The data obtained suggested a greater vulnerability in female subjects (Table 3), in particular in post-menarche ones. A comparison between the 11-year-old and 13-year-old male students showed that the scores in all the EDI – 2 scales and the frequency of dysfunctional eating behaviours (with the exception of binge eating) tended to decrease as the age increased (Table 4). An opposite trend appeared in the female sample. In order to assess the impact of the menarche factor (regardless of the age variable) we compared the pre-post puberty girls separately in each age group (11, 12, 13 years old). In all the subsets considered, the post-menarche girls obtained higher values in the BMI, in some EDI - 2 scales (in particular, Drive for thinness, Body dissatisfaction and Enteroceptive awareness) and, only in the 12-year-olds group, a significant presence of abnormal eating behaviours (Tables 5, 6, 7) was observed. Post-puberty girls seem to distinguish themselves for those personality features which relevant literature often indicates as correlates or risk indicators of eating disorders. Thus it seems that body changes are faster and experienced less dramatically by the male sample. We do not mean to consider the menarche as a traumatic experience in itself. Our hypothesis is that while the event is not the direct cause of a hyper-attention to eating, it is used by 'predisposed' subjects in such a way as to become a traumatic event (Cotrufo, 2005).

In our opinion, these data are interesting since they seem to confirm the time link between the body changes occurring during puberty and the development of the symptoms of anorexia, as several scholars of adolescence have stated (Bruch, 1973; Laufer, 1984; Gordon, 1980).

Table 2. Socio-demographic characteristics, BMI distribution and eating behaviours of the sample (N=2657)

	N	%
N	2657	
Gender		
Male	1345	50.6%
Female	1312	49.4%
Age	12.13 ± 0.78 [a]	
11 years old	675	25.4%
12 years old	964	36.3%
13 years old	1018	38.3%
BMI-for-age	21.76 ± 4.27[a]	
Underweight	29	1.1%
Normal weight	1397	52.6%
Overweight	646	24.3%
Obese	584	22.0%
Abnormal eating behaviours		
Drive for thinness ≥ 14	371	14.0%
Diet	818	30.9%
Binge eating	1048	39.5%
At least twice a week	196	18.8%
Loose control during episodes	84	42.9%
Compensatory Strategies	230	8.7%
At least twice a week	56	28.3%
Weight control	1609	60.6%

[a] Values are means ± standard deviations

Table 3. The comparison between males and females in the individual EDI-2 scales and eating behaviors (N = 2657)

				Average scores	
EDI 2 scales	U	z	p	Males (N=1345)	Females (N=1312)
Drive for thinness	672 433.50	-10.68	.000	4.65	7.19
Bulimia	840 372.00	-2.27	.023	2.08	1.79
Body dissatisfaction	711 151.50	-8.62	.000	6.79	9.34
Ineffectiveness	777 439.00	-5.33	.000	4.28	5.12
Perfectionism	810 303.50	-3.66	.000	5.15	4.57
Interpersonal distrust	785 632.50	-4.91	.000	4.83	4.25
Interoceptive awareness	754 093.50	-6.51	.000	4.40	5.59
Maturity fears	840 704.50	-2.11	.035	7.75	8.06
Asceticism	859 985.00	-1.13	.255	4.19	4.29

Table 3. (Continued)

EDI 2 scales	U	z	p	Average scores: Males (N=1345)	Average scores: Females (N=1312)
Impulse regulation	859 406.50	-1.06	.285	5.22	4.98
Social insecurity	813 294.50	-3.47	.001	5.19	4.60
Body Mass Index (BMI)	843 208.00	- 1.94	.052	21.95	21.58
Eating Behaviours	χ^2	df	p	Males	Females
Diet	19.193	1	.000	27.0%	34.8%
Binge eating	28.231	1	.000	44.5%	34.4%
Compensatory strategies	1.383	1	.240	9.3%	8.1%
Weight control	34.980	1	.000	55.0%	66.2%

Table 4. The comparison between the 11 and 13 years old male subjects in the individual EDI-2 scales and eating behaviours (N = 889)

EDI 2 scales	U	z	p	Average scores: 11 years old (N=348)	Average scores: 13 years old (N=541)
Drive for thinness	76 913.50	-4.65	.000	5.54	4.01
Bulimia	91 048.00	-.87	.382	2.26	2.10
Body dissatisfaction	88 048.50	-1.59	.112	7.25	6.48
Ineffectiveness	81 793.00	-3.32	.001	4.95	3.95
Perfectionism	77 415.00	-4.49	.000	6.02	4.77
Interpersonal distrust	77 017.50	-4.60	.000	5.54	4.36
Interoceptive awareness	78 433.50	-4.22	.000	5.40	4.00
Maturity fears	76 893.50	-4.62	.000	8.61	6.90
Asceticism	78 700.00	-4.16	.000	4.80	3.88
Impulse regulation	84 896.50	-2.37	.017	5.83	4.95
Social insecurity	92 160.00	-.53	.596	5.46	5.18
Body Mass Index (BMI)	78 852.00	-4.15	.000	21.18	22.50
Eating Behaviours	χ^2	df	p	11 years old	13 years old
Diet	15.998	1	.000	34.5%	22.3%
Binge eating	9.510	1	.002	40.8%	51.4%
Compensatory strategies	8.991	1	.003	13.3%	7.2%
Weight control	6.500	1	.001	59.2%	50.5%

Alongside the high prevalence among females it is important to remark that there are also males who develop these disorders. Five to ten percent of the subjects with anorexia nervosa (Oyebode et al., 1988) and 10-15% of those with bulimia nervosa are estimated to be males (Carlat and Camargo, 1991).

Table 5. Differences between pre- and post-menarche girls in the individual EDI-2 scale and eating behaviours in the female 11 year olds

EDI 2 scales	U	z	p	Average scores 11 year olds: Pre-menarche (N=244)	Average scores 11 year olds: Post-menarche (N=75)
Drive for thinness	7 516.00	-2.34	.019	7.07	8.96
Bulimia	7 959.00	-1.99	.046	1.02	1.60
Body dissatisfaction	7 001.00	-3.08	.002	8.04	11.01
Ineffectiveness	7 743.00	-2.02	.043	4.87	6.27
Perfectionism	8 836.50	-.45	.652	5.12	4.99
Interpersonal distrust	8 780.00	-.53	.595	4.70	4.43
Interoceptive awareness	7 471.00	-2.41	.016	5.17	6.84
Maturity fears	8 179.00	-1.39	.163	9.11	8.41
Ascetism	8 298.50	-1.22	.220	4.27	4.81
Impulse regulation	8 354.50	-1.15	.251	4.56	5.43
Social insecurity	7 768.50	-1.99	.047	4.40	5.33
Body Mass Index (BMI)	6 535.50	-3.70	.000	20.09	22.05
Eating Behaviours	χ^2	df	p	Pre-menarche	Post-menarche
Diet	2.945	1	.086	35.7%	46.7%
Binge eating	.684	1	.408	25.8%	30.7%
Compensatory strategies	.040	1	.842	7.4%	8.1%
Weight control	.859	1	.354	70.5%	76.0%

Table 6. Differences between pre- and post-menarche girls in the individual EDI-2 scale and eating behaviours in the female 12 year olds

EDI 2 scales	U	z	p	Average scores 12 year olds: Pre-menarche (N=192)	Average scores 12 year olds: Post-menarche (N=312)
Drive for thinness	24 462.50	-3.47	.001	5.47	7.32
Bulimia	28 303.50	-1.11	.264	1.56	1.88
Body dissatisfaction	23 965.50	-3.77	.000	7.72	10.21
Ineffectiveness	28 895.50	-.66	.504	4.94	4.97
Perfectionism	28 072.50	-1.19	.234	4.07	4.49
Interpersonal distrust	28 757.50	-.75	.449	4.34	4.21
Interoceptive awareness	26 794.50	-1.99	.046	4.92	5.51
Maturity fears	28 208.00	-1.10	.271	8.37	7.89
Asceticism	27 963.00	-1.26	.207	4.02	4.24
Impulse regulation	26 422.50	-2.18	.029	4.31	5.08
Social insecurity	28 251.00	-1.07	.282	4.77	4.40
Body Mass Index (BMI)	19 504.00	-6.58	.000	20.28	22.57

Table 6. (Continued)

EDI 2 scales	U	z	p	Average scores 12 year olds Pre-menarche (N=192)	Post-menarche (N=312)
Eating Behaviours	χ^2	df	p	Pre-menarche	Post-menarche
Diet	8.458	1	.004	22.4%	34.6%
Binge eating	.310	1	.578	29.7%	32.1%
Compensatory strategies	5.104	1	.024	4.2%	9.6%
Weight control	5.634	1	.018	60.9%	71.2%

Table 7. Differences between pre- and post-menarche girls in the individual EDI-2 scale and eating behaviours in the female 13 year olds

EDI 2 scales	U	z	p	Average scores 13 year olds Pre-menarche (N=64)	Post-menarche (N=412)
Drive for thinness	10 498.00	-2.63	.008	5.72	7.76
Bulimia	12 149.00	-1.06	.288	1.70	2.28
Body dissatisfaction	10 965.00	-2.14	.032	8.08	10.05
Ineffectiveness	12 986.50	-.19	.846	5.11	5.16
Perfectionism	11 131.00	-2.01	.044	3.84	4.51
Interpersonal distrust	11 617.00	-1.54	.123	4.56	3.88
Interoceptive awareness	10 510.50	-2.62	.009	4.58	6.09
Maturity fears	11 714.50	-1.44	.150	8.05	7.35
Asceticism	12 006.00	-1.16	.246	3.92	4.41
Impulse regulation	10 504.00	-2.64	.008	4.14	5.54
Social insecurity	11 915.50	-1.24	.213	5.03	4.52
Body Mass Index (BMI)	10 027.50	-3.08	.002	20.74	22.37
Eating Behaviours	χ^2	df	p	Pre-menarche	Post-menarche
Diet	6.219	1	.013	23.4%	39.7%
Binge eating	.182	1	.670	45.3%	42.5%
Compensatory strategies	.487	1	.485	6.3%	9.0%
Weight control	.679	1	.410	56.3%	61.7%

In a population of 100,000 subjects, Hoek et al. (2003) have recorded an incidence rate of 0.8% (female/male ratio = 27/1) for bulimia and below 0.5% for anorexia. Other research works seem to show a greater prevalence as compared to the past (Carlat et al., 1997; Nelson et al., 1999; Kjelsas et al., 2004).

Despite the apparent lack of studies on male anorexia, in the literature there are references to documents dating back to 1689, when Richard Morton described the case of a young 16-year-old boy affected by "a total lack of appetite", though showing no symptoms that could associate his gradual loss of weight to some organic pathology (Morton, 1694).

Since the 1960s several research works have been carried out with the aim of investigating the typical characteristics of male anorexia and exploring in depth the gender differences relating the prevalence of such disorders. In males and in females alike, the onset of the disorder occurs during adolescence or early adulthood, and the clinical characteristics are also very similar in the two groups, with the obvious exception of the symptom of amenorrhea (Olivardia et al., 1995; Keel et al., 1998; Braun et al., 1999; Woodside et al., 2001).

A major research area has focused on investigating the relationship existing between sexuality and male anorexia.

A comparison between a sample of 27 anorexic or bulimic males and one of 142 anorexic or bulimic females showed that the males appeared to have more problems than females in terms of sexual isolation, sexual inactivity and acceptance of their homosexuality (Herzog et al., 1984).

It is also estimated that the percentage of anorexic males who have experienced or entertain homosexual relationships ranges between 14% and 42% (Robinson and Holden, 1986; Fichter and Daser, 1987; Schneider and Agras, 1987). The study carried out by Carlat et al. (1997) on 135 subjects diagnosed with ED showed that 27% of the sample had a bisexual or homosexual sexual orientation and 32% described a total loss of interest that had been going on for at least one year before the initial assessment. It must be remembered that the normal percentage of gays in the American male population is estimated to range between 3% and 6% (Laumann et al., 1994; Seidman and Rieder, 1994).

The hypothesis that the presence of EDs in males is the expression of an incomplete heterosexuality does not find confirmation in all the works in the literature. A comparison between a sample of 25 males diagnosed with ED according to the criteria of the DSM – IV, one of females diagnosed with BN and a control sample did not show any significant differences in sexual orientation between the groups (2 homosexuals and 2 bisexuals in the ED group and 1 bisexual in the control group; Olivardia et al., 1995). However, it must be borne in mind that these are the results of minor studies, observing smaller samples than in research done earlier on.

In numerous cases, empirical evidence shows male homosexuals as having a greater risk of developing an ED (Yager et al., 1988; Strong et al., 2000; Russell and Keel, 2002; Kaminski et al., 2005; Feldman and Meyer, 2007). In a research carried out in 2003, Yelland and Tiggemann compared a group of 52 male homosexuals with a control group of heterosexual males and a group of 55 heterosexual females. The results show concern about physical appearance and psychological characteristics typically associated with EDs which make the sample of homosexual males more similar to the group of heterosexual females than to that of the control males. The homosexuals differed from the control sample remarkably, also with respect to the impulse to increase their muscular mass.

A longitudinal study on a sample of 2924 adolescents highlighted how a homosexual sexual orientation and sexual experiences with people of the same sex at the age of 14-19 seem, at a 5-year distance, to be important predictors of bulimic behaviours (Wichstrom, 2006).

It is worth remarking that homosexual orientation in women does not seem to be an equally important risk factor in the development of EDs. A comparison between a sample of 212 heterosexual males and 182 females, one of 81 homosexual males and 38 females and one sample of 131 bisexual males and 144 females, showed a great difference between male homosexuals and male heterosexuals with respect to body dissatisfaction (27.8% vs. 12.0%), the adoption of compensating strategies such as self-induced vomiting (11.7% vs. 4.4%), the frequency of restricting behaviours (8.9% vs. 5.5%) and binge eating (25.0% vs. 10.6%). The sample of homosexual females showed a smaller body dissatisfaction as compared to heterosexual females (French et al., 1996). In other studies, no significant differences appeared between heterosexual and homosexual women with respect to the presence of dysfunctional eating attitudes and behaviours (Hefferman, 1996; Moore and Keel, 2003).

In an interesting research work carried out by Meyer et al. (2001) on a group of 100 university students (40 homosexuals and 60 heterosexuals), the results showed – for the whole sample and for the group of homosexuals alone – significant correlations between the scores obtained at the EAT and the "Femininity" scale of the Bem Sex Role Inventory, and between the "masculinity" scale and healthy eating behaviours. The authors conclude that, unlike the masculine attitude, femininity is an important risk factor in the onset of an ED. Other authors have analysed the role of femininity in eating disorders with largely similar results (Murnen and Smolak, 1997; Behar et al., 2003; Cotrufo et al., 2007).

The last fifteen years have witnessed a growing interest in a "new", mainly male pathology, i.e. reverse anorexia (RA) (Pope et al., 1993). The clinical picture of this disorder, later named muscle dimorphic disorder (Pope et al., 1997), is characterised by the presence of a pathogenic idea whereby the subject is never satisfied with his/her muscle size, despite muscle hypertrophy. This idea leads to a perseverance in attempting to increase the muscular mass through physical exercise, namely weightlifting (Phillips et al., 1997; Hildebrandt et al., 2006), the adoption of dysfunctional eating behaviours such as high-proteing diets and strategies to counter the increase in body fat (Kleiner et al., 1994), the use of vitamin supplements and the intake of large doses of anabolising steroids. The latter behaviour seems to be present in 46% of subjects with reverse anorexia (Olivardia et al., 2000) and in 44% of bodybuilders (Blouin and Goldfield, 1995). In addition to the complications deriving from the intake of these substances, the disorder also damages the subject's social and working activities (Pope et al., 2000; Olivardia, 2001).

Although the studies aimed at monitoring comorbidity between reverse anorexia and eating disorders highlight the resemblance of some traits (Davis and Scott-Robertson, 2000; Olivardia et al., 2000; Goldfield et al., 2006), no studies are available to date which can explain this similarity in empirical terms.

Conceptually, RA is included in the body dysmorphic disorder, and the concern for not being muscular enough may be determined by a distorted perception of one's body image (H.G. Pope et al., 1997; Olivardia et al., 2001; C.G. Pope et al., 2005).

Even though there are no epidemiologic works indicating the spreading of this disorder (Olivardia, 2001), it is believed that 5% of males who do body building suffer from RA (Pope et al., 1997) and that 9% of the subjects with body dysmorphism concentrate their feeling of ineffectiveness on the muscles (Pope et al. 2000).

In 1997 Pope (et al.) formulated a few diagnostic criteria which would make it possible to formulate this diagnosis. Another very important element must be added, in our opinion which, if confirmed empirically, would contribute to the understanding of the whole symptom pattern. The majority of these subjects has sexual problems which they link to the ineffectiveness of their physical appearance, and in particular to their masculinity. In a research carried out by Mangweth et al. (2001) a group of male body builders was compared with a group of males with mental anorexia and a control group. The results obtained showed that 4% of the body builders and 10% of the subjects diagnosed with anorexia showed a bisexual or homosexual sexual orientation, while 32% and 43% respectively reported a loss of sexual drive (vs. 7% in the control group).

Considering the experience of impotence and ineffectiveness as the main pathogenic factor, it is thus assumed that, like male anorexics, also subjects with reverse anorexia are carriers of a weak or troublesome male identity, which seems to view the increase in muscular mass as a form of compensation (Cotrufo, 2005). This argument, that has been put forward in theoretical terms (Klein A.M., 1993), has not yet been the subject of sufficiently reliable empirical studies.

Is it possible to attempt a discussion of the data we have reported? Can this empirical evidence be included in a theoretical construct which may give these figures a meaning?

The epidemiological data indicate that between the 1960s and 1970s the spreading of AN increased as compared to the previous centuries, that EDs are pathologies that set in during puberty and that they are 'feminine' rather than 'female' pathologies. What happened to western adolescent girls in the second half of the 20th century?

At first, AN concerned the middle and upper classes in western societies, then it spread to the lower classes and eventually, two or three decades later, to developing societies. On the basis of these considerations, many authors thought that a link between social transformations and the ED onset might be identified. The English psychologist Gordon, who analysed in depth the issue of the social spreading of anorexia (Gordon, 1990) made some observations that we consider extremely important. He highlights some psychological features that he considers as characteristic of anorexia and can actually be found in these female patients, namely an ambivalence concerning autonomy and self-esteem, the pursuit of success and the impulse to take control (in this respect Gordon talks of a generalised self-control). He maintains that these psychological problems can only be understood if they are placed in a wider perspective, following the pattern of development of a psycho-social identity. Gordon believes that, if the cultural expectations concerning an individual change, then "symptoms of identity confusion will be frequent. [...] These disorders [anorexia and bulimia] represent the extreme expression of the radical change of social expectations concerning women, which has taken place on a large scale since the middle of the 20th century, and especially in the 1960s. In a relatively short timeframe young women have found themselves facing a number of new pressures for them to pursue success, competitiveness and independence". Following Devereux (1978), the author believes that when a phenomenon becomes as widespread as an epidemics it means that those who suffer from an acute form of the disorder become unaware carriers of a diffuse cultural crisis. He puts forward the hypothesis that the sense of ineffectiveness typical of pre-anorexic females, is somehow compensated by eating restrictions, which seem to give the anorexic a sense of power never experienced before. In this perspective, the anorexic habit of dietary restriction would serve as a sort of 'compensation' that women of this time produce to cope with a sense of ineffectiveness - a sort of defence, then.

The issues mentioned by the English author raise quite often in the clinical relationship with anorexic female patients. In particular, meetings with these patients highlight their great determination and their absolute unwillingness to distance themselves from the main symptom, dietary restriction. In addition to that, as stated by the Kestembergs (1974), exercising this control on hunger produces a sort of pleasure per se, *the pleasure of feeling hungry*, the pleasure of feeling a need to respond to and at the same time of feeling that she has the necessary psychic resources not to *surrender*, but to control the hunger pangs. According to Gordon, the special feeling of the girl who will become an anorexic is not peculiar to *that* girl, but characterises modern women in general. He also describes the age of the great onset, adolescence, as the time in which a little girl must give up her fantasies about becoming as strong and powerful as a boy and, when there has already been a sexual experience that has brought her to an ever greater loss of self-esteem, she will carry on with her plan of a body without curves and able to express an absolute power of control. Actually, even considering the connection highlighted by some authors (Vandereycken and van Deth, 1994), this power of control over the "needs" of the body makes it possible to liken anorexia to the ascetic practices of time past. These practices consisted in constantly mortifying the requests coming from the body in order to reach God purified from the sins of the flesh: it seems that anorexic girls of our time re-propose, following the example of Catherine of Siena, a mind-body dualism which is expressed through the power of the former over the latter. Actually, if anorexia spread starting from the 1960s, voluntary abstention from eating is present in all ages and in all cultures. Think, for example, of Buddhist monks, or the Hindu Sadhus who have made a vow to renounce the body's needs and wander naked, with no other belonging than a small bowl to beg for the food needed to survive. The rite of Ramadan in Islamic cultures also testifies to the importance of the vow of renunciation to the body's needs as an expression of faith and devotion to the divine. What I wish to stress through these brief historical notes is the presence in human culture of fasting, voluntary abstention from eating, together with sexual abstention, as a major element of penitence and purification, of an asceticism aimed at showing a preference for the spiritual aspects of life as compared to the bodily ones: the expression of how mind and spirit exercise their supremacy over the profane requests of the body. The principal symptom of anorexia, forced eating restriction, used to be a prerogative of specific categories of people, who adopted these behaviours as the expression of their ability to control the impulses originating in the body; people who put themselves in a condition of supremacy over the physical need of hunger and who, in different ways, showed some sort of spiritual devotion. What happened in the second half of the 20th century that caused the spreading of this ascetic behaviour as far as to involve, in subclinical forms, 15% of all adolescent girls?

In the course of the 20th century, the role of the woman has changed much more than it had in the whole of the history of humanity. Starting from the Suffragette demonstrations early in the century and the human rights movements between the 1960s and 1970s the texture of society has gone through a great deal of change, through smooth and gradual, or sudden and more violent processes. These changes have given the women in western societies new spaces, new roles and, above all, greater opportunities of expression. The feminist movement then gave a further contribution to giving women a new social dimension. Today women think of themselves, of the future, of their career possibilities and the fulfilment of their expectations in a way that is very similar to men's. This leap is very often evident within families, which tend to highlight the cultural differences and the different social positions held by mothers and daughters.

Before that time, a woman's interests revolved mainly around her husband and children, and her personal gratification depended for the most part on their achievements. Her work consisted in making their life as untroubled as possible, so that they might invest their time in activities of growth which would have an indirect impact on the whole family. Today women do not project their gratification onto their husbands, but try to achieve it directly in a daily competition with men on grounds which until a few years ago were precluded to them. This woman has thus become more dynamic, has got rid of the apron, has left the kitchen and the home to enter, often quite successfully, the world of professions. This new, dynamic and competitive dimension finds one of its most significant symbolic expressions in the rejection of the classical feminine 'shape', meaning the buxom and maternal look prevailing in the previous years.

This new woman, this competitive woman, wishing to be recognised as an autonomous element of society, this woman in search of a direct visibility rather than one deriving from the quality of her marriage, has also a new aesthetic model. Her appearance no longer has to convey the idea of 'good wife' but rather one of strength, efficiency, dynamism and competitiveness.

The issue of beauty deserves further attention, however. We do not believe that the aim of an anorexic woman is to become prettier; society, however, does *attribute* this aim to the anorexic woman – and this is the focus of Devereux's notion of ethnic disorder. We would not then read our patient's yearning in positive terms – what she wants to do and be – but rather in negative terms – what she mustn't do and, above all, be. In this constant endeavour to become skinny there is no room for aesthetic pleasure; an anorexic woman usually shows no interest in the other sex and does not wish to be physically liked. The bodily level is disowned completely; if some wish to be liked still exists, it concerns the spiritual, moral or performance level – definitely not the physical one.

An anorexic does not want to be thin to be pretty; she wants to be thin *not to be physically in the world*; she does not want to be seen as a beautiful, desirable or exciting woman, but she wants to feel as a person with an iron willpower, able to make sacrifices which ordinary people struggle with. Once again, it seems that we should pay attention to the issue of the anorexic behaviour as a sort of defence from an emergency concerning the sense of ineffectiveness.

The anorexic's ineffectiveness is compensated by the symptoms of anorexia, which surface in all their dramatic nature when the restricting eating behaviour gives way to occasional bulimic episodes of binge eating. This is the case when the patient comes into direct contact with what was to be disowned: *a body carrier of desire and a psyche unable to manage it.*

At this point it becomes impossible, in our opinion, not to associate eating desire with sexual desire. It is fair to assert that in human cultures the action of eating does not mean only feeding and sustaining the biological organism. The fact that the hunger stimulus to self-preservation is fulfilled or frustrated in concrete reality, the fact that it is a mother (with all the related relational implications) that originally takes care of this need, and the fact that this need is linked to the sense of taste which transforms it into a *sensual*, and thus erotised, need, make nourishment of the human race *other* than what it is for other animal species. In the history of humanity, the hunger stimulus, the food object and the taste pleasure have taken on meanings that, being metaphors of the stimulus-object-pleasure chain, have perverted the original self-preserving nature of the hunger stimulus and have caused it to take on an-*other* meaning. This 'shifting' from the self-preserving biological order to the drive-based psychic order has been dealt with elsewhere (Cotrufo, 2005) and constitutes, in our opinion, an important tool to look at mental anorexia.

Freud mentions the term anorexia for the first time in his Draft G to Fliess, in which he writes "The food neurosis called 'anorexia' can be compared to melancholia. The well-known *anorexia nervosa* of girls seems to me (based on accurate observations) to be a melancholy which appears in cases of an as yet incomplete sexuality [...] *Loss of hunger: in sexual terms, loss of libido*" (Freud, 1895). Even the etymology of the word takes us to the same conclusions as Freud's. The etymology of anorexia is *an-orexia*, which means lack of hunger. A deeper etymological analysis, however, shows that *orexia* derives from the Indo-European word *orégein*, which means to look for, to hold out one's arms, to yearn. In this sense, appetite is no longer limited to hunger, but involves the person as a whole and his/her appetites as search, relation and yearning. The anorexic therefore becomes a subject who doesn't search, doesn't hold out her arms, has no appetites and doesn't yearn. In this sense, *lack*, widely and dramatically shown also by her physical appearance, becomes the *core* of the anorexic experience and seems to reflect very well the clinical and psychic reality of our patient.

Binswanger comments on the description made by Janet about one of his patients, Nadia: "The appearance of menstruation, the growth of hair on the pubis, the development of the breasts, almost drove her mad. Until the age of 20 she kept pulling her hair out of the pubis. Since puberty, her general conditions have worsened constantly, and it is at that time that she stopped eating normally and together with others. In every mannery, in the way she dresses and in the way she arranges her hair, Nadia tries to hide her own sex (like Ellen West had been doing until the age of 18), and makes every possible effort to look like a male student. Janet believes that it is not possible to talk of homosexuality in this case, because Nadia would be equally ashamed of being a boy; she would like to be sexless altogether, or better, patently without a body, because all its parts would raise the same feeling inside her; the rejection of food would therefore be but a very peculiar manifestation of this single feeling" (Binswanger, 1944). According to Janet, Nadia's entire pathology can be explained by one single morbid feeling which he calls *honte du corps*.

What happens to a woman during adolescence? Puberty entails very evident body changes, especially in women. We could take into account two interacting factors, one exogenous and one endogenous. Feminine shapes – the breasts, the hips – make the (ex-)little girl sexually desirable. The looks of boys of her age, and not only, bring the girl to face a world of relations that is different from the one she was experience no longer than a few months before.

The endogenous component concerns the same changes that lead to greater attention to the body's stimuli. With regard to this, I would suggest to take into consideration Laplanche's hypothesis. He believes that "*what must be said is by all means astonishing*: in human sexuality and its development, *what is acquired occurs before what is inborn*, it does not build on it. This is very important, especially for adolescent psychology, since at the time when instinct appears, the ground is already completely *occupied* by the drive and its support, the phantom. Hence the idea of a mingling, during puberty, of drive and instinct" (Laplanche, 1993). This concept, whose logic contains some paradoxical aspects, is, in actual fact, paradoxically obvious. It is an enlightening element to understand the 'drama' of puberty in human beings. Children's sexuality, with its characteristics of perversion and polymorphism (Freud, 1905), in Laplanche's view has nothing to do with the biological sexual instinct of reproduction, which only appears at a later time, during puberty, when internal and external genitals mature. This sexual instinct becomes part of and, above all, must be represented within a space that is not empty, but is a *saturated space of psychism*, full of representations and phantoms of the pre-sexual sexual. In this perspective, then, it finds the place taken by drive, and it is with the latter that it has to interact. The desiring and desired body, as a sexual and mature body, makes the conflicting nature of children's sexual fantasies even more coactive because now it is possible to move to act out. In this perspective, the psychic work of organising and holding back overflowing drives can become even more difficult. In the sexually desiring adolescent the pre-oedipal and oedipal dynamics emerge again, and sexual excitement, which had been relegated in a state of latency, surfaces once again, this time in a more abrupt way since it is supported by a mature body that could make acting-out possible. Following this reasoning, the readers with some clinical experience of anorexia must have remarked how that girl seems to remain in a state of latency, as if the moment of puberty itself had been disowned. Actually, a typical characteristic of female sexuality is passivity, meaning the natural passive-feminine disposition which, before being a psychic trait, basically derives from the female anatomy. By passivity we mean the female disposition to being an object (of penetration) and, later, to becoming a carrier of (active) desire which, however, is realised through a passive disposition. Well, female passivity (and I wish to remind that in psychoanalytical theory the female's drive aim is passive by definition) falls in a social context that rejects this disposition altogether. The readers themselves may turn up their noses at this statement about femininity. This radical rejection imposes on the girls of our day to reject sexual desire *tout court*, as it is a passive aim, a passivity which today's society rejects while it rewards active, dynamic women; a passivity which in psychic terms translates into that paralysing feeling of ineffectiveness mentioned by all the clinical studies on EDs and viewed as one of the main causes for the aetiology of anorexia.

We stated that the symptoms of anorexia, in their relation with the ascetic dimension, are the expression of a response to a deep-set feeling of ineffectiveness. This seems to be even more coactive during puberty, since sexual instinct strengthens sexual drive, making the girl feel the need to hold it back. The skinny body and the disappearance of the period become the marks of a *non*-accomplished puberal transformation, of a *disowned* sexual maturity. The anorexic body talks: it tells the spectator, enraptured by the power evoked by hunger endurance, that this woman has no time and no maturation, she is not subject to transformations and, above all, she has no need whatsoever.

REFERENCES

Abraham, S., and O'Dea, J.A. (2001). Body mass index, menarche, and perception of dieting among peripubertal adolescent females. *International Journal of Eating Disorders*, *29*, 23-28.

Ackard, D.M., and Peterson, C.B. (2001). Association between puberty and disordered eating, body image, and other psychological variables. *International Journal of Eating Disorders*, *29*(2), 187-194.

Altug, A., Elal, G., Slade, P., and Tekcan, A. (2000). The Eating Attitudes Test (EAT) in Turkish university students: relationship with sociodemographic, social and individual variables. *Eating and weight disorders, 5*, 152-160.

American Psychiatric Association (1994). *Diagnostic and statistical manual of mental disorders* (4th ed.). Washington, DC: Author.

Behar, R., De la Barrera, M., and Michelotti, J. (2003). Clinical characteristics and gender identity among eating disordered patients subtypes. *Revista Medica de Chile, 131*(7), 748-758.

Beren, S.E., Hayden, H.A., Wilfley, D.E., and Grilo, C.M. (1996). The influence of sexual orientation on body dissatisfaction in adult men and women. *International Journal of Eating Disorder, 20*(2), 135-141.

Biswanger, L. (1944). Der fall Ellen West. In *Schizophrenie* (1957), Naske: Pfullingen.

Blouin, A.G. and Goldfield, G.S. (1995). Body image and steroid use in male bodybuilders. *International Journal of Eating Disorders, 18*, 159-165.

Braun, D.L., Sunday, S.R., Huang, A., and Halmi, K.A. (1999). More males seek treatment for eating disorders. *International Journal of Eating Disorder, 25*(4), 415-424.

Bruch, H. (1973). *Eating Disorders, Obesity, Anorexia Nervosa and the Person Within*. New York: Basic Bosok.

Carlat, D.J., and Camargo, C.A. Jr. (1991). Review of bulimia nervosa in males. *The American Journal of Psychiatry, 148*(7), 831-843.

Carlat, D.J., Camargo, C.A. Jr., and Herzog, D.B. (1997). Eating disorders in males: a report on 135 patients. *The American Journal of Psychiatry, 154*(8), 1127-1132.

Chen, H., and Jackson, T. (2007). Prevalence and sociodemographic correlates of eating disorder endorsements among adolescents and young adults from China. *European Eating Disorders Review: The journal of the Eating Disorders Association.*

Cotrufo, P., Barretta, V., Monteleone, P., and Maj, M. (1998). Full-syndrome, partial-syndrome and subclinical eating disorders: an epidemiological study on female students in Southern Italy. *Acta psychiatrica Scandinavica, 98*, 112-115.

Cotrufo, P., Gnisci, A., Caputo, I. (2005). Psychological characteristics of less severe forms of eating disorders: an epidemiological study among 259 female adolescents. *Journal of Adolescence,* 28, 147-154.

Cotrufo, P. (2005). *Anoressia del Sessuale Femminile. Dal Caos alla Costituzione del Limite.* Milano: Franco Angeli Ed.

Cotrufo, P., Cella, S., Cremato, F., and Labella, A.G. (2007). Eating disorders attitude and abnormal eating behaviours in a sample of 11-13 year-old school children: The role of body transformation. *Eating and Weight Disorders, 12*(4), 154-160.

Crow, S.J., Agras, W.S., Halmi, K., Mitchell, J.E., and Kraemer, H.C. (2002). Full syndromal versus subthreshold anorexia nervosa, bulimia nervosa, and binge eating disorder: A multicenter study. *International Journal of Eating Disorder, 32*, 309-318.

Dancynger, I.F., and Garfinkel, P.E. (1995). The relationship of partial syndrome eating disorders to anorexia nervosa and bulimia nervosa. *Psychological Medicine, 25*, 1019-1025.

Davis, C., and Scott-Robertson, L. (2000). A psychological comparison of females with anorexia nervosa and competitive male bodybuilders: body shape ideals in the extreme. *Eating Behaviors, 1*(1), 33-46.

Davis, S.M., and Lambert, L.C. (2000). Body image and weight concerns among Southwestern American Indian preadolescent schoolchildren. *Ethnicity and Disease, 10*, 184-194.

Davison, K.K., Markey, C.N., and Birch, L.L. (2003). A longitudinal examination of patterns in girls' weight concerns and body dissatisfaction from ages 5 to 9 years. *International Journal of Eating Disorders, 33*, 320-332.

Devereux, G. (1978). *Saggi di etnopsichiatria generale.* Roma: Armando.

Dietz, W.H. (1998), Health conseguences of obesity in youth: childhood predictors of adult disease. *Pediatrics, 101*, 518-525.

Eagles, J.M., Johnston, M.I., Hunter, D., Lobban, M., and Millar, H.R. (1995). Increasing incidence of anorexia nervosa in the female population of Northeast Scotland. *The American journal of psychiatry, 152*, 1266-1271.

Eapen, V., Mabrouk, A.A., and Bin-Othman, S. (2006). Disordered eating attitudes and symptomatology among adolescent girls in the United Arab Emirates. *Eating Behaviors*, 7(1), 53-60.

Elal, G., Altug, A., Slade, P., and Tekcan A. (2000), Factor structure of the Eating Attitudes Test (EAT) in a Turkish university sample. *Eating and Weight Disorders*, *5*(1), 46-50.

Esposito-Del Puente, A., Contaldo, F., De Filippo, E., Scalfi, L., Di Maio, S., Franzese, A., Valerio, G., and Rubino, A. (1996). High prevalence of overweight in a children population living in Naples (Italy). *International Journal of Obesity*, *20*, 283-286.

Fairburn, C.G., and Walsh, B.T. (2002). Atypical eating disorders (eating disorders not otherwise specified). In C.G. Fairburn, and K.D. Brownell (Eds.), *Eating disorders and obesity* (pp. 171-177). London: The Guilford press.

Feldman, M.B., and Meyer, I.H. (2007). Eating disorders in diverse lesbian, gay, and bisexual populations. *International Journal of Eating Disorder, 40*(3), 218-226.

Fichter, M.M., and Daser, C. (1987). Symptomatology, psychosexual development and gender identity in 42 anorexic males. *Psychological Medicine*, *17*, 409-418.

French, S.A., Story, M., Remafedi, G., Resnick, M.D., and Blum, R.W. (1996). Sexual orientation and prevalence of body dissatisfaction and eating disordered behaviors: a population-based study of adolescents. *International Journal of Eating Disorders*, *19*(2), 119-126.

Freud, S. (1895). Minuta G. La melanconia. In OSF: Vol. 2. Torino: Boringhieri.

Friedman, M.A., Wilfley, D.E., Pike, K.M., Striegel-Moore, R.H., and Rodin, J. (1995). The relationship between weight and psychological functioning among adolescent girls. *Obesity research, 3*, 57-62.

Garner, D.M. (1991). *Eating Disorder Inventory – 2. Professional manual.* Odessa, FL: Psychological Assessment Resources.

Gentile, K., Raghavan, C., Rajah, V., and Gates, K. (2007). It Doesn't Happen Here: Eating Disorders in an Ethnically Diverse Sample of Economically Disadvantaged, Urban College Students. *Eating Disorders*, *15*(5), 405-425.

Ghazal, N., Agoub, M., Moussaoui, D., and Battas, O. (2001). Prevalence of bulimia among secondary school students in Casablanca. *L'Encephale, 27*, 338-342.

Goldfield, G.S., Blouin, A.G., and Woodside, D.B. (2006). Body image, binge eating, and bulimia nervosa in male bodybuilders. *Canadian Journal of Psychiatry*, *51*(3), 160-168.

Gordon, R.A. (1990). *Anorexia and bulimia. Anatomy of a social epidemic.* Oxford: Basil Blackwell Ltd.

Hausenblas, H.A., Symons Downs, D., Fleming, D.S., and Connaughton, D.P. (2002). Body image in middle school children. *Eating and weight disorders, 7*, 244-248.

Heffernan, K. (1996). Eating disorders and weight concern among lesbians. *International Journal of Eating Disorder, 19*(2), 127-138.

Herzog, D.B., Norman, D.K., Gordon, C., and Pepose, M. (1984). Sexual conflict and eating disorders in 27 males. *The American Journal of Psychiatry*, *141*(8), 989-990.

Hildebrandt, T., Schlundt, D., Langenbucher, J., and Chung, T. (2006). Presence of muscle dysmorphia symptomology among male weightlifters. *Comprehensive Psychiatry, 47*(2), 127-135.

Hoek, H.W., and Van Hoeken, D. (2003). Review of the prevalence and incidence of eating disorders. *International Journal of Eating Disorders, 34*, 383-396.

Kaminski, P.L., Chapman, B.P., Haynes, S.D., and Own, L. (2005). Body image, eating behaviors, and attitudes toward exercise among gay and straight men. *Eating Behaviors, 6*(3), 179-187.

Keel, P.K., Klump, K.L., Leon, G.R., and Fulkerson, J.A. (1998). Disordered eating in adolescent males from a school-based sample. *International Journal of Eating Disorders, 23*(2), 125-132.

Kestemberg, E., Kestemberg, J., and Decobert, S. (1974). *La fame e il corpo*. Roma: Astrolabio.

Kiziltan, G., Karabudak, E., Unver, S., Sezgin, E., and Unal, A. (2006). Prevalence of bulimic behaviors and trends in eating attitudes among Turkish late adolescents. *Adolescence*, *41*(164), 677-689.

Kjelsas, E., Bjornstrom, G., and Gotestam, K.G. (2004). Prevalence of eating disorders in female and male adolescents (14-15 years). *Eating behaviors, 5*, 13-25.

Klein, A.M.(1993). *Little big men: bodybuilding subculture and gender construction*. Albany: State University of New York Press.

Kleiner, S.M., Bazzarre, T.L., and Ainsworth, B.E. (1994). Nutritional status of nationally ranked elite bodybuilders. *International Journal of Sport Nutrition, 4*(1), 54-69.

Knez, R., Munjas, R., Petrovecki, M., Paucić-Kirincić, E., and Persić, M. (2006). Disordered eating attitudes among elementary school population. *Journal of Adolescent Health, 38*(5), 628-630.

Laplanche, J. (1993). *Problematique VII. La sexualité humaine. Biologisme et biologie.* Paris : Le Plessis-Robinson.

Lask, B., and Bryant-Waugh, R. (1994). *Childhood onset anorexia nervosa and related eating dsorder*. Lawrence Erlbaum.

Laufer, M. and Laufer, M. E. (1984). *Adolescence and Developmental Breakdown. A Psychoanalytic View.* New Haven and London: Yale University Press.

Laumann, E.O., Gagnon, J.H., Michael, R.T., and Michaels, S. (1994). *The Social Organization of Sexuality: Sexual Practices in the United States*. USA: University of Chicago Press.

Lorenzo, C.R., Lavori, P.W., and Lock, J.D. (2002). Eating attitudes in high school students in the Philippines: a preliminary study. *Eating and weight disorders, 7*, 202-209.

Madanat, H.N., Hawks, S.R., Novilla, M.L. (2006). A comparison of disordered eating attitudes and behaviors among Filipino and American college students. *Eating and Weight Disorders*, *11*(3), 133-138.

Mangweth, B., Pope, H.G. Jr, Kemmler, G., Ebenbichler, C., Hausmann, A., DeCol, C., Kreutner, B., Kinzl, J., and Biebl, W. (2001). Body image and psychopathology in male bodybuilders. *Psychotherapy and Psychosomatics*, *70*, 38-43.

Mayville, S.B., Williamson, D.A., White, M.A., Netemeyer, R.G., and Drab, D.L. (2002). Development of the Muscle Appearance Satisfaction Scale: a self – report measure for the assessment of Muscle Dysmorphia symptoms. *Assessment*, *9*(4), 351-360.

Meyer, C., Blissett, J., and Oldfield, C. (2001). Sexual orientation and eating psychopathology: the role of masculinity and femininity. *International Journal of Eating Disorder, 29*(3), 314-318.

Moore, F., and Keel, P.K. (2003). Influence of sexual orientation and age on disordered eating attitudes and behaviors in women. *International Journal of Eating Disorder, 34*(3), 370-374.

Morton, R. (1694). *Phthisologia or a Treatise of Consumptions*, London: Smith and Walford.

Murnen, S.K., and Smolak, L. (1997). Femininity, masculinity, and disordered eating: a meta-analytic review. *International Journal of Eating Disorders*, *22*(3), 231-242.

Nelson, W.L., Hughes, H.M., Katz, B., and Searight, H.R. (1999). Anorexic eating attitudes and behaviors of male and female college students. *Adolescence, 34*, 621-633.

Nobakht, M., and Dezhkam, M. (2000). An epidemiological study of eating disorders in Iran. *International Journal of Eating Disorders, 28*, 265-271.

Nunes, M.A., Barros, F.C., Anselmo Olinto, M.T., Camey, S., and Mari, J.D. (2003). Prevalence of abnormal eating behaviours and inappropriate methods of weight control in young women from Brazil: a population-based study. *Eating and weight disorders, 8*, 100-106.

O'Dea, J.A., and Abraham, S. (1999). Onset of disordered eating attitudes and behaviors in early adolescence: interplay of pubertal status, gender, weight, and age. *Journal of adolescence, 34*, 671-679.

Olivardia, R. (2001). Mirror, mirror on the wall, who's the largest of them all? The features and phenomenology of muscle dysmorphia. *Harvard Review of Psychiatry*, *9*(5), 254-259.

Olivardia, R., Pope, H.G. Jr, and Hudson, J. I. (2000). Muscle dysmorphia in male weightlifters: A case – control study. *American Journal of Psychiatry*, *157*, 1291-1296.

Olivardia, R., Pope, H.G. Jr., Mangweth, B., and Hudson, J.I. (1995). Eating disorders in college men. *The American Journal of Psychiatry*, *152*(9), 1279-1285.

Oyebode, F., Boodhoo, J.A., and Schapira, K. (1998). Anorexia nervosa in males. Clinical features and outcome. *International Journal of Eating Disorder, 7*, 121-124.

Phillips, K.A., O' Sullivan, R.L., and Pope, H.G. Jr (1997). Muscle Dysmorphia. *Journal of Clinical Psychiatry, 58*, 361.

Pope, C.G., Pope, H.G., Menard, W., Fay, C., Olivardia, R., and Phillips, K.A. (2005). Clinical features of muscle dysmorphia among males with body dysmorphic disorder. *Body Image*, *2*(4), 395-400.

Pope, H.G. Jr, Gruber, A.J., Choi, P., Olivardia, R., and Phillips, K.A. (1997). Muscle Dysmorphia. An underrecognized form of body dysmorphic disorder. *Psychosomatics, 38*, 548-557.

Pope, H.G. Jr, Katz, D.L., and Hudson, J.I. (1993). Anorexia nervosa and "reverse anorexia" among 108 body builders. *Comprehensive Psychiatry, 34*, 406-409.

Pope, H.G. Jr, Olivardia, R., and Phillips, K. (2000). *The Adonis Complex: The Secret Crisis of Male Body Obsession*. New York: Free Press.

Ricciardelli, L.A., and McCabe, M.P. (2001). Children's body image concerns and eating disturbance: a review of the literature. *Clinical psychology review, 21*, 325-344.

Robinson, P.H., and Holden, N.L. (1986). Bulimia nervosa in the male: a report of nine cases, *Psychological Medicine, 16*, 795-803.

Rolland, K., Farnill, D., and Griffiths, R.A. (1997). Body figure perceptions and eating attitudes among Australian schoolchildren aged 8 to 12 years. *International Journal of Eating Disorders, 21*, 273-278.

Rosenvinge, Jan H., Borgen, J.S., and Borresen, R. (1999). The prevalence and psychological correlates of anorexia nervosa, bulimia nervosa and binge eating among 15-years-old students: a controlled epidemiological study. *European Eating Disorders Review, 7*, 382-391.

Russell, C.J., Keel, P.K. (2002). Homosexuality as a specific risk factor for eating disorders in men. *International Journal of Eating Disorders, 31*(3), 300-306.

Sancho, C., Arija, M.V., Asorey, O., and Canals, J. (2007). Epidemiology of eating disorders: A two year follow up in an early adolescent school population. *European Child and Adolescent Psychiatry, 16*(8), 495-504.

Sands, R., Tricker, J., Sherman, C., Armatas, C., and Maschette W. (1997). Disordered eating patterns, body image, self-esteem, and physical activity in preadolescent school children. *International Journal of Eating Disorders, 21*, 159-166.

Sasson, A., Lewin, C., and Roth, D. (1995). Dieting behavior and eating attitudes in Israeli children. *International Journal of Eating Disorders, 17*, 67-72.

Schneider, J.A., and Agras, W.S. (1987). Bulimia in males: a matched comparison with females. *International Journal of Eating Disorder, 6*, 235-242.

Schur, E.A., Sanders, M., and Steiner, H. (2000). Body dissatisfaction and dieting in young children. *International Journal of Eating Disorders, 27*, 74-82.

Seidman, S.N., and Rieder, R.O. (1994). A review of sexual behavior in the United States. *The American Journal of Psychiatry, 151*, 330-341.

Shisslak, C.M., Crago, M., McKnight, K.M., Estes, L.S., Gray, N., and Parnaby, O.G. (1998). Potential risk factors associated with weight control behaviors in elementary and middle school girls. *Journal of Psychosomatic Research, 44*, 301–313.

Shroff, H., and Thompson, J.K. (2004). Body image and eating disturbance in India: media and interpersonal influence. *International Journal of Eating Disorders, 35*, 198-203.

Striegel-Moore, R.H., Mc Mahon, R.P., Biro, F.M., Schreiber, G., Crawford, P.B., and Voorhess, C. (2001). Exploring the relationship between timing of menarche and eating disorder symptoms in black and white adolescent girls. *International Journal of Eating Disorders, 30*, 421-433.

Strong, S.M., Williamson, D.A., Netemeyer, R.G., and Geer, JH. (2000). Eating disorder symptoms and concerns about body differ as a function of gender and sexual orientation. *Journal of Social and Clinical Psychology, 19*, 240-255.

Suhail, K., and Zaib-u-Nisa (2002). Prevalence of eating disorders in Pakistan: relationship with depression and body shape. *Eating and Weight Disorders, 7*(2), 131-138.

Uzun, O., Güleç, N., Ozşahin, A., Doruk, A., Ozdemir, B., and Calişkan, U. (2006). Screening disordered eating attitudes and eating disorders in a sample of Turkish female college students. *Comprehensive Psychiatry*, *47*(2), 123-126.

Vander Wal, J.S., and Thelen, M.H. (2000). Eating and body image concerns among obese and average-weight children. *Addictive behaviors, 25*, 775-778.

Wichstrøm, L. (2006). Sexual orientation as a risk factor for bulimic symptoms. *International Journal of Eating Disorder, 39*(6), 448-453.

Williamson, S., and Delin, C. (2001). Young children's figural selections: accuracy of reporting and body size dissatisfaction. *International Journal of Eating Disorders, 29*, 80-84.

Woodside, B.D., Garfinkel, P.E., Lin, E., Goering, P., Kaplan, A.S., Goldbloom,,D.S., and Kennedy, S.H. (2001). Comparisons of Men With Full or Partial Eating Disorders, Men Without Eating Disorders, and Women With Eating Disorders in the Community. *The American Journal of Psychiatry, 158*, 570-574.

Yager, J., Kurtzman, F., Landsverk, J., and Wiesmeier, E. (1988). Behaviors and attitudes related to eating disorders in homosexual male college students. *The American Journal of Psychiatry*, *145*(4), 495-497.

Yelland, C., Tiggemann, M. (2003). Muscularity and the gay ideal: body dissatisfaction and disordered eating in homosexual men. *Eating Behaviors*, *4*(2), 107-116.

Zini, A., Siani, R., Sandri, M., Soardo, F., Siciliani, O. (2007). Partial syndromes in eating disorders: a prevalence study on a sample of Italian adolescents. *Eating and Weight Disorders*, *12*(3), 125-131.

In: Eating Disorders in Adult Women
Editor: Julian N. Fuchs

ISBN 978-1-60456-673-4

Chapter 4

MODERN HOLY ANOREXIA: HOW ADVERTISING EXPLORES AND DISSEMINATES ASCETIC IDEALS

Fernanda Baeza Scagliusi**, *Barbara Hatzlhoffer Lourenço, Adriana Allegretti Barreto, Priscila de Morais Sato, Marle Alvarenga and Táki Athanássios Cordás

Bulimia and Eating Disorders Program (AMBULIM)
Institute of Psychiatry – Clinics Hospital, University of São Paulo
Rua Dr. Ovídio Pires de Campos, 785. Zip code: 05403-010
São Paulo, SP – Brazil

ABSTRACT

The construction of Western social structures has been highly influenced by religious ideals, especially those related to Christianity. Ascetics are among the most remarkable ones, and have an important role by stimulating simplicity and self-discipline in the detriment of physical pleasures. Such features can be easily identified in the life story of Middle Age anorexic saints, such as Catherine of Siena and Mary Magdalene of Pazzi. Their search for sin redemption, spiritual purification and reconnecting with God was made through a system of moral values and practices where penitence and suffering prevailed. Nowadays, thinness has been, especially among women, overvalued as a basic attribute of beauty and success. This has been widely spread by the media, which use ascetic precepts as a tool to build and keep the "ideal woman" image in modern society. Therefore, the current study aimed to recognize and analyze ascetic and religious messages that are used in advertising directed to adult women. We found that many beauty rites that have been socially scattered and accepted reproduce forbidden rules. The ancient chastity dedicated to a religious god is now replaced by the oral chastity for the

* Corresponding author: Fernanda Baeza Scagliusi. E-mail: fernanda.scagliusi@gmail.com. Address: Bulimia and Eating Disorders Program (AMBULIM). Institute of Psychiatry – Clinics Hospital, University of São Paulo. Rua Dr. Ovídio Pires de Campos, 785. Zip code: 05403-010. São Paulo, SP – Brazil.Telephone number: 55 11 3069 6975.

god of beauty, aiming to reach self-control. By transferring the feminine guilt from sex to eating, food consumption is not experienced by women as a pleasure, but merely as a way to satisfy nutritional needs. The dilemma between food production and consumption is reflected on advertising, which are conflicting, since they deliver concomitantly the ideas of controlling, dieting and overeating. Therefore, there is a conflict between redemption and sin, salvation and temptation, where eating appears as a desire that does not comply with good manners nor is socially accepted, though inevitable. Finally, the widely spread image of the ideal woman as well as this feeling of guilt may lead to the lack of acceptance of body shape and size. This generates the adoption of restrictive practices in order to fulfill current patterns and also creates a cycle that frequently leads to eating disorders.

1. Introduction

The term *religion* is originated in the Latin word *religio*, which indicates, firstly, a set of rules, observances, warnings and interdictions, without referring to the current meaning of ceremonials, myths, divinities or religious expressions (Silva 2004). Various explanations were proposed for the etymology of *religio*. Cicero suggested a bond with *relegere* (to reread), making evident a habit of religious individuals, who pay great attention to subjects related to gods, relentlessly rereading holy writings. Lactance and Servio defended an association with *religáre*, to reconnect, emphasizing the tie, the connection with deities, and stating a feeling of pertaining (Houaiss 2001).

There is no consensus about the most adequate definition for religion, but it is generally accepted that this concept is attached to well-defined historical and social contexts, and has been built along with the West culture, being strongly linked to Christianity's ascension. In spite of the fact that every known cultures comprises religious manifestations, some civilizations that share cultures apart from the Western post-classic ones might not have specific vocables to designate religion (Silva 2004; Engler 2004).

Therefore, the concept of religion should consider the wide variety of religious phenomena. According to Engler (2004), the sacred is a common component in all religions, even though its existence cannot be confirmed.

In most cases, religion can be defined as a set of beliefs that are expressed as service and adoration to a god, who pertains to a divine environment. As a way to establish a relationship with the supreme, believers are obedient to this god. This relationship is guided by commands proceeding from scriptures considered holy, which particularize, according to their contents, rituals and moral codes that are usually filled with symbolisms and has to be followed (Lowenberg et al. 1974). Nevertheless, it is necessary to point out that the belief in a supernatural or transcendental reality does not satisfy all religious cultures, and that the faith in only one god would exclude some segments from the religion's definition, as Buddhism and an assortment of polytheisms (Silva 2004).

The diverse religions perform vast influence in our habits and choices, affecting our conduct in different scales. Among these, there is the religious fundamentalism movement, which is present in every religion and is based on a literal interpretation of holy scriptures (Griffin and Berry 2003). Fundamentalists are the most conservative followers of a sect, and they believe that their religious precepts and principles are dogmatic, i.e., infallible and absolute truths.

Among sundry religions, Hinduism, Buddhism, Islamism, Judaism and Christianity are probably the main contemporary religious segments. All of them establish associations with human eating habits. Lowenberg et al. (1974) state that food abstinence and/or offering, for example, assume devotion and respect features in various creeds. As a result, it is possible to presume that human diet can be strongly characterized by religious traditions.

Hinduism is one of the most ancient religions and it worships numerous gods that are considered manifestations of a supreme being, designated Brahman, the Universal Spirit. The Hindu universe is cyclic and encompasses the principle that nothing is totally destroyed, but, instead, transformed. A system of castes and ideas of reincarnation and destiny distinguish this religion, in which the present state of life is considered a straight consequence of past lives' attitudes. Orthodox followers support the idea that Brahman is present everywhere and, for that reason, every life is sacred and must be preserved. Thus, the most devoted Hindus are strictly vegetarians and follow antiviolence rules described in a holy writing, the Code of Manu (Lowenberg et al. 1974).

According to Lowenberg et al. (1974), Hindus of every castes value cows as sacred animals. They should touch and feed cows whenever this is possible. The kitchen is a holy place in a Hindu house, and food preparation and consumption must involve reverence, because food contains parts of Brahman. Milk, *ghee* (a kind of butter) and coconut are considered sacred food. Besides cow's meat, the ingestion of onion, garlic, turnip, poultry, tomato and lentil is forbidden. Some fasting days are observed, with the practice of absolute fasting or abstinence of cooked food.

In a certain way, Buddhism originates from Hinduism. Buda, the Enlightened, has taught principles that consider suffering as inherent to the human condition. He also showed origin of suffering and healing. The Karma concept explains that the human being is the result of his attitudes, and implies acquiring merit and progressing. Buddhist monks' efforts to acquiring merit are crucial to this religion, since they completely depend on voluntary contributions of both food and clothes. Their vows include the commitment of limiting food consumption after mid-day to tea and coconut milk, with no further meals until the next day. For that reason, many Buddhist families use to skip lunch in order to send their food to monks. Other influences of Buddhism on food consist in recommending reduced consumption of alcohol and toxic products, as these harm the human body integrity (Lowenberg et al. 1974).

In the other hand, Islamism is a religion and a way of living as well. Allah is considered the only and true God, to whom all humankind should submit. Islamism is based on five pillars: faith, prayer, donation, fasting and pilgrimage to the city of Mecca. Lowenberg et al. (1974) said that, during the month of Ramadan, Moslems fast daily from sunrise to sunset as a way for sin remission. Only children, aged and sick people, pregnant and feeding women, as well as travelers, are exempt from that practice. The latter three, however, should compensate the fasting days lost as soon as they are able to do it.

The Koran, sacred scripture, classifies pure and proper foods for consumption. Animals dead for sickness, strangling or for having been beaten to death are forbidden. Pork, blood, wine and other intoxicating beverages are also proscribed. In certain regions, people can't say the word "swine". The way animals are slaughtered must be observed to guarantee the legitimacy of food. There are also Islamic traditions about how to eat. Among them, the habits of thanking God for the meals, eating with the right hand and wearing no shoes while doing it.

In the case of Judaism, the sacred scripture is the Torah. With regard to dietary habits, the observed rules establish bond with the religious beliefs that had transformed separate tribes into a unified people, which is considered chosen for the only and true God and should fight the idolatry and the polytheism. The will of God is represented by the differences found in nature, derived from the process of creation, and must be respected by maintaining such distinctions and forbidding the hybrid. Thus, the Torah distinguishes pure and impure animals. Pure animals ruminate and have divided hooves, simultaneously. Such characteristics assure that, in detriment of the consumption of meat, these animals don't hunt and, in contrast, eat foods of vegetable origin, which were the food granted to them by God. Aquatic animals, in turn, must have fins and scales, which excludes, for example, the consumption of shellfish and crustaceous in general. The ingestion of meat from animals that died for natural causes or illness is not allowed. The same applies to the blood ingestion, which is considered the soul and life of the animal and, therefore, should be offered to God only. The use of internal fat of animals is a taboo. As a result, soap for washing dishes must be free of these. There are restrictions to the consumption of meat and dairy in the same meal, as well as to prepare these different products with the same tools, as a way to hinder a culinary incest, based on: *"You shall not boil a kid in its mother's milk"*. The scriptures establish appropriated intervals of time for a Jew eat meat and dairy (Lowenberg et al. 1974).

The most orthodox Jews consider food control as a proof of their love for to God and a part of their lifestyle. The kosher food is the one allowed by the scriptures, processed and prepared in a way that is considered correct. A rabbi must accompany the slaughter of the animal to ensure the purity of kosher meat, which should be treated to completely remove the blood.

Lowenberg et al. (1974) also showed that the Jewish sacred days have important symbolism involving the food of the believers. They must prepare in advance all food for the Sabbath, their resting day, from Friday sunset to Saturday sunset. The Yom Kippur is a day of complete fasting. Only children below 13 years old are exempted. The Pesach festival, which represents the liberation of the Jews, prohibits the use of flour and fermented products, since fermentation represents a human interference, and suggests the use of a special bread, not fermented; the matzo.

The most widespread religion in the world, Christianity, presents some subdivisions that characterize the religious beliefs and customs of its followers. It identifies, in general, Protestants, Orthodox and Roman Catholics.

Among Protestants, the Mormons, followers of the Church of Jesus Christ of the Latter Day Saints, have specific food practices as an integral part of their religious beliefs (Lowenberg et al. 1974). The Seventh-day Adventist Church, which believes in the return of Christ to the Earth, has remarkable influence in the environment of hospitals, schools and various organizations sponsored by it. Adventists follow the principles of Protestantism, believing, additionally, in the prophecies of Mrs. White, a woman who got important position in the structure of this church. The Bible is the supreme law and the Ten Commandments are followed literally.

Lowenberg et al. (1974) analyzed that a healthy life is widely valorized among Adventists. They believe that the best diet is the vegetarian, prescribed by God: the more simple it is, the better will the body perform. Much of the Seventh-day Adventists are egg-dairy-vegetarian. Meat products are rejected because they are classified as dirty and impure, capable of causing various diseases and accentuating human being's animal characteristics, making him less sympathetic to other people needs. Stimulants such as tea, coffee, alcoholic drinks and smoking are considered harmful. Water is the best drink, and must be ingested preferably at ambient temperature and never at the meals. In general, the food should not be too spicy so as not to injure the stomach. Breakfast should be substantial, lunch presents itself as the largest of meals and dinner must be mild, not overloading the gastrointestinal tract. Snacks are discouraged so that the food is well digested and absorbed; thus, meals must take place at five to six hours of interval.

The Orthodox Christians are located primarily in the Middle East, the Balkans, at northwest of the Mediterranean and in Russia. The Greek Orthodox Church preaches numerous days of fasting, distributed throughout the year to prove that man's soul can guide his body. These periods may last up to 40 days. The days of fasting are characterized by the prohibition of the consumption of animal products. Older devotees refrain themselves from using olive oil, a basic food of the regional diet. This means therefore great sacrifice and devotion to God (Lowenberg et al. 1974).

The Easter is the most important celebration for the Orthodox Christians. Before the fasting that preceding it, there is a period of preparation to make houses clean from all forbidden foods. The consumption of lentils soup and lamb at this time of the year involves various religious meanings, such as the memory of the tears of the Virgin Mary, the blood of Christ who saved the world and the belief in his resurrection. The communion – important event within Christianity, which believes that body and blood of Jesus are present – is made by Orthodox Christians with bread prepared with the purest ingredients. Funeral ceremonies also add foods to the rituals: when boiled, the whole grain of wheat (named koliva) symbolizes the resurrection of Christ and must be offered to the deceased (Lowenberg et al. 1974).

The Roman Catholic Church preaches, for example, the abstention of red meat consumption during the Holy Friday, in memory of Jesus' death. In past decades, this habit was recommended on all Fridays, and days of fasting were also advised (Lowenberg et al. 1974). Although they are present in most religions, ascetic ideas are even more emphasized in Catholicism. The importance of controlling what you eat, that is, what nourishes your body, carries a duality between body and soul, hedonism and asceticism.

According to this reasoning, although it is a necessary condition for human survival, the body is seen as a prison of the soul. This is why many religious practices are intended for the purification of the body through asceticism. The only individual way for transcending existence is based on spirituality. Therefore, the attachment to the pleasures of the flesh makes spiritual elevation impossible to be achieved. Thus hedonism, which preaches are the search for body pleasures and pain suppression as a way of life, can not lead to soul salvation.

The predominance of Christianity in the West is mostly represented by the Catholic Church. Considering the great impact of religion on the human life, it is important to analyze the historic influence of this church and its religious precepts in food, and how that relationship is manifested today in a world full of advertising and consumerism. As a result, we must pay attention to the possible interference of this context in eating disorders predisposition.

2. Bibliographic Review

2.1. Anorexic Saints

Despite being considered a contemporary disease, there is major evidence that anorexia as it is today is a continuous of a behavior common to medieval saints, who were used to practice self-imposed fasting. A woman in the Middle Ages could use religious fasting as a way to getting rid of her duties and/or exercising control over others, rejecting an undesired marriage, avoiding sex or even praying to reach blessings for her relatives. The purpose of fasting saints was to be in communion with God, without pursuing a beauty ideal. They could even overcome clergy authorities, become teachers and counselors and even reform the existing the rules of the Church (Weinberg et al. 2005).

Therefore, while the issues of contemporary anorexia nervosa involve genetic and biological factors, as well as psychological and family aspects, it is possible to find a relationship between the female faster saints of the Middle Ages and the current anorexics (Weinberg et al. 2005). St. Catherine of Siena, St. Mary Magdalene of Pazzi and St. Rose of Lima illustrate the situation observed in young women of the Middle Ages who practiced fasting for such long periods as to be considered miraculous.

Catherine Benincasa (1347-1380) belonged to a family of craftsmen of Siena, Italy, dedicated to wool dyeing. She was a beloved, admired and spoiled child. Researchers say that at six years old Catherine had his first vision in which she saw Jesus sitting in a beautiful throne on the roof of a church. From there onwards, she had changed and a severe authority over herself and others replaced her former graciousness.

At the age of 12, she began to worry about her future marriage, and when she discovered that she had been promised to her widow brother-in-law, Catherine became desperate and had her hair cut. She decided then to join the Mantelatas, aged single women or widows, who lived at home under very strict rules, completely devoted to praying, working and caring for poor and ill people.

For three years she has been in spiritual retreat, talking only to her family about essential subjects and leaving house to go to the church exclusively. She adopted bread and uncooked herbs as her only food and used to vomit whenever forced to eat further. She reduced her sleeping time, used cilicium and an iron chain to mortify her body three times, and also she exposed herself to frequent boiling water jets during the bath.

At the age of 20, she left her spontaneous reclusion and came back to the community life. At the same time she devoted herself completely to the political-religious activity that has built her reputation: the reform of the Church. Although Catherine did not eat any food nor take drinks at that time, she was always very active. That makes people suspicious about the devil's presence. Her impact on others was comparable to that of the 20th century anorexic women: admiration, fear, suspicion and even hatred, while everyone wanted to control her.

When she was 33 years old, she wrote a letter stating that she suffered from pains in the body and, shortly afterwards, she could not walk anymore. She died on June 29, 1380 and was declared saint by Pope Pius II in 1461. She was also declared patron saint of Italy by Pope Pius XII in 1939. She was chosen among several other saints as a model to follow mainly because of the rigidity of her asceticism, among other reasons. Authors such as Raimbault, Eliacheff, Bindaud and Frendrik define the behavior of St. Catherine of Siena, characterized by prolonged fasting, hyperactivity, modification of the body and self-flagellation, as typical of the current anorexics (Weinberg and Cordás 2006).

Mary Magdalene of Pazzi (1566-1607) was born in Florence and had his first mystical ecstasy when she was 12 years old. At the age of 16 she joined the Carmelite of Saint Mary of Angels' monastery. There are reports that Mary Magdalene of Pazzi had been influenced by the ideas and writings of Catherine of Siena. Her baptism name was Catherine (a tribute from her parents to St. Catherine of Siena), later changed to Mary Magdalene, because St. Catherine of Siena used to consider Mary Magdalene as a model to be followed, since she fasted during 33 consecutive years after the death of Christ.

Cordás and Weinberg (2002a) reported that in 1585, Mary Magdalene of Pazzi restricted her diet to bread and water, except on Sundays, when she used to eat remnants of food left by the other sisters, saying that she followed God's orientation. When forced by her superiors to eat better, she began to cause vomit. Sometimes she was found eating quickly and hidden. She also started sleeping few hours and taking cold water baths as a way to punish and prevent herself from devil temptations. When she passed by the store-room, according to her reports, the devil opened the drawers and shelves, seducing her with its "culinary treasures". Perhaps the prolonged fasting and the voracity episodes of Mary Magdalene of Pazzi correspond nowadays to the behavior of a purging-subtype anorexic.

Saint Rose of Lima (1586-1617), when a child, was very obedient and hardworking, and spent several hours on the altar. After reading about of St. Catherine of Siena's life, she took her as a model, devoting herself to mortifications and fasting three times a week. She also had her hair cut (as did Catherine) and didn't matter to mistreat her hands with heavy work. She strove with her parents for ten years for not to marry until she achieved their permission to continue in her life dedicated to God.

At the age of 15, she has made a promise that she was loyal to until death: not to eat meat and ingest only bread and water for the rest of her life. She presented signs of hyperactivity, reduced her hours of sleep and increased working hours. The fact that she could become an object of desire for some people made Rose submit herself to mortification aiming at eliminating any beauty traits.

When he was 20 years old, she joined the Sisterhood of the Third Order of St. Dominic of Penance, where she increased the frequency and severity of her penitence. She used to use an iron belt around waist, a crown of thorns hidden under a row of roses and spent days without food. When she could not stand up anymore, she laid down in a bed built by her, made of mincing glass, thorns and stones.

According to Weinberg et al. (2005), the imitative behavior of Rose towards Catherine of Siena is a further indication of the outbreak of anorexics saints in the Middle Ages. This behavior can also be seen in many young anorexics today, which, sometimes, develop the disease as result of a prior contact with others ill persons.

These cases lead to emphasizing the relation between the behavior of female anorexics saints with ascetic ideals, which aim at voluntary avoiding physical pleasures and stressing simplicity and self-discipline. Thus, under a rigid system of moral and religious values, there is the intention of neutralizing what is considered wrong in society, through the practice of penitence and suffering. That would be the way to get redemption of sins, spiritual purification and reconnection with God (Huline-Dickens 2000; Griffin and Berry 2003).

However, the act of surviving without any food has ceased to be considered a miracle. The old ways of practicing piety have given place to charity, education and caring the poor.

Self-imposed fasting started to be interpreted as a sign of witchcraft and demonic possession (Griffin and Berry 2003). In addition, prolonged fasting started to be seen by doctors as a pathological symptom, that is, the miracle virgins were viewed as hysterics patients.

By the end of the nineteenth century, the doctors that were studying the anorexia nervosa were limited to the physical aspects of the disease. Only with the rise of dynamic psychiatry the emotional aspects of the disease were analyzed. Sigmund Freud (1856-1939) connected anorexia to hysteria, saying that one of the most common symptoms of hysteria is a combination of anorexia and vomiting, and explained the disease as a neurotic behavior that expresses undeveloped or suppressed sexuality. Pierre Janet (1859-1947) associated the disease to an obsessive-compulsive framework, in which the behavior of anorexics derives from the "belief to be ugly and ridiculous", "cannot be loved" and "do not be like everyone". Although these two authors believe that the appetite had symbolic meanings in the psyche of the subject, Freud understood the anorexia as disgust for food and Janet as refusal (Weinberg and Cordás 2006).

Moreover, let us remind that back from the first centuries of Christianity, female sexuality has been repressed as guilt of religious nature (Wolf 1991). One can observe it clearly in female anorexic saints. The Calvinist moral has strengthened that view, as it stressed the connection between food and sexuality and strongly preached against palate's sensual temptations. It is worth noticing that for human beings oral and sexual pleasures relate in several ways, such as during the feeding in the first months of life and in oral erotic practices, which mix the functions of organs of nutrition and the provision of sensual rewards. This fusion of sex and food is common to many cultures (Carneiro 2005). Thus, since sexuality involves also the oral satisfaction, the control of appetite is part of any woman's education (Cordás and Weinberg 2002b).

In the light of that, the food refusal represents a refusal to pleasure, or even to sexuality. Meager bodies resulting from food restriction show weakness and infantilism, and affirm a protest to grow (Carneiro 2004). According to Cordás and Weinberg (2002b), the body is the basis of perception and organization of human life, both in biologically and socially sense. This makes clear the meaning of each body as the intermediary through which we build ourselves in the world.

Anorexia nervosa is a good example of the relationship between diets and moral, as well of the significance of the body and the sexuality as privileged *loci* of moral problems. As noted today, women imprisoned in models of "perfection" cease to live their lives fully, including their sexuality (Goldenberg 2005).

2.2. Current Connections of Religious Attitude with Eating Disorders

Eating disorders show multifactorial etiology (Morgan et al. 2002). In general, the biopsychosocial model is adopted to integrate the variety of factors that contribute to the development of eating disorders. This model encircles social and cultural aspects, familial influences and individual risk factors as possible predisposing, triggering and maintaining characteristics of adverse eating behaviors (Polivy and Herman 2002).

Influences and factors related to eating disorders can converge under innumerous possible ways, making their particular combination in a given individual almost unique and scarcely generalizable. Body dissatisfaction retains great relevance in eating disorders development (Stice and Shaw 2002), since many causes commonly associated with these diseases are manifested through this element. Some examples of these causes are family and peer pressures, teasing, mass media influences and individual psychological influences. However, as Polivy and Herman (2002) propose, the actual occurrence of eating disorders also depends on if and how the individual understands body weight and shape as the answer to the problems of identity and control.

Low self-esteem, negative affect, depression and anxiety are precursors and prominent characteristics of eating disorders. Additionally, there are other factors, such as the habit of dieting to lose weight, the idealization of thinness (markedly in a culture of food abundance), contact with disordered attitudes and behaviors, and cognitive distortions, including perfectionism, impulsive patterns and obsessive thoughts. As well, genetic and neuroendocrine aspects, and stressful life events (interpersonal experiences like emotional or sexual abuse, illnesses, pregnancy) play a role during the emergence of an eating disorder (Polivy and Herman 2002; Johnson et al. 2006; Morgan et al. 2002; Silberg and Bulik 2005).

At the present context, religious influences work as sociocultural and psychological factors in the development of eating disorders, differently from the evident linkage observed between the religion and the prolonged voluntary abstinence from food endorsed by anorexic saints. Although conclusive evidence is not available so far, Huline-Dickens (2000), reviewing studies about religious themes and anorexia nervosa, noticed that anorexic individuals were more often fundamentalists. It was also reported that the degree of weight loss was associated with the level of importance of religion to patients, especially among Anglicans, in whom ascetic ideals were prevailing. Another research analyzed by this author demonstrated higher prevalence of eating disorders in patients of Jewish and Catholic backgrounds than in general population, which can express a probable relationship with food's importance in these religions. Puritans support the constant exercise of vigilance and self-control, with restrictions on spontaneity and sensuality, as well as evidence the burden of guilt and are driven to efficiency and achievement, in a sort of ideas substantially similar to the practices of modern anorexics.

Huline-Dickens (2000) mentions that eating disordered patients employ religious language and symbolism. Moreover, biographies of contemporary individuals with anorexia nervosa describe subjective religious experiences, including, for example, the belief that hunger purifies desire. Families with an anorexic member usually are characterized by rigidity and over-protectiveness, with strong ethical and religious codes. These families also continuously demand loyalty, expecting women to be sensitive, devoted and self-sacrifing. Patients conform to the family ascetic norms and strive to better themselves socially. Plus, they can fulfill a function of salvation, guaranteeing bigger stability to their families.

When religious values closely connect with family structures, a reiteration of men and women roles in society occurs, ratifying the differences between genders. Inclusively, this is a particularly interesting panorama throughout the period of adolescence, in which, during the search for the meaning of life and the establishment of relationships outside domestic environment, there is higher susceptibility to renovating ideas – which can be of a religious scope.

In accordance to what was declared by Saint Paul, *"I do not permit a woman to teach or to have authority over a man; she must be silent. For Adam was formed first, then Eve. And Adam was not the one deceived; it was the woman who was deceived and became a sinner"* (1 Timothy 2:12-14), it is possible to verify that this culture traditionally imposes to women higher levels of guilt, passivity and weakness. Furthermore, the original sin, committed by a woman, derived from the violation of an alimentary rule that was accompanied by the simultaneous awareness of sexuality, along with gluttony and haughtiness – considering that, after the ingestion of the forbidden fruit in disobedience from God, Adam and Eve recognized and were embarrassed about being naked (Carneiro 2005). In addition, given that they are considered to be the main causes of evil and sin, women display more feelings of frustration, anger, hostility and self-punishment, and hence these feelings can possibly generate syndromes like depression and eating disorders, exhibited in a more recurrent basis by this specific population segment (Huline-Dickens 2000).

However, it has to be highlighted that even individuals who do not follow or are barely involved to religious creeds are susceptible to these ideals, since both Catholic faith and Protestant precepts made asceticism influence, in a noteworthy scale, the moral values and the growth of Western industrialized civilizations. Ascetic concepts and judgments, consequently, are generously inserted in social structures, filling the "collective unconscious".

As we establish a parallel between holy anorexia and anorexia nervosa, it is reasonable to demonstrate that, as well as the anorexic saints felt sublime for denying their bodies through self-starvation and extreme emaciation, the modern anorexics also report feelings of power and resistance when adopting these conducts. To both, the others, who do not oppose to corporal needs, do not have the required strength to refuse these appeals, which are vitals for survival. The difference consists in the fact that the anorexic saints used to credit this power to God, while the modern anorexic credit it to themselves, i.e., to the individual. This is very representative of the present days, in which the individualism preponderates (Jarry 1998). In either case, women wish to reach control over their lives by obtaining highly valued aspects in each society. Thus, anorexic saints pursued spiritual perfection, fasting and other forms of self-denying whilst modern anorexics intend to acquire physical perfection, thinness and self-control. Notwithstanding, in both situations, they are never satisfied with the efforts implied to achieve their ideals – holiness or emaciation (Huline-Dickens 2000).

The dislocated role of religion in the currently eating disorders conjuncture is, therefore, understood. In detriment of the service for a religious god, modern anorexics wish to attend to a god of beauty and consumption, idealizing thinness as a reason for life and happiness.

2.3. Current Society: Capitalism and Consumerism

Capitalism is defined as an economic system based on private property and freedom of commerce and industry, aiming primarily at making profit. As a result of this strong power in contemporary society, the consumerism receives great prominence, because, according to Paixão (2006), the power of consumption is the propellant of profit and dictates the rules for each one's role within capitalist social pyramid.

Consumerism is the act of consuming products and services, often without conscience. The role of consumerism in society is very important for the understanding of several problems that affect the population today (Griffin and Berry 2003). Many people believe that it is the great reason for immobilizations and also a vehicle for narcissisms through its esthetic, social and moral stimulus, appearing as the big fundamentalism of our days (Paixão 2006).

According to Griffin and Berry (2003), the advertising has an essential role in the culture of consumerism, analyzing that, sometimes, it may influence the purchase of a product.

2.4. The Importance of Advertising and the Construction of Woman's Social Role

The word *propaganda* comes from the concept of *propagare*, a gardening technique consisting of encraving new sprouts of plants in the earth to obtain new ones. It was first used by the Catholic Church in the *Congregation de Propaganda Fide*, in 1633, with the meaning of an artificial and cultivated diffusion of an idea (Carrascoza 2004). The concept of propaganda also relates to public, religious, institutional and commercial contents. The *advertising* concept, by the other hand, is within the definition of propaganda and relates to commercial messages only. Advertising uses linguistic and stylistic resources to convince the target audience. Since the commanding authority is absent, the source of the message uses a subtle manipulation in order to seduce and persuade the receiver (Carvalho 2001).

In the present industrial and consumption society, advertising plays a very significant role and can even be a transforming factor of the audience behavior and thoughts. The advertising message is an essential tool to disseminating modern ideals. It carries progress, renovation and development granted by technology. As a paradox to the chaotic global scenario, advertising announcements show a "dream world" that discloses what has to be used and bought, by reconciling the principles of pleasure and reality (Carvalho 2001).

Our consumption society drives an inversion of Copernicus universe, where objects gravitated around the humankind. Instead, nowadays humans gravitate around the objects. Owning objects and products becomes synonym of happiness and success. Advertising plays a role in this new model, since without it objects would only be consumption items. Once transformed into myths, however, they acquire attributes that belong to the human condition (Carvalho 2001).

Using specific language resources, the advertising text reflects traits of the modern capitalist society. Consequently, the advertising speech works as a transforming tool whenever words cease to be informative only and acquire strength to persuade. The messages presume an existential emptiness in each human being and offer a product that promises to fulfill the individual's self (Carvalho 2001).

Although it takes different configurations, the advertising text ranges between two canons: the Apollonian and the Dionysian, using Nietzsche's terminology. Those two lines of persuading are complementary and each one can predominate in an advertising text, depending on target public, product profile and announcer's intentions. The Apollonian aspect relates to individual aspirations. It appeals to rationality and considers the ideals of the target public. Its basic premise is happiness. Through a deliberative discourse, made of proposition, argumentation and conclusion, the Apollonian texts raise and discuss real facts through specific topics, with explicit opinions. The Aristotelic, logic-formal speech, which is basic for the Apollonian attitude, explores circularity, repeated statements, presence, authority and comparisons as persuasive arguments. The Dionysian speech, however, is driven by the irrational to reach the emotions. Its speech uses the first or third person and delivers a subtle counseling. The main resources of the Dionysian text are illustrations, examples, citations and figures that touch the ludic and fanciful perception of the audience (Carrascoza 2004).

Women have a significant representation among the consumers targeted by commercial advertising. Women are very susceptible to advertising messages since their image has been by many ways built and sold socially. From the industrial revolution onwards, women have been controlled either materially or by stereotypes. Therefore they depend more than men on cultural models and are more likely to be influenced by these (Wolf 1991). The consumption society identifies and reinforces the feminine role that has been the historical product of a patriarchal society. For that reason, most of the advertising announcements is directed to the feminine public, under a clear appeal: in order to be successful, women must always look beautiful and as young as possible. Mostly, advertising campaigns directed to women show success, vanity, lookings and family (Carvalho 2001).

Advertising announcements build contexts that seem to be naturally true. That is done by connecting products to images, values and beliefs culturally established and accepted long time ago. The media also helps disseminating and reinforcing several myths related to women, by reproducing and maintaining social meanings about certain appropriate roles. Therefore, advertising reflects not the real one, but an ideal woman: beautiful, young, thin, white, elegant and rich (Silva 1997).

Women pictured by beauty advertising announcements are surrounded by myth. Their beauty pattern has a symbolic value, unattainable by most of the real women. To take advantage of that, the advertising language talks to each woman's desires to seduce her inner universe. That is how it persuades and drives to the consumption of products that are often useless, but are conceptually important for their social acceptance (Silva 1997).

As a result from utilizing an idealized beauty to selling products, publicity has caused bodies fragmentation. Advertisement explores different body parts by establishing patterns for each one of these and creating "a beauty image like a puzzle". This fragmentation reinforces the concept of the feminine body as an object, by building and changing it to sell it as one more product (Formiga 2002).

Feminine images are a way of defining femininity as conceived culturally. This conception is the basis for the advertising speech about women. Those images are not always favorable to women as individuals, once social patterns do not reflect real images, but visual stereotypes. This model also involves behavior patterns, since esthetic judgments always come along with ethical assumptions (Silva 1997).

According to Wolf (1991), the decrease of religious authority nowadays opens a gap to a new gospel standing for the beauty church. Based on religion, the consumption appeal separates women into two groups, the "elected ones" (models and other women who fit the established beauty patterns) and the "cursed ones" (women whose beauty differ from the cultural ideals).

The beauty rituals displace the original sin, from being born mortal, to being born a woman. The female consumer buys not only the product, but also a hidden speech, which also includes searching for soul pureness through cleanliness and body care. No young woman should feel that it is too soon to worry about "ugliness" signs: the single fact of existing as a woman means being in deterioration. Current beauty patterns are so unreal that despite the best possible looking a woman has, she always feels deteriorated. The effect of selling this condition is equivalent to the religious doctrine, upon which guilt feelings are necessary for a believer to donate for the church maintenance. In the same way, a woman will only spend with "repairs" if she feels she is deteriorating (Wolf 1991).

Beauty rites also reproduce many of the prohibitions of the religious fundamentalism in relation to sexual appetite through an equivalent taboo related to oral appetite. When the sexual revolution created a new generation of women, sexually available, it became urgent to relocate feminine guilt. The women who kept themselves chaste for a religious god are nowadays chaste to a beauty god. In the past, sexual intercourse should intend procreation, not pleasure. Presently we face a similar situation where food consumption should provide biological needs, letting aside the pleasure that it brings along (Wolf 1991).

2.5. Religious Language in Advertising

Advertising plays an important role in the overall media, from television, radio, magazines and traditional newspapers, to the most recent vehicles, such as internet. Aiming at capturing the audience in an increasingly subtle manner, and permeating with significant impact all aspects of human life, the media develop very sophisticated approaches. Consequently, interpreting the real meaning of advertising messages becomes a complex task, which has to consider both the text and the non-verbal messages.

Based on the above, the following examples will emphasize the religious and moral contents of advertising messages related to eating behaviors and attitudes. These advertisings were made by Brazilian professionals and they are available in the *Clube de Criação de São Paulo* (Sao Paulo Creative Club) website, founded in 1975 by professionals to protect and enhance creativity of Brazilian advertising. The objective of this analysis is to uncover cultural ideas and values that are based on asceticism. We do not intent to affirm that the companies and professionals cited wanted to turn the world an ascetic place, we rather think that these values are so strong in our culture that they are used even in advertising. The names of the products or brands were omitted or replaced by XXX.

2.5.1. Gluttony Sinners

By stating in the center of an advertisement *"For gluttony sinners, heaven is here"*, a steak house invites those who enjoy the act of eating to a presumed paradise. However, the image that comes with the title changes completely the meaning of "heaven". A large red and cloudy back, as well as an eye-catching band of fire that emerges from the bottom of the advertising message, bring the idea of hell. The image includes a silver and black fork that may be interpreted as the devil's trident and/or horns. For all that, we can identify its Dionysian character.

At the bottom of this advertisement, the logotype of the steak house are next to the motto *"Meat is sacred here"*, which challenges religious precepts that sometimes consider meat as impure and dirty. The meat they refer to is not only the food, but may also be associated to the pleasures of the human flesh, only accepted in an environment like hell. In addition, the connection between the eating pleasure and sinning becomes clear, because barbecue consumers are immediately viewed as sinners. Thus, the game chosen by the food industry to sell its products becomes apparent in a world where food has a negative connotation.

2.5.2. Chocolate without Guilt

In a predominant brown back of an advertisement of a brand of shampoos and conditioners, it can be read: *"We have finally found out a chocolate that she consumes without guilt. New chocolate shampoo and conditioner XXX"*. The image of shampoo and conditioner bottles is surrounded by many chocolate scrapings, and it is near the text described above. This Apollonian message is obviously directed to the feminine public. Using the consumer identification as an advertising tool, the contents of this announcement suppose that every woman feels guilty for liking and eating chocolate. Even though this is not an advertisement of food, the message perpetuates this widely internalized thought of contemporary society, projecting and preserving women's oral chastity and denial of pleasure.

2.5.3. The Sacred Time

An advertisement from a barbecue restaurant affirms: *"Meat is a temptation. So is dessert. And people still say that the meal is a sacred time"*. The first two sentences of the text are highlighted in red, while the last sentence is written in brown, a more understated color. This message is placed side by side with an oversize photo of a chocolate cake.

The idea of meal as a holy time comes from religious principles. However, the barbecue restaurant challenges it. Its advertising shows Dionysian and Apollonian features and states that both meat and dessert are temptations, which, in religious vocabulary, means they are considered dirty inner impulses directed to sin and to evil.

Nevertheless, the disproportional image of the dessert in this announcement attracts great attention and incites or, at least, stimulates consumers to order it, disrespecting what would be judged as a correct and acceptable alimentation. In a society of food abundance, the pleasure involved in the act of eating is once again explored and censured in a contradictious way. Thus, advertising becomes a vehicle to spread this frequently made association between food and religious moral.

2.5.4. You are What You Eat

At the right bottom side of an advertisement from a Brazilian brand of toasts it is read: "If there is something that 99% of people carry from childhood is the love for chocolate. Who can resist? It is too good. The thing that is not good at all is to abuse, to substitute healthy foods for too much sugar and fat. The XXX toasts help you keeping good shape and health, preserving all flavor. Light and crispy, they combine with everything you can think of, including a clear conscience".

In the right side of the announcement, this text is arranged in wavy lines, adjacent to a small image of the product inside its package and below a bigger and enlightened photograph of two light toasts with honey. These two toasts are next to the slogan: "XXX's toasts. Living light is way much tasty".

The explicative text shown above clearly used Apollonian characteristics as a way to persuade consumers, making them chose a "light life" that is "so much better". It explores consumer's rationality and a reductionist and solely biological concept of an ideal alimentation, using a deliberative speech, with appropriate proposition, argumentation and conclusion. The beginning of the text discloses a common experience to the reader, in order to create identification. Besides that, it explicitly states its opinion, which it repeats with the circularity inherent to advertisement words and images.

The left side of the advertising announcement shows a drawing of a woman who seems to feel uncomfortable within her own body. This one has the round shape of a chocolate candy. Because of that, the meaning of "You are what you eat", located near this drawing, is taken to the extreme, and puts in evidence a heavy body, full of sugar, obese. The woman color mixes with the environment in which she is inserted and her body shape is perceived as the main feature. Her face is frightened and shows some suffering, probably because of excessive chocolate ingestion. This feeling may be justified in the ascetic base of social and personal beliefs. These emphasize the biologic view of alimentation and forbid the pleasure that should come with it. In contraposition, the toast, light and thin, is at an enlightened place, it illuminates itself the space around, and represents the way towards a healthy and good life.

2.5.5. It is not Immoral

Another example of the XXX's integral toast publicity campaign states again the ideal to strive for. The motto is *"Living light is way much tasty"*, and, this time, the text makes use of an essentially Dionysian language, with a big emotional appeal. A text asserting *"It is not immoral, it is not illegal and it is not fatty. But it is as tasty as if it were"* is placed at the left side of the announcement and, similarly to what was described in item 2.5.4, the main light focus irradiates from the toast, placed at the right side. Again, two toasts with honey are illuminated and the product is given a redemptory role.

The wavy writing of the text reinforces the idea of lightness that is sold with the toast. At the same time, putting weight on has been placed at the same level of illegality and immorality, that is, something not accepted socially, leaving traits of prejudice against obese individuals.

The advertising announcement infers that tasty food is undoubtedly immoral, illegal and fatty. So, it reproduces religious and ascetic precepts, which condemn any way of pleasure.

sumindo-se como algo n engordar foi colocado no mesmo patamar da ilegalidade e da imoralidade,

2.5.6. The Last Temptation

We are going to present a more extreme example of advertisement. This piece was not approved by the manufacturer of the product. Although the piece was not approved, it is available at the *Clube de Criação de São Paulo* (Sao Paulo Creative Club) website. This advertisement of an ice cream shows an electric chair in a dark room. An empty ice-cream bowl is beside the chair. In the bottom side only, one can read *"The last temptation"*. The use of an image practically without text to touch consumers and the implicit counseling define this advertisement as clearly Dionysian.

The ice cream is presented as the last and irresistible wish of the convicted, which emphasizes the utmost importance of the product. It is also interesting that the word "temptation" was used, instead of "wish". If the word "wish" had been used, the message would be: "this ice-cream is so good that if you had to eat only one thing before you die you would choose it". The use of the word "temptation" relocates the pleasure context into the guilt context. Other crucial issue is that the consumption of ice-cream is the last of the temptations this person had. Because of the fact that the person is a criminal, one can read this sentence as "the last sin" or "the last crime". Is eating such a bad thing? In a society so concerned with beauty and conservation of the body, advertising and selling a food viewed as "naughty and unnecessary" is complicated. Probably that is the reason why the announcers here presented could choose this approach. They appear to be saying: "Yes, you know that this food is an indulgence, because you don't need it in order to keep your body fit and functional. Yes, it can make you fat. But it is good… Come on, what is a little sin?". What else can they say in a society that does not accept the pleasure of eating *per se*?

Finally, it is interesting to notice that in this case the guilt for eating was annulled by the execution that followed. If we consider the typical thoughts of anorexic individuals (both in holy anorexia and anorexia nervosa), this logic reproduces the search for redemption justified by the preference to dying instead of "sinning". The act of eating and the consequent and natural weight gaining are so unacceptable that leaving the terrestrial body and disconnecting from flesh becomes a necessary solution ("I would rather to die than sinning", "I would rather die than being fat").

2.6. Association with Eating Disorders

Capitalist system and consumerism markedly exert influences on all aspects of life, including the interaction with eating habits and attitudes. In concordance to what was previously explained, this interference is adequately represented by the importance of mass media and advertising in this environment, intensified with the modernization and the advent of globalization that have greatly affected familiar and social dynamics (Rathner 2001).

Capitalism and Western way of life afforded an ample gamut of options and possibilities to the individual, culminating in an ambivalence and ambiguity situation that encumbers the actual decision-making. Movements as nationalism, racism, xenophobia and religious fundamentalism are examples of attempts of fight against inherent traits of modernity: uncertainty and obscurity.

Contiguous to this scenario, Rathner (2001) affirms that it is admissible to indicate that modernization offered progressive management, surveillance and regulation of the human body via market forces, which succeeded in spreading the thin ideal to all social stratums throughout time, especially when women's job and study opportunities were enlarged. At the same time, it is remarkable that food works as the first and major delineator of the moral behavior of a given individual, who are supposed, since childhood, to adapt to rules delimiting how much, where, how and when somebody has to eat, to obtain self-control (Carneiro 2005).

So, the dilemma between production and consumption, particularly in respect to foodstuff, is typical in the West and is also reflected in communication messages that are equally conflicting and concomitantly divulge ideas of controlling and eating restraint and ideas of overeating. Applying the religious facet observed among the examples of advertising shown, this confrontation happens between redemption and sin, salvation and temptation, evidencing the act of eating as a desire that does not comply with good manners nor is socially accepted, though inevitable.

Aiming a population with higher than average weight and, besides, employing thinner models and strongly moralistic messages, the media can execute an indirect effect in predisposition of eating disorders and contribute to body image preoccupations, provoking a disordered eating pattern, notably among women (Griffin and Berry 2003). According to Andrade and Bosi (2003), the perfect body ideal currently designated by our society and broadcasted by the mass media incites women, essentially during adolescence, to huge body dissatisfaction, constantly hating themselves due to some "extra" kilograms and abusing of extremely restrictive diets and intense exercises as a way to compensate "extra" calories, attempting to correspond to the up- to-date cultural model.

In some cases, publicity uses beauty models that tend to occupy the extreme limit of the obsessive search for the perfect body, disfiguring then the tenuous parting line between the healthy care with body and the insidious installation of narcissistic diseases. The human body is transformed into a site of rituals that induce individuals to refute their basic requirements, throwing themselves in a vicious circle involving restrictive diets, prolonged fasting and rigid controls about food ingestion, body and body image (Andrade and Bosi 2003). Nonetheless, it must be emphasized that consumers create a circular relationship with the media, bearing in mind that a message coded in image is sold only by means of consumer's acceptance (Rathner 2001).

Subsequently, in this sense, it is significant to elucidate that when we opt for the consumption of some food we are subordinated to the act of incorporation, i.e., to send this food beyond boundaries between external and internal limits of our body. Both in the biological aspect and in the view of representations and creeds, incorporation entails the transformation of man into what he eats (Fischler 1988). Thus, the incorporation principle can be understood as an endeavor to establish control over body, mind and, afterward, over identity, taking into account that every food encloses effects in human organism. Each act of incorporation is relevant for denoting, concurrently, a risk to our own identity and a chance or hope to become more than what we actually are.

Likewise, incorporation mechanism is valid to subjects related to consumerism and advertising. Nowadays, this concept can be applied to the products selection and ulterior purchase. These products are gifted with characteristics that can influence human body, redefining it. When a person buys a product, she or he expects that this product will change her or him. The act of buying makes the person "somebody" in a world that lives for consumerism. Also, the act of "having something" causes a feeling of "belonging". For example, one may belong to a group that only uses glasses from the *griffe* X or to a group that only drinks diet sodas.

As Fischler (1988) suggested, at the same time incorporation nourishes the notion of collective identity – the specificity of foods chosen to be eaten (or products to be consumed) is essential to provide a feeling of pertaining and to stipulate differences in relation to other groups, resembling cases of patients with eating disorders. Simultaneously, this classification of foods (and products) in line with a culture expresses a view of world and grants a meaning to man and his universe, being, inclusively, endowed with a religious dimension, more accurately in the etymologic aspect of this word (*religáre*, to reconnect: connection, tie).

Consonant with currently extensively divulged values, human body becomes, in this manner, another product to be recreated or purchased, in the illusion of infinitive malleability. Consumers face a confused religious paradigm that is intermixed to the language of advertisements and the social reality. This paradigm shows up as an additional preponderant factor to the institution of self-control over image, personality and individual beliefs, and, as a result, over eating choices and attitudes, delineating, finally, the vulnerability to eating disorders.

3. Conclusion

The influence of Christianity in the West was powerful enough to mark historically the relationship between man and his diet. From a field in which rules and observances of biblical scriptures used to practice direct request in eating habits and attitudes of diverse young females in the Middle Ages, religion has been consolidated up to now as an important socioeconomic and cultural factor, plenty internalized and able to induce beliefs and judgments.

Essential gear of capitalist system, advertising acts as a perpetuator of cultural ideals that embrace those related to diet, body and beauty. Regarding these specific principles, there is an imperative influence of asceticism, preponderantly among the female public. Because of the propagation of unattainable beauty and thinness models, body dissatisfaction is fomented and then makes feasible the adoption of restrictive practices for adjusting human body to the current patterns, creating a cycle that frequently discharges in the development of eating disorders.

In conclusion, it is possible to affirm that the impetus to serve a religious god was transferred to a context in which another god, the god of beauty, is venerated. Moreover, some values that are endorsed by the religion remain important: the denial of pleasure and the need for self-control over the body. Western culture allowed women to have sexual pleasure, but oral pleasure is still a taboo. The sin of the flesh has been, along time, symbolized by food. Nowadays, eating is a sin itself. Although other influences (as economics ones) are obviously important to this matter of fact, religion continues to accomplish an important role in the dissemination of ascetic patterns, interposed in collective unconscious and well-incorporated by the language used in advertising. In view of that, finally, a situation of increasing vulnerability to the development of eating disorders is generated.

4. References

Andrade, A., and Bosi, M. L. M. (2003). Mídia e subjetividade: impacto no comportamento alimentar feminino [*Media and subjectivity: impact on female feeding behavior*]. Revista de Nutrição, 16, 117-125.

Carneiro, H. F. (2004). Transtornos alimentares ou um impasse dietético? [*Feeding disorders or a dietary impasse?*]. Psicologia em Revista, 10, 270-287.

Carneiro, H. S. (2005). Comida e sociedade: significados sociais na história da alimentação [*Food and society: social meanings in feeding's history*]. História: Questões and Debates, 42, 71-80.

Carrascoza, J. L. A. (2004). Razão e sensibilidade no texto publicitário: como são feitos os anúncios que contam histórias [*Reason and sensibility in the advertising text: how announcements that tell stories are made*]. São Paulo: Futura.

Carvalho, N. (2001). Publicidade: a linguagem da sedução [*Advertising: the language of seduction*] (3rd ed.). São Paulo: Ática.

Cordás, T. A., and Weinberg, C. (2002a). Santas anoréxicas na história do Ocidente: o caso de Santa Maria Madalena de Pazzi [*Anorexic saints in Western history: the case of Saint Mary Magdalene of Pazzi*]. Revista Brasileira Psiquiatria, 24, 157-158.

Cordás, T. A., and Weinberg, C. (2002b). Clorose: a efêmera doença das virgens [*Chlorosis: the virgins' ephemeral disease*]. Revista de Psiquiatria Clínica, 29, 204-206.

Engler, S. (2004). Teoria da religião norte-americana: alguns debates recentes [*Theory of North-American religion: some recent debates*]. Revista de Estudos da Religião, 4, 27-42.

Fischler, C. (1988). Food, self and identity. Social Science Information, 27, 275-292.

Formiga, S. (2002). Um corpo que cai: a reificação dos corpos pela publicidade [*The reification of bodies by advertising*]. Gênero, 2, 61-74.

Griffin, J., and Berry, E. M. (2003). A modern day holy anorexia? Religious language in advertising and anorexia nervosa in the West. European Journal of Clinical Nutrition, 57, 43-51.

Goldenberg, M. (2005). Gênero e corpo na cultura brasileira [*Gender and body in Brazilian culture*]. Psicologia Clínica, 17, 65-80.

Houaiss, A. (2001). Dicionário Houaiss da língua portuguesa [*Houaiss Portuguese dictionary*]. Rio de Janeiro: Objetiva.

Huline-Dickens, S. (2000). Anorexia nervosa: some connections with the religious attitude. British Journal of Medical Psychology, 73, 67-76.

Jarry, J. L. (1998). The meaning of body image for women with eating disorders. Canadian Journal of Psychiatry, 43, 367-374.

Johnson, J. G., Cohen, P., Kasen, S., and Brook, J. S. (2006). Personality disorder traits evident by early adulthood and risk for eating and weight problems during middle adulthood. International Journal of Eating Disorders, 39, 184-192.

Lowenberg, M. E., Todhunter, E. N., Wilson, E. D., Savage, J. R., and Lubawski, J. L. (1974). Food, man, and religion. In: Food and man (2nd ed., pp. 193-231). New York: John Wiley and Sons.

Morgan, C. M., Vecchiatti, I. R., and Negrão, A. B. (2002). Etiologia dos transtornos alimentares: aspectos biológicos, psicológicos e sócio-culturais [*Etiology of eating disorders: biological, psychological and sociocultural determinants*]. Revista Brasileira de Psiquiatria, 24, Suppl 3, 18-23.

Paixão, T. O. (2006). Do consumismo às possibilidades de construção da cidadania. Ribeirão Preto [*From consumerism to the possibilities of citizenship's construction*]. Presented at GT 03 – Advertising, Propaganda e Marketing of South-Eastern Intercom.

Polivy, J., and Herman, C. P. (2002). Causes of eating disorders. Annual Review of Psychology, 53, 187-213.

Rathner, G. (2001). Post-communism and the marketing of thin ideal. In: M. Nasser, M. Katzman, and R. A. Gordon (Eds.), Eating disorders and cultures in transition (pp. 93-104). Hove, East Sussex: Brunner-Routledge.

Silberg, J. L., and Bulik, C. M. (2005). The developmental association between eating disorders symptoms and symptoms of depression and anxiety in juvenile twin girls. The Journal of Child Psychology and Psychiatry, 46, 1317-1326.

Silva, E. M. (2004). Religião, diversidades e valores culturais: conceitos teóricos e a educação para a cidadania [*Religion, diversities and cultural values: theoretical concepts and the education for citizenship*]. Revista de Estudos da Religião, 2, 1-14.

Silva, M. L. (1997). Publicidade e ideologia: um estudo dos anúncios de produtos de beleza em Nova [*Advertising and ideology: a study of beauty products' advertisements in Nova magazine*]. Rio Grande do Sul. [Dissertation, Faculdade dos Meios de Comunicação Social da Pontifícia Universidade Católica do Rio Grande do Sul].

Stice, E., and Shaw, H. E. (2002). Role of body dissatisfaction in the onset and maintenance of eating pathology: a synthesis of research findings. Journal of Psychosomatic Research, 53, 985-993.

Weinberg, C., and Cordás, T. A. (2006). Do altar às passarelas: da anorexia santa à anorexia nervosa [*From altar to catwalks: from holy anorexia to anorexia nervosa*]. São Paulo: Annablume.

Weinberg, C., Cordás, T. A., and Munoz, P. A. (2005). Santa Rosa de Lima: uma santa anoréxica na América Latina? [*Saint Rose of Lima: an anorexic saint in Latin America?*]. Revista de Psiquiatria do Rio Grande do Sul, 27, 51-56.

Wolf, N. (1991). The beauty myth: how images of beauty are used against women. New York: Morrow.

In: Eating Disorders in Adult Women
Editor: Julian N. Fuchs

ISBN 978-1-60456-673-4

Chapter 5

CONSENT, CAPACITY AND HUMAN RIGHTS FOR OLDER WOMEN WITH ANOREXIA NERVOSA

Terry Carney[1]
University of Sydney, Sydney, Australia

ABSTRACT

Typically anorexia nervosa is diagnosed as a condition of teenage girls where the rates of mortality and morbidity are very high and recovery rates very low. This chapter discusses the condition as experienced by older women who have either lived with anorexia during adolescence and as young women or who have been diagnosed later in life. The discussion will traverse issues of consent to treatment or its refusal, capacity to provide consent, and the application of human right protections arising from various human rights instruments.

A. INTRODUCTION

Severe anorexia nervosa principally affects women, with an onset at a young age (Dresser, 1984), though it also affects some men (Touyz, Kopec-Schrader and Beumont, 1993) and its onset can be delayed to middle or older age (Berry and Marcus, 2000). Its chronicity, high mortality and treatment resistance are legendary. There is both a stock of people who have built up extensive histories of experiencing anorexia nervosa and what the medical and other service systems offer, as well as a steady flow of 'first time' presentations.

The core precept of western medicine and bioethics, which privileges 'consent' to treatment above nearly all other considerations, is particularly fraught in anorexia nervosa cases, since the need to consider granting consent does not arise in the minds of AN sufferers. While both new and longer-standing groups of AN suffers often present as quite articulate and rational, apart from their 'anosognosia'—the 'pocket' of inability to accept the gravity of the condition or the urgency of treatment (Beumont and Carney, 2003; further:

---

[1] Professor of Law, Faculty of Law, University of Sydney, Sydney, Australia.

Vandereycken, 2006: 353ff)—it does not necessarily follow that similar answers should be given to an older chronic sufferer to the questions of consent, capacity and human rights implications of whether or not to respect treatment refusals, as compared to the young adolescent (Draper, 2003).

This Chapter takes Australian law and experience and some international examples to argue that in the case of an older, or chronic sufferer of AN, greater respect should be given to decisions not to participate in certain treatment regimes, given their maturity and accumulated life experiences ('maturity of experience') with regard to their condition. In Part B, it is suggested that the concept of 'insight', rightly criticised for being too vague and rubbery to reliably serve as a proxy for patient 'capacity' to decide for themselves, may have one saving grace: in the hands of professional and sophisticated gatekeepers of the use of coercion in treatment, it may permit life experience and patient 'maturity' to be reflected in decisions made about their treatment. In Part C it will be suggested that, while human rights standards may point weakly in the same direction, they have less purchase at the *substantive* level (beyond favouring restricted use of coercion in treatment), but nevertheless may make an important *procedural* contribution—requiring that legal processes for overriding treatment decisions of AN patients should provide the time and resources (or the 'reflective decisional space') in which a more sophisticated and nuanced 'insight' analysis can find expression.

B. Thinking About 'Capacity-to-Decide' for Older/ Chronic Sufferers of AN

Any distinction in favour of according greater respect for the treatment choices of older or chronic sufferers of AN ultimately rests on a preference for a contextual, rather than an abstract 'cognitive' approach to capacity.

1. Does 'Quality of Life' Carry Greater/ Determinative Weight for Chronic AN?

Both Dresser and Draper have argued in favour of respecting competent decisions by *chronic* sufferers to reject treatment or food, subject to showing the ability to grasp, retain, weight and rationally process information (Dresser, 1984: 357, 373; Draper, 2000: 126).

Thus Heather Draper argues that It is right for clinicians to treat all *new* referrals ... as potential recoveries. This means that if the patient comes close to death, they should be fed even if they say that they do not want this intervention…I would argue that this is justified because the refusal may not be autonomous (Draper, 2003: 284).

However chronic sufferers develop deeper understandings of their quality of life, which may be relevant to assessing (and respecting) the competence of such longer-standing suffers' objections to further treatment, because the length of time that one has to cope with an illness adds invaluable information about the 'informed' aspect of one's decisions about it, and adds greater weight to the view that there is a quality of life judgement to be made here, and not just one about whether or not to feed (ibid).

This richer or more multi-layered approach gains credence from Tan et al's qualitative interviews revealing levels of complexity, variation and ambiguity/uncertainty associated with how anorexia patients 'thought' about their condition; thought patterns which were sharply at odds with the simplistic 'intellectual' form taken by legal tests of competence, which hinge on 'understanding and reasoning'. Their case data revealed that:

> anorexia nervosa can have complex and variable effects on concentration, beliefs, and thought processing, without affecting their ability to perform well on [a standard test of competence]. At the same time, they also report alterations of values, ranging from the typical values attached to fatness, to much broader changes in values such as devaluation of other aspects of life, unusual values, and integration of anorexia nervosa into the personal identity (Tan, Stewart, Fitzpatrick and Hope, 2006: 279)

Most would accept that an inability to appreciate the true dimensions of one's own condition (true anosognosia) removes capacity to insist that the law respects a decision to reject treatment (Torrey and Kress, 2004: 87). But as Tan et al observed from their AN interviews, things are often less much less clear-cut than this, such as where the person grasps and accepts all aspects of the analysis of a situation, other than its *salience* to that person (Tan, Stewart, Fitzpatrick and Hope, 2006: 271-72). And greater respect might be thought to be due to a person's current objection to treatment where it is congruent with opinions pre-dating their illness, than when it is at odds with previous views (ibid, 278).

2. Is 'Insight' a Better Test of Capacity?

The definition and application of capacity to consent as a basis for acceptance (or imposition) of medical regimes of 'close management' (ie tough clinical regimes), or under involuntary committal laws, is elusive (Carney, Tait, Saunders, Touyz and Beumont, 2003).

So elusive that, in AN cases, as indeed in mental health more generally, proxy concepts like 'lack of insight' subsume the legal test (Diesfeld, 2003; Freckelton, 2003b; Perkins, 2003a: 127; Perkins, 2003c). Victorian Mental Health Review Board ('MHRB') rulings in anorexia cases illustrate this. Denials or equivocation about having AN or an adequate weight (*Re EC* (2001): 7), or weak explanations like forgetting to take enough food when camping (*Re ET*, 2001: 6), were given short shrift. But the same fate awaited some applicants even when they did accept their condition and the need for treatment, because the insight was deemed too recent, or was too conditional, to constitute *real* evidence of capacity for informed decision-making about their condition (*Re DM* (2002): 11-12; *Re KJ* (2001: 8)).

Resort to such amorphous and value-laden concepts in mental health can be criticised on various grounds, including facilitating practices of reasoning 'backwards' from a conclusion in order to justify committal orders, as found in studies of British mental health tribunals (Perkins, 2003c; 2003a; 2003b), or as being too indeterminate. Insight also operates as a proxy vehicle for encapsulating conclusions grounded in *value* choices (Freckelton, 2003a: 327-29; Vine, 2003: 122-23); value choices which are often contentious, providing a vehicle for the rationalisation by mental health tribunals of the 'play it safe' approach of authorising involuntary treatment in AN cases, as we have previously found (Carney, Tait, Saunders, Touyz and Beumont, 2003).

On the other side of the ledger, it can be validly argued that traditional tests of legal 'capacity' place too much store in rather *superficial* enquires about a person's understandings of the 'broad nature and effect' of treatment; thus degenerating into little more than intellectual tests of abstract abilities of comprehension. 'Insight' has therefore been commended as carrying the *potential* of engaging in *deeper* inquiries into a patient's 'perceptions', should decision-makers take their responsibilities seriously (rather than use it as a short-cut), thus better tapping the essence of mental illness and conditions like anorexia nervosa (Torrey and Kress, 2004: 84).

3. Is a 'Relational' or Family-Based Approach Preferable?

To North American readers, brought up on mental health laws which distinguish between authority to involuntarily detain and the quite separate issue of involuntary treatment, it may seem passing strange that, with one exception (Tasmania), Australian mental health laws confer automatic authority to treat all involuntarily detained patients. The main device struck for determine ng to override an objection in that State, a statutory health attorney, is also at odds with general US preferences for strong liberal philosophies (Carney, 2008b), instead adopting the more communitarian slant found in the nearly 40 US States with 'family consent laws' for people who have not executed durable powers of attorney, though the scope of those powers are usually more limited (West, 2004: 124-25).

Tasmania has been an exception in Australian mental health, by providing that mental health committal did not carry an automatic right to treat, leaving that to the Guardianship Tribunal (as too in Arizona), or to the 'person responsible', though this may be abandoned soon (DHHS, 2007: 14-18). While empowering family members through the 'person responsible' may better comport with community cultural values (Carney, 2008a) by valorising family over the individual, the Japanese experience gives pause for caution.

In Japan, where the family already exercise extensive authority to invoke involuntary mental health care (Weisstub and Carney, 2006), commentators have contemplated widening the existing adult guardianship role of local social service authorities (Doran, 2002: 374-75; Arai, 2003; Carney, 2004) to enable initiation of compulsory treatment for anorexia nervosa, specifically in order to relieve the burden which this places on family members (Kondo, Takaoka, Ikawa and Niwa, 2004). On the other hand, as our research has suggested, guardianship tribunals may make a better fist of assessing the complexities of 'competence' than do mental health tribunals (Carney, Tait, Touyz, Ingvarson, Saunders et al., 2006).

Within the US, psychiatric advance directives have been popular ever since Congress passed the Patient Self Determination Act in 1990 (Papageorgiou, King, Janmohamed, Davidson and Dawson, 2002; Atkinson, Garner and Gilmour, 2004). Health Care Powers of Attorney have also been popular, since they often apply more vacuous 'best interests' guidelines (in place of or in competition with substituted judgement tests) which allow more wriggle room for decisionmakers to take account of family interests (Kim, Scheyett, Elbogen, Van Dorn, McDaniel et al., 2007). However rates of compliance with wishes tend to be low among professionals. For advance directives regarding treatment, for instance, stakeholder views are quite divided (Atkinson, Garner and Gilmour, 2004; Kim, Scheyett, Elbogen, Van Dorn, McDaniel et al., 2007), with up to half of some US psychiatrists indicating that they would exercise statutory powers to 'over-ride' objections to treatment (Swanson, McCrary, Swartz, Van Dorn and Elbogen, 2007).

C. Rights Analyses of Anorexia

In light of German jurisprudence doubting extensive use of coercion in the treatment of anorexia nervosa—other than within the context of adult guardianship constraints (Laakmann, Ortner, Kamleiter, Ufer, Frodl et al., 2006; Thiel and Paul, 2007)—there is keen interest in possible human rights implications. Here the record is a mixed one: *process rights* (such as to speedy hearings, favourable burdens of proof, or access to documents and legal representation) have fared tolerable well (Zuckerberg, 2007), but *substantive* rights (such as not to be detained solely on the basis of clinical opinions) have fared poorly (Arboleda-Florez and Weisstub, 2008).

1. The Emerging 'Persuasive-Dialogue' Model of Australian Human Rights Law

Unlike virtually every other western legal system Australia does not have a national Bill of Rights. Victoria's *Charter of Human Rights and Responsibilities Act 2006* (Vic), and the Australian Capital Territory *Human Rights Act 2004*, are the only jurisdictions to have enacted (non-entrenched) human rights protections (Carney and Beaupert, 2008), embracing a cluster of civil rights covering freedom, respect, equality and dignity (VEOHRC, 2007). These are 'negative' rights, derived from the *International Covenant on Civil and Political Rights* (1966) ('ICCPR'), rather than economic, social and cultural rights, like the right to health found in Article 12 of the *International Covenant on Economic, Social and Cultural Rights* (1966) ('ICESCR'). While the 'interdependence and indivisibility' of these two sets of rights is one of the fundamental principles of the human rights framework (Alston, 1995: 94), it is only in a very few areas that overseas human rights court rulings have interpreted rights like that to freedom from arbitrary deprivation of liberty, to very thinly found government obligations to comply with minimum standards of care, and even then they are confined to detained prisoners rather than people subject to compulsory measures (Fennell, 1999; Prior, 2007). While that may change should the Tasmanian Government accept the Tasmanian Law Reform Institute Report proposal for *inclusion* of economic, social and cultural rights (Tasmania, 2007: Rec 15, pp 118-122), there is little comfort in terms of possible *rights* of AN patients to treatment or support resources.

The enforcement regimes under the Victorian and ACT Charters deliberately favour the 'educative' strategy over the 'litigious', by concentrating on fostering dialogue and soft suasion towards rights compliance (Williams, 2006). Rights are not enforceable by individuals in isolation from the decisions of public bodies, or of the courts and tribunals when interpreting the law, and do not carry *new* monetary or other remedies (Evans and Evans, 2006). Rights compliance is a combination of monitoring by the relevant Human Rights Commissions (Vic , ss 41-42; ACT, s 41) and a narrower set of remedies which may be pursued in court. The object is to change the *culture of decision-making* by taking account of human rights precepts, through the 'interpretive provision' of reading ambiguous legislation to render it compliant (Vic Charter, s 32; ACT Charter, s 30), the obligation for 'public authorities' to comply with human rights, or through declarations of 'incompatibility' (ACT s 32) or 'inconsistent interpretation' (Victoria s 36). Once in issue, the rights are not unlimited, but are subject to 'reasonable limits' able to be justified in a 'free and democratic society based on human dignity, equality and freedom' (Vic s 7(2); ACT s 28), elaborated under s 7(2)(a)-(e) of the Victorian Charter, paying regard to certain stipulated factors, such as the nature and purpose of the right and any limitation of it.

The Victorian Charter provides for a more direct route to resolve any dispute as to statutory construction relating to the Charter. If a question of human rights law arises during court or tribunal proceedings, the matter may be referred to the Supreme Court on application by a party to the proceedings (s 33). In Victoria, the remedy is a 'declaration of inconsistent interpretation' (s 36), requiring the relevant Attorney General to table a written response within 6 months of its issue (Vic, s 37; similarly ACT s 33). Declarations of incompatibility under the equivalent British statutory construction provision have been infrequent (15 instances since October 2000, with another 5 reversed on appeal: Clayton, [2007]: 13) but three were mental health cases (Gledhill, 2007: 385), and in other instances the courts have re-interpreted legislation so as to render it compatible with human rights.

The human rights of greatest potential interest are those to freedom from arbitrary deprivation of liberty and to a 'fair hearing' (s 24(1)). Others with obvious, although less clear cut implications, in the mental health context are the right to freedom from torture (and experimentation and treatment without consent: s 10), the right to be treated humanely when deprived of liberty (s 22(1) [dealing with '[h]umane treatment when deprived of liberty' provides that '[a]ll persons deprived of liberty must be treated with humanity and with respect for the inherent dignity of the human person']) and the right to freedom from discrimination and equal protection of the law (s 8).

2. Possible Australian Bases for Human Rights Challenges/Guidance

Section 21 of the Victorian *Charter,* dealing with the right to liberty, prompt advice of grounds for detention and speedy review of its lawfulness, is the most obvious basis for assessing whether compulsory treatment for anorexia nervosa is inconsistent with Charter principles.[2]

The entitlement to prompt advice about the basis for preliminary detention is widely recognised in mental health provisions requiring that patients be promptly provided with information about their rights and pending MHT review proceedings (see, MHA Vic, s 18; MHA NSW, ss 74, 76, 77; MHA ACT, s 50). However implementation of this right is entrusted to hard-pressed mental health service staff, and is especially challenging in situations where literacy skills are weak, or translation is unable to be provided or personally checked for comprehension (Carney and Beaupert, 2008). Thus, despite the apparent statutory protections for provision of written and oral statements of patient's rights, it was found in

[2] This provision precludes deprivation of liberty except 'on grounds established by law and in accordance with procedures established by law'; requires prompt notice to be given of the reasons for the deprivation; and effectively provides for the writ of habeas corpus in making provision for prompt determination of the lawfulness of any deprivation of liberty by a court.

2001 that 30% of patients did not know they could access information before the Board or appeal their involuntary status, that many found it difficult to access such information, and that about half did not know about legal representation (Auditor-General, 2002).

Speedy review of admission is most in jeopardy under mental health laws in jurisdictions such as Victoria Tasmania, South Australia and Western Australia,[3] where *clinicians* make initial admissions and, as in Vic and WA, up to 8 weeks is allowed to elapse before MHT review of admissions (MHA Vic s 30(1); MHA WA, ss 48 and 138(2)).[4] South Australian clinicians authorise up to 6 weeks detention before review (MHA SA, s 12), while Tasmania allows 1 month (MHA Tas s 52). By contrast, NT orders must be reviewed within 7 days (*Mental Health and Related Services* Act (NT) ('MHA NT'), ss 39(1), 45(3) and 123), while NSW, insists on review of admissions by a Magistrate 'as soon as practicable' after a second medical opinion confirms the original basis for admission (MHA NSW s 27(d)).

The comparable provisions of the *European Convention*, Articles 5(1) and (4), founded the British ruling that 'routinely delaying' reviews for 8 weeks breached the 'prompt presentment' principle (Gledhill, 2007: 398; *R(C) v ... MHRT* [2002] 1 WLR 176, [2001] Mental Health L Rep 110). Breach of the speedy hearing rule was one of the three cases awarded damages (Clayton 2007: 26), a remedy not available as such under the Victorian charter (Evans and Evans, 2006: 274ff). The *Mental Health Act 1983* (UK) was also found to be inconsistent with human rights principles for effectively requiring *patients* to show that their detention was not warranted, placing the burden of proof for release on the applicant (Bindman, Maingay and Szmukler, 2003: 91; Gledhill, 2007: 385-89). Collateral rights credited to European Court of Human Rights rulings in cases like *Megyeri v Germany* (1993) 15 EHRR 584, or UK Human Rights interpretations, include extending legal representation even to patients who do not request it (Coats, 2004), and periodic review hearings (Davidson, McCallion and Potter, 2003: 41).

3. Towards a More 'Reflective Process' of Legal Review?

While mental health reviews are automatically scheduled in Australia, legal representation is heavily rationed, generally on a 'merits basis' and is quite rare (5-10% in Victoria: Lesser, 2007: 12), though in NSW all involuntarily *hospitalised* patients are now provided with a legal aid advocate at initial hearings by the magistrate, and by the MHT. However scarcity of funding has not been accepted overseas as an excuse. Thus the operational reason of having too few medical members to enable prompt listings did not excuse the breach found in *R(KB and others) v MHRT* ([2002] (EWHC (Admin) 639; [2003] Mental Health L Rep 1), and a lack of adequate case-management software failed to excuse

---

[3] MHA Vic ss 9, 12, 12AC, 14 [clinicians may make a CTO for an involuntary patient]; MHA Tas, s 29; Mental Health Act 1993 (SA) ('MHA SA'), s 12; Mental Health Act 1996 (WA) ('MHA WA'), s 43.

[4] However, the Victorian Board attempts to schedule hearings sooner than the 8 week limit. 'Mental health inquiries' must discharge if the grounds are not satisfied, but otherwise authorise orders for initial involuntary observation or treatment (or both) for up to 3 months (s 35(5)(c)), or release on a CTO or into the hands of a 'primary carer': ss 35(5), (b), (a) respectively. Prior to their expiration the Tribunal must review any application for extension (ss 37(1)(a), (2)) and do so every 3 months thereafter during the first 12 months (s 37(1)(b)) and then 6 monthly: s 37(1)(c). Under the Mental Health (Treatment and Care) Act 1994 (ACT) ('MHA ACT'), other than in emergencies, involuntary treatment can only commence by way of a tribunal order.

the breach found in *R(B) v MHRT* ([2002] EWHC (Admin) 1533; [2003] Mental Health L Rep, 19).

The right to a 'fair' hearing by 'a competent, independent and impartial court or tribunal' following a 'fair and public hearing', may also be in severe jeopardy in mental health settings at present. Procedural standards such as to natural justice and patient access to documents are incorporated in the legislation (Watchirs, 2000; Rees, 2003). However the latter are not unqualified rights, and may express too widely the power to withhold where information is judged to be 'harmful' (cf the wider exceptions condemned in Nth Ireland: Davidson, McCallion and Potter, 2003: 42), even though European jurisprudence has favoured clinical practices (Gostin, 2000; Bindman, Maingay and Szmukler, 2003: 92). And the hearings themselves may be much too brief, and in jurisdictions where multi-member hearings are dispensed with (or dispensable), too superficial to honour human rights principles for a 'fair' hearing (further: Carney and Beaupert, 2008). In essence there is substance to Bruce Winick's complaint about the 'basic dishonesty' of superficial or 'peripheral' processes of mental health review which fail to engage the clinical evidence founding committal (Winick, 2005: 145).

The difficulty in mounting a human rights critique on many other grounds is the generally 'pro-therapy' cast to much of the remaining jurisprudence. Thus there is no requirement for the committal process to be founded in other than appropriate clinical opinions about a person's condition, and even admissions based on non specialist opinions of general physicians appear to pass muster (Zuckerberg, 2007: 515). Treatability, or the availability of treatment to the person detained, are likewise not required (ibid, 516). Failure to fully engage with the 'least restrictive alternative', in the absence of other compelling considerations, may be slightly more productive (ibid, 517), but in AN cases the risk of death or morbidity will leave little room for maneuver there.

This leaves the MI Principles requiring 'informed consent' to treatment, subject to various exceptions such as being found 'incapable' by a competent authority (such as a MHT or GT), or an 'unreasonably withheld' consent couple with a competent authority finding that it is in the best interests of the person to treat without consent (ibid, 518).

4. Lessons from German Human Rights Jurisprudence Restricting Resort to Coercion?

Germany has recently explored the tension between a strong constitutional protection of individual rights under the *Basic Law* (Grundgesetz) and possible use of adult guardianship as a response to extreme cases of anorexia nervosa (Laakmann, Ortner, Kamleiter, Ufer, Frodl et al., 2006; Thiel and Paul, 2007).

Article 2(2) of the Federal Constitution (Basic Law) provides that a person's right to life and physical integrity is 'inviolable' and may be interfered with only pursuant to law, while Article 104(1) stipulates that individual freedom may only be restricted pursuant to specific legal authority and conformity to prescribed procedures. Adult guardianship is also a federal matter, under section 1896(1) of the Federal Statute Book (Bundesgesetzbuch): §1896, para 1,

1BGB11, page 1580.[5] This states that a legal guardianship order can be made when somebody of full legal age is unable to partially or wholly care for themselves due to a psychological illness or a physical, intellectual or mental disability (Laakmann, Ortner, Kamleiter, Ufer, Frodl et al., 2006: 36). Finally, section 1906(1) of the *Civil Code* (Bürgerliches Gesetzbuch) imposes a 'best interests' restraint on the exercise by a guardian of the power to admit their ward to a period of involuntary hospitalisation or treatment,[6] and section 1906(2) insists on obtaining judicial orders for all such committals (immediately after the admission in the case of an emergency). Mental health (and related) committals, however, are authorised under the laws of the different German Länder ('States') which confine admissions narrowly to a mental illness that would lead to the concrete and direct endangering of that person or another person (Thiel and Paul, 2007: 130).

In recent years the German courts have ruled that compulsory hospitalisation—or in some cases, forced feeding'—is constitutionally acceptable provided it passes a test of 'proportionality' (ibid, 130). Thus in the case *AZ:2W 17/02*, decided on 25 January 2002, the appellate court for Schleswig decided that the lower court had been in error in concluding that a person with terminal anorexia nervosa could not be hospitalised under §1906(1) of the German *Civil Code*. The lower court had reasoned that an admission would be 'redundant' since forced feeding did not come within the parameters of the guardianship power. The appellate court rejected that reasoning and found that forced hospitalization was constitutional provided that it was not disproportionate, a question to be judged by the appellate court, paying regard to whether the patient's condition had worsened and whether her situation was life threatening (in which case intervention would not be disproportionate). Most recently the Federal Court of Justice (*AZ: XII ZB 236/05*) endorsed the proportionality test, but indicated that, while a simple hospitalisation pursuant to the guardianship provisions would be proportionate to the loss of liberty at stake, a higher threshold applied when compulsion was also used,[7] either to retain the person in hospital or to impose treatment such as force feeding.

This German reconciliation of individual rights and the imperative to intervene or treat is of interest not only because the 'proportionality' test resonates with the human rights jurisprudence on which the Victorian and ACT human rights laws are based (Williams, 2006) but because the test in many ways mimics the ethical rationale for unconsented 'stomach-pumping' of an emergency overdose admission which we have previously endorsed for AN cases, and founds a 'light touch' German clinical practice of confining coercion to a few cases, exposed for short periods of time (Laakmann, Ortner, Kamleiter, Ufer, Frodl et al., 2006: 39-46), and encouraging the use of patient-clinician 'contracts (ibid 43).

---

[5] As in Australia, patients below the age of majority are dealt with under other laws, in this case, German family law (Laakmann, Ortner, Kamleiter, Ufer, Frodl et al., 2006: 39).

[6] §1906(1) provides that the hospitalization of a ward of the guardian (when associated with a restriction on the ward's liberty) is only allowed if it is in the best interests of the ward due to the fact that:

1) his or her mental illness or intellectual or mental disability places the ward in danger of either suicide or considerable physical harm; or
2) A health examination, treatment or medical intervention is necessary and would not be pursued without the involvement of the guardian and the ward cannot recognize the need for intervention or cannot act with their own judgment because of a mental illness or intellectual or mental disability. [our emphasis].

[7] Citing Thiel, A, Röttgers, HR, "Zwangsbehandlung von psychisch kranken Menschen nach dem Betreuungsrecht." Psychiat Prax, 2006, 33, 196-201.

D. Conclusion

The ethical and other limits in the construction of mental health laws (Carney, 2008b) largely replay themselves in debates about the role of law in treatment of AN (Carney, Tait, Touyz, Ingvarson, Saunders et al., 2006: 19-29).

The expansive (or classical liberal) expression of the liberty of the subject is best realised through binding psychiatric advance directives ('PADS'), which authentically transmit the values of a person for better or for worse. At the other end of the philosophical spectrum lie the paternalist readings best expressed by way of a 'best interests' (or as argued here, an 'insight') test.

The problem with the first is that empirical evidence shows that the professionals relied on to faithfully honour PADS are deeply divided (and conflicted) between the positions of fully respecting autonomy of choice even if it leads to death, respecting autonomy *except* when it leads to death, or the utilitarian liberal position of respecting autonomy only when no significant harm is entailed (Atkinson, Garner and Gilmour, 2004: 678). The problem with best interests tests are that, as Hillary Rodham (Clinton) memorably wrote over a quarter of a century ago, they are both a 'slogan in search of a definition' and 'empty vessels into which …values and perceptions are poured' (Rodham, 1973). Even the supposed 'middle ground' test of 'substituted judgment (attempting to step into the person's shoes and apply their values) is problematic. As Louise Harmon wrote a decade and a half ago, this too is ultimately a 'fiction' (Harmon, 1990).

This Chapter has explored a more pragmatic resolution to these dilemmas so far as the older, chronic sufferer of AN in concerned. In developing the argument for according greater presumptive weight to respecting their choices about treatment, it was suggested that Draper and others correctly identify the gravamen of the claim as residing in their 'maturity of experience' concerning their condition, a body of material and values which cannot readily be accommodated in legal decisionmaking without some 'open-textured' ingredient of decisions about capacity (such as the concept of 'insight') and a 'reflective decisional space' in which such matters can competently by explored when deciding whether or not to override patient choice. While human rights standards may confer few *substantive* rights for older AN patients (other than leaning in the direction of restricting the use of coercion in treatment), they may strengthen the *procedural* claim for courts and tribunal to be given the hearing time, advocacy services and other resources which contribute to the creation of that reflective decisional space in which a more sophisticated and nuanced 'insight' or other open-textured analysis can find expression.

Bibliography

Cases

Re EC (2001). *Re EC.* Unreported Statement of Reasons of the Victorian Mental Health Review Board, 17 July 2001 (Meadows, Newby and Gidley).

Re ET (2001). *Re ET.* Unreported Statement of Reasons of the Victorian Mental Health Review Board, 29 November 2001 (O'Shea, Healy and Hall).

Re DM (2002). In the appeal and review of DM an involuntary patient at Royal Melbourne Hospital. Unreported Statement of Reasons of the Victorian Mental Health Review Board, 22 February 2002 (Newby and Wood, McSherry dissenting).

Re KJ (2001) In the review of KJ an involuntary patient at Monash Medical Centre. Unreported Statement of Reasons of the Victorian Mental Health Review Board, 14 August 2001 (Meadows, Gallois and Gidley).

References

Alston, P. (1995). 'Disability and the International Covenant on Economic, Social and Cultural Rights'. In: T. Degener and Y. Koster-Dreese (ed) *Human Rights and Disabled Persons: Essays and Relevant Human Rights Instruments*. Dordrecht, Martinus Nijhoff Publishers.

Arai, M. (2003). 'Guardianship for Adults: A new safety net in Japan'. A paper delivered at the conference: *Society for Legal Guardianship 'Japan-Australia Adult Guardianship Workshop'*, Sydney, 29 September 2003.

Arboleda-Florez, J. and D. Weisstub, Eds. (2008). *Mental Health Rights: The relation between constitution and bioethics*. Autonomy and Human Rights in Health Care: An international perspective. Dordrecht, The Netherlands, Springer.

Atkinson, J., H. Garner and H. Gilmour (2004). 'Models of Advance Directives in Mental Health Care: Stakeholder views'. *Social Psychiatry and Psychiatric Epidemiology,* 39(8): 673-680.

Auditor-General (2002). *Mental Health Services for People in Crisis.* Auditor General, Victoria, Melbourne.

Berry, E. and E. Marcus (2000). 'Disorders of Eating in the Elderly'. *Journal of Adult Development,* 7: 87-99.

Beumont, P. and T. Carney (2003). 'Conceptual Issues in Theorising Anorexia Nervosa: Mere matters of semantics?' *International Journal of Law and Psychiatry,* 26(6): 585-598.

Bindman, J., S. Maingay and G. Szmukler (2003). 'The Human Rights Act and Mental Health Legislation'. *British Journal of Psychiatry,* 182(2): 91-94.

Carney, T. (2004). 'Aged Capacity and Substitute-Decisionmaking in Australia and Japan'. *LawASIA Journal,* 2003/4: 1-21.

Carney, T. (2008a). 'Culture, Community or Rights: Securing health in a post-modern, privatised world'. In: D. Weisstub and G. Pintos (ed) *Autonomy and Human Rights in Health Care*. Dordrecht, The Netherlands, Springer. 36: 155-172.

Carney, T. (2008b). 'The Mental Health Service Crisis of Neoliberalism—An antipodean perspective'. *International Journal of Law and Psychiatry,* 31(#): forthcoming.

Carney, T. and F. Beaupert (2008). 'Mental Health Tribunals: Rights drowning in un-"chartered" health waters? ' *Australian Journal of Human Rights,* 14(1): forthcoming.

Carney, T., D. Tait, D. Saunders, S. Touyz and P. Beumont (2003). 'Institutional Options in Management of Coercion in Anorexia Treatment: The Antipodean experiment'. *International Journal Law and Psychiatry,* 26(6): 647-675.

Carney, T., D. Tait, S. Touyz, M. Ingvarson, D. Saunders and A. Wakefield (2006). *Managing Anorexia Nervosa: Clinical, Legal and Social Perspectives on Involuntary Treatment*. New York, Nova Science.

Clayton, R. ([2007]). 'The Human Rights Act Six Years On: Where are we now'. *European Human Rights Law Review*: 11-26.

Coats, J.W. (2004). 'Mental Health Review Tribunals and Legal Representation - Equality of arms? ' *Psychiatric Bulletin,* 28: 426.

Davidson, G., M. McCallion and M. Potter (2003). *Connecting Mental Health and Human Rights.* Northern Ireland Human Rights Commission, Belfast.

DHHS (2007). *Review of the Mental Health Act 1996: A discussion paper.* Tasmanian Department of Health and Human Services, Hobart.

Diesfeld, K. (2003). 'Insights on "Insight": The impact of extra-legislative factors on decisions to discharge detained patients'. In: K. Diesfeld and I. Freckelton (ed) *Involuntary Detention and Therapeutic Jurisprudence*. Aldershot, Ashgate: 359-382.

Doran, I. (2002). 'Elder Guardianship Kaleidoscope: A comparative perspective'. *International Journal of Law, Policy and the Family,* 16: 368-398.

Draper, H. (2000). 'Anorexia Nervosa and Respecting a Refusal of Life-prolonging Therapy: A limited justification'. *Bioethics,* 14(2): 120-33.

Draper, H. (2003). 'Anorexia Nervosa and Refusal of Nasogastric Feeding: A reply to Simona Giordano'. *Bioethics,* 17(3): 279-289.

Dresser, R. (1984). 'Feeding the Hunger Artists: Legal issues in treating anorexia nervosa'. *Wisconsin Law Review,* [1984]: 297-374.

Evans, S. and C. Evans (2006). 'Legal Redress under the Victorian Charter of Human Rights and Responsibilities'. *Public Law Review,* 17(4): 264-281.

Fennell, P. (1999). 'The Third Way in Mental Health Policy: Negative Rights, Positive Rights and the Convention'. *Journal of Law and Society,* 26(1): 103-127.

Freckelton, I. (2003a). 'Involuntary Detention Decision-Making Criteria and Hearing Procedures: An opportunity for therapeutic jurisprudence in action'. In: K. Diesfeld and I. Freckelton (ed) *Involuntary Detention and Therapeutic Jurisprudence*. Aldershot, Ashgate: 293-337.

Freckelton, I. (2003b). 'Mental Health Tribunal Decisionmaking: A therapeutic jurisprudence lens'. *Psychiatry, Psychology and Law,* 10(1): 44-62.

Gledhill, K. (2007). 'Human Rights Instruments and Mental Health Law: The English experience of the incorporation of the European Convention on Human Rights'. *Syracuse Journal of International Law and Commerce,* 34: 359-403.

Gostin, L. (2000). 'Human Rights of Persons with Mental Disabilities: The European Convention of Human Rights'. *International Journal of Law and Psychiatry,* 23(2): 125-59.

Harmon, L. (1990). 'Falling Off The Vine: Legal Fictions and the Doctrine of Substituted Judgment'. *Yale Law Journal,* 100(1): 1-71.

Kim, M.M., A.M. Scheyett, E.B. Elbogen, R.A. Van Dorn, L.A. McDaniel, M.S. Swartz, J.W. Swanson, et al. (2007). 'Front Line Workers' Attitudes towards Psychiatric Advance Directives '. *Community Mental Health Care Journal*: in press.

Kondo, T., K. Takaoka, N. Ikawa and N. Niwa (2004). 'Law Relating to Compulsory Treatment of Patients with Anorexia Nervosa'. *International Medical Journal,* 11(4): 281-284.

Laakmann, G., M. Ortner, M. Kamleiter, S. Ufer, T. Frodl, B. Goldstein-Muller, M. Jager, et al. (2006). 'Treatment of Vitally Endangered Anorexia Nervosa Patients Based on Guardianship Laws'. *Nervenarzt,* 77(1): 35-6, 38-40, 43-9.

Lesser, J. (2007). *Review and Decision Making for Persons with a Serious Mental Illness: Achieving Best Practice* The Winston Churchill Memorial Trust of Australia, Melbourne.

Papageorgiou, A., M. King, A. Janmohamed, O. Davidson and J. Dawson (2002). 'Advance Directives for Patients Compulsorily Admitted to Hospital with Serious Mental Illness'. *British Journal of Psychiatry,* 181: 513-519.

Perkins, E. (2003a). *Decision-Making in Mental Health Review Tribunals.* London, Policy Studies Institute.

Perkins, E. (2003b). 'Mental Health Review Tribunals'. In: K. Diesfeld and I. Freckelton (ed) *Involuntary Detention and Therapeutic Jurisprudence*. Aldershot, Ashgate: 221-239.

Perkins, E. (2003c). 'A New Tribunal?' *Psychiatry, Psychology and Law,* 10(1): 113-121.

Prior, P. (2007). 'Mentally Disordered Offenders and the European Court of Human Rights'. *International Journal of Law and Psychiatry* 30(6): 546-557.

Rees, N. (2003). 'International Human Rights and Mental Health Review Tribunals Obligations'. *Psychiatry, Psychology and Law,* 10(1): 33-43.

Rodham, H. (1973). 'Children Under the Law'. *Harvard Educational Review,* 43(4): 487-514.

Swanson, J.W., V. McCrary, M.S. Swartz, R. Van Dorn and E.B. Elbogen (2007). 'Overriding Psychiatric Advance Directives: Factors Associated with Psychiatrists' Decisions to Preempt Patients' Advance Refusal of Hospitalization and Medication '. *Law and Human Behavior,* 31(1): 77-90.

Tan, J., A. Stewart, R. Fitzpatrick and T. Hope (2006). 'Competence to Make Treatment Decisions in Anorexia Nervosa: Thinking processes and values'. *Philosophy, Psychiatry, and Psychology,* 13(4): 267-282.

Tasmania (2007). *A Charter of Rights for Tasmania.* Tasmania Law Reform Institute, Hobart.

Thiel, A. and T. Paul (2007). 'Compulsory Treatment in Anorexia Nervosa'. *Psychotherapie, Psychosomatik, Medizinische Psychologie,* 57(3-4): 128-135.

Torrey, F. and K. Kress (2004). *The New Neurobiology of Severe Psychiatric Disorders and Its Implications for Laws Governing Involuntary Commitment and Treatment.* University of Iowa,

Touyz, S., E. Kopec-Schrader and P. Beumont (1993). 'Anorexia Nervosa in Males: A report of 12 cases'. *Australian and New Zealand Journal of Psychiatry,* 27: 512-517.

Vandereycken, W. (2006). 'Denial of Illness in Anorexia Nervosa - A Conceptual Review: Part 1 Diagnostic significance and assessment; Part 2 Different forms and meanings '. *European Eating Disorders Review,* 14(5): 341-351; 352-368.

VEOHRC. (2007, Thursday 8 November 2007). 'The Victorian Charter of Human Rights and Responsibilities Explained.' <http://www.humanrightscommission.vic. gov.au/ human% 20rights/the%20victorian%20charter%20of%20human%20rights%20and%20responsibilities/> (accessed Thursday 8 November).

Vine, R. (2003). 'Decision-making by Psychiatrists about Involuntary Detention'. In: K. Diesfeld and I. Freckelton (ed) *Involuntary Detention and Therapeutic Jurisprudence.* Aldershot, Ashgate: 113-132.

Watchirs, H. (2000). *Application of Rights Analysis Instrument to Australian Mental Health Legislation.* Department of Health and Aged Care, Canberra.

Weisstub, D. and T. Carney (2006). 'Forensic Mental Health Law Reform in Japan: From criminal warehousing to broad-spectrum specialist services? ' *International Journal of Law and Psychiatry,* 29(2): 86-100.

West, C. (2004). 'Gay and Lesbian Partners are Family Too: Why Wisconsin should adopt a family consent law'. *Wisconsin Women's Law Journal,* 19: 119-140.

Williams, G. (2006). 'The Victorian Charter of Human Rights and Responsibilities: Origins and scope'. *Melbourne University Law Review,* 30(3): 880-905.

Winick, B.J. (2005). *Civil Commitment: A Therapeutic Jurisprudence Model.* Durham, North Carolina, Carolina Academic Press.

Zuckerberg, J. (2007). 'International Human Rights for Mentally Ill Persons: The Ontario experience'. *International Journal of Law and Psychiatry,* 30(6): 512-529.

In: Eating Disorders in Adult Women
Editor: Julian N. Fuchs
ISBN 978-1-60456-673-4

Chapter 6

An Integrative Perspective over Dissociation and Eating Disorders in Women

Ehud Bodner[1] and Iulian Iancu[2]
1 The Interdisciplinary Department of Social Sciences, Bar - Ilan University 52900 Ramat-Gan, Israel
2 Rehovot Mental Health Center, Remez Str. 80, Rehovot 76449, Israel

Abstract

Although there is no psychological existence without the body, there are times when psychological motivations and defensive maneuvers take over basic bodily functions. Dissociation is considered as a psychological mechanism that enables such taking over (Axelsen and Sveaass, 1994; Orbach et al., 1997) or enables distance from one's troubling experience. An extreme use of dissociation can lead to complete disregard of painful memories and emotions, neglecting elementary bodily functions, and to full ignorance of painful sensations (Orbach, 1994; Orbach et al., 1997). Then, a vicious cycle may ensue, in which less attention is ascribed to basic bodily needs, more importance is tied to psychological motivations, and then again, less consideration is paid to bodily needs, and so on. This mechanism is suggested to play a major role in the etiology of eating disorders (Iancu et al., 2006). By dissociating one's thoughts from the physical discomfort caused by endless dieting and intensive exercising, patients with eating disorders (Fairburn and Harrison, 2003) manage to eat less and exercise more. In this chapter we will present an integrative perspective on the relationship between dissociation and eating disorders in women. We will commence with a short description of eating disorders. Then, we will review studies that evaluated dissociation in patients with eating disorders. Subsequently, we will discuss physiological processes in women (menstruation, pregnancy, birth) that may teach them to dissociate themselves from physical discomfort and pain. Following that, we will describe several psychological characteristics of women regarding eating disorders that differentiate them from men. We will explain the impact of these psychological tendencies on the ability of women with eating disorders to dissociate themselves from their bodily needs. Finally, we will discuss the clinical implications of our integrative perspective on the treatment of women with eating disorders. Specifically, we will discuss preventive efforts of eating disorders in women:

namely educational efforts, identification of high risk individuals, and hypnotherapy of women with eating disorders.

1. Eating Disorders

The prevalence of eating disorders has been reported to increase in recent decades (Becker, Grinspoon, Klibanski, and Herzog, 1999; Lucas, Beard, O'Fallon, and Kurland, 1991, Lucas, Crowso, O'Fallon, and Melton, 1999). Eating disorders are much more prevalent in women (Fairburn and Harrison, 2003), and during the last decades have especially increased in young women (Becker, Grinspoon, Klibanski, and Herzog, 1999). These conditions are associated with significant morbidity and mortality, suffering for the individual and family, and severe economic implications (Fairburn and Harrison, 2003).

In our modern society, women are under constant social pressure to be slim. Women ascribe more importance than men to their body shape and weight, and are more occupied with counting calories (Fairburn and Harrison, 2003). The tremendous importance attributed to being slim causes some of the women to break their relations with others, to concentrate on weight and food, and to develop eating disorders. These women concentrate on the over-valued idea of becoming slim, develop behavioral habits that are performed automatically and with a diminished attention to bodily sensations (e.g., binge eating, deliberate vomiting, massive physical exercises), and thereby gain a sense of control. Unfortunately, the tendency of women with eating disorders to seek help declines when they feel in control over their weight (Fairburn and Harrison, 2003).

A higher prevalence of women is evident in three out of the four diagnostic categories (DSM-IV, 1994), of eating disorders – i.e., anorexia nervosa, bulimia nervosa, and binge eating (Barry, Grilo, and Masheb, 2002; Nielsen, 2001; Pawluck and Gorey, 1998; Rastam, Gillberg, and Garton, 1989). In anorexia nervosa, the incidence is 19 per 100,000 per year in females and 2:100000 in males. In Bulimia nervosa it is 29 per 100000 in females and 1:100000 in males. Seventy five percent of the patients with binge eating are women. Only atypical eating disorder demonstrates a similar ratio between men and women.

Anorexia is mostly common in girl adolescents (Pawluck and Gorey, 1998) and is characterized by a significant weight reduction and a distorted body image. The disorder includes a disruption in menstruating and additional physical complications. It also includes excessive gymnastics and purification behaviors (e.g., self-initiated vomiting and use of laxatives). These symptoms may be followed by difficulties in regulating their mood, concentration problems and nervousness. It can also go along with anxiety and depressive symptoms, a decrease in sexual drive and an obsessional preoccupation with body weight. Patients lose their interest in their environment and become isolated and withdrawn. They think they are fat and aim at reducing weight. They do not consider the unpleasant physical sensations which follow their disorder (e.g., weakness, dizziness, fatigue) as warning signals, but as a clear sign for their success in competing against themselves (i.e., reducing more weight in less time) or against others (i.e., reducing more weight than others).

Bulimia nervosa (Palmer, 2004) is prevalent in female adolescents, but can also occur in women above the age of thirty. These patients ascribe a lot of importance to weight reduction and to body weight. Therefore, it is no wonder that some of the anorectic patients develop bulimia. In bulimia nervosa, the efforts to limit food consumption fail, and control over eating is sought but not achieved. In bulimics, the body weight fluctuates around the normal, due to the binge eating and to the attempts to reduce amounts of food. It is the binge eating and not the reduced weight, which characterizes this disturbance. Accordingly, the consumed food amounts can reach a peak of 2000 kcals (Rosen, Leitenberg, Fisher, and Khazam, 1986). There is also a type of bulimia nervosa which includes purification behaviors (Mitchell, Hatsukami, Pyle, Eckert, and Boutacoff, 1987). In addition, bulimia includes substance misuse and self-injurious behaviors (Paul, Schroeter, Dahme, and Nutzinger, 2002). These aforementioned behaviors are also habitually performed (Hutchinson, Gow, and Jamieson, 2007).

Patients who suffer from atypical eating disorders (Ricca, Mannucci, Mezzani, et al., 2002) have suffered from anorexia nervosa or from bulimia nervosa in the past, or will suffer from these disturbances in the future. Therefore, it is no wonder that this group of disturbances combines components which are similar to the two abovementioned disturbances (Fairburn and Harrison, 2003), such as heavy restriction of food consumption, excessive exercise, binge eating and a subnormal and even lowered body weight. Regarding their cognitive focus, some concentrate on controlling over food amounts and some on the maintenance of their body weight.

Binge eating (Eddy, Keel, Dorer , et al., 2002) usually occurs in elder age groups, in comparison to the other three previous disturbances. Some of these patients suffer from a preliminary tendency towards binge eating and therefore, also suffer from overweight. This is a much less serious disturbance and its spontaneous recovery is considerably higher.

Eating disorders are considered as a dangerous psychiatric disturbance (Nielsen, 2001). The mortality rate of women who suffer from anorexia nervosa reaches 10 percent in a period of 10 years. Eating disorders are also chronic disorders. In a follow-up after women who suffered from bulimia nervosa (Herzog, Hopkins, and Burns, 1993), about a third to a half have suffered from bulimia, or from a severely atypical eating disorder five and even 10 years after the disturbance had started. A similar prognosis is relevant for patients with atypical eating disorders (Fairburn and Harrison, 2003). These patients tend to develop anorexia nervosa or bulimia nervosa during a period of three years after the beginning of their disturbance.

Fairburn and Harrison (2003) argue that currently, there is not enough knowledge to present a casual model, supported by empirical evidence, which combines the various factors responsible for eating disorders (Fairburn and Harrison, 2003). Nevertheless, they mention some of the etiological factors, such as: (1) Genetic predisposition to develop anorexia nervosa and bulimia nervosa; (2) Range of environmental risk factors; (3) Low self-esteem combined with obsessional and perfectionistic personality tendencies, and (4) Over-sensitivity of the woman to her body due to a heightened frequency of overweight in some of the patients' parents and because of an early menstruation. They also discuss the existence of neglect or abuse in some of the families of these patients and the social pressure on women to lose weight (Fairburn and Harrison, 2003).

Another explanation for many of the behaviors that characterize eating disorder patients is based on their tendency to use dissociation (Everill, Waller, and MacDonald, 1995). In the next section we will discuss the link between dissociation and eating disorders in women and elaborate on the connections between early sexual abuse, borderline personality disorder and eating disorders in women.

2. Dissociation and Eating Disorders

Dissociation. Dissociation is described as a disintegration of consciousness, memory, identity, and sensation and is considered a defense mechanism against intolerable trauma (Braun, 1988; Zlotnick et al., 1996). Dissociative disorders and experiences are frequently related to childhood neglect and abuse history (Putnam et al., 1996; Chu and Drill, 1990; Tutkun, 1998).

Many studies have demonstrated the higher dissociative abilities of women with eating disorders. Demitrack, Putnam Brewerton, Brandt, and Gold (1990) showed that the anorexics and bulimics scored significantly higher than controls on the Dissociation Questionnaire (DIS-Q; Vanderlinden, Van Dyck, Vandereyeken, Vertommen, and Verkes, 1993), and on the Dissociative Experiences Scale (DES; Bernstein and Putnam, 1986). Similar findings were reported by Schumaker, Warren, Schreiber, and Jackson (1994) who compared 26 anorexic and 18 bulimic patients to controls on the Riley Questionnaire of Experiences of Dissociation (QED; Riley, 1988) and found that the eating disorder patients reported higher scores. Grave, Oliosi, Todisco, and Vanderlinde (1997) compared obese binge eaters to healthy obese individuals and found higher dissociative scores among the binge eaters on the DIS-Q. Vanderlinden, Spinhoven, Vandereycken, and Van Dyck (1995) compared 51 eating-disorder women patients (bulimics, mixed anorexics and anorexics) on several dissociative and hypnotic measures. They found both dissociation and hypnotizability scores to be higher for the bulimics than for the mixed anorexics, who, also scored higher than anorexics (see Hutchinson, Gow and Jamieson, 2007).

Traumatic experiences. It is the disturbance in body image and the disruption in body sensation (e.g., the increase in pain tolerance) which link the process of dissociation to eating disorders (Nagata, Kiriike, Iketani, Kawarada, Tanaka, 1999; Vanderlinden, Spinhoven, Vandereycken, and van Dyck, 1995). The disturbance in body image in patients with eating disorders seems to be related to an early traumatic experience, usually sexual abuse (e.g., Murray, Macdonald, and Fox, 2008; Allison, Grilo, Masheb, and Stunkard, 2007). For example, 25% of a large group of eating disorder patients (N = 98) reported traumatic events. This subgroup had significantly higher scores on the DIS-Q (Vanderlinden et al., 1993), compared with normal controls and high degree of dissociative experiences combined with amnesia to a similar degree as in a group of patients with dissociative disorders. Grave, Rigamonti, Todisco, and Oliosi (1996) compared the rate of traumatic experiences and DIS-Q score between 103 female patients with eating disorders and 112 high school graduating students serving as controls. The highest trauma rate was among patients with bulimic symptoms. In addition, whereas 20 patients (19.4%) demonstrated pathological dissociative experiences only 3.6% in the control group demonstrated such symptoms. Favaro and Santonastaso (1995) examined 491 female college students and found more frequent abuse experiences in women with eating disorders (but no differences on the DIS-Q scores).

Early traumatic experiences can be triggered in patients with eating disorders by a late trauma. Tobin, Molteni, and Elin (1995) described a subgroup of patients with anorexia nervosa and bulimia nervosa symptoms that were triggered by a medical trauma (e.g., injury, cancer, surgery) which occurred after age 30. This subgroup had a relatively good premorbid professional and marital adjustment, but suffered from severe sexual and physical abuse by family members in their childhood. The authors described the following pathological manifestations in these patients: dissociated disturbance that included dissociated mood and multiple personality disorder, self-destructive behavioral episodes that repeat early trauma, and avoidance of food.

Borderline personality disorder. Another condition which is related to eating disorders is borderline personality disorder. Borderline personality disorder is widely mentioned as a comorbid clinical diagnosis for eating disorder patients with a history of sexual abuse (Davis, Claridge, and Cerullo, 1997; Herzog et al., 1993). Steiger et al. (1992) found that women who suffer from both high body dissatisfaction and borderline traits display an elevated profile of eating disturbances. The existence of sexual abuse in childhood and of self-injurious behaviors in borderline personality patients yielded a substantial body of research that established a triad of relationships between eating disorders symptomatology, sexual abuse and borderline personality (Davis et al., 1997; Steiger et al., 1992; Waller, 1994). Waller (1994) examined a series of 115 eating-disordered women, and found a secondary diagnosis of borderline personality disorder to be associated with a reported history of sexual abuse in these women. The association was specifically with early childhood sexual abuse (first experienced before age 14). Davis et al. (1997) and Claridge, Davis, Belhouse and Kaptein (1998) found that borderline personality can significantly predict weight preoccupation in women.

Suicide and self-injurious behaviors. The increased dissociation in women with both eating disorders and a history of sexual abuse, is related to their tendency to perform self-injurious behaviors or to commit suicide. Claes, Vandereycken, and Vertommen (2006) describe a great deal of similarity between self-injurious behaviors and eating disorders: (1) Like eating disorders which are more prevalent in women (Fairburn and Harrison, 2003), self-injurious behaviors are 1.5 to 3 times more frequent in women (e.g., Robinson and Duffy, 1989; Yates, 2004). (2) A disturbed body image which produces behaviors that harm the body is evident both in eating disorders (Fairburn and Harrison, 2003), and in self-injurious behaviors (Tameling and Sachsse, 1996). (3) Many studies describe sexual abuse in childhood as one of the etiological reasons for eating disorders (e.g., Claes and Vandereycken, and Vertommen, 2006; Miller, McCluskey-Fawcett, Irving, 1993; Murray, MacDonald, and Fox, 2008) and for self-injurious behaviors in female patients (Diekstra, 1993). High rates of self-injurious behaviors have been reported in women with eating disorders, mostly in bulimics (e.g., Claes, Vandereycken, and Vertommen, 2006; Welch and Fairburn, 1996). In addition, the risk of suicide is particularly pronounced among patients with Anorexia nervosa (Berkman, Lohr, and Bulik, 2005).

Pain tolerance. The aforementioned similarities between suicidal and self-injurious behaviors and eating disorders, and the prevalence of dissociation among eating disorders patients (Hutchinson, Gow and Jamieson, 2007) can be explained by the ability of patients with eating disorders to tolerate pain (Claes, Vandereycken, and Vertommen, 2006). High pain tolerance is suggested as a physiological trait that enables dissociation from bodily sensations which are followed by acts of self harm. High pain tolerance was observed both in suicidal individuals (Orbach, 1994; Orbach et al., 1997), and in patients with self-injurious behaviors (Tameling and Sachsse, 1996). Tolerance for pain was also found in eating disorder patients (Pirke, Pahl, Schweiger, and Warnhoff, 1985; Stein et al., 2003), and in particular, among patients suffering from eating disorders and self-injurious behaviors (Claes, Vandereycken, and Vertommen, 2001, 2006).

Orbach (1994) and Orbach and colleagues (1997) argued that the ability of suicidal individuals to dissociate themselves from their body increases their tolerance for pain and thereby makes the suicidal act possible for them. They exposed 38 suicidal inpatients and 29 controls, aged 14-19, to series of thermal pain stimuli and measured its effect by means of a Thermal Sensory Analyzer (TSA). They compared dissociative tendencies, pain thresholds and tolerance for pain among these suicidal inpatients with the same measures in 29 nonsuicidal inpatients, and 34 control participants. The suicidal participants demonstrated significantly higher thresholds and higher tolerance for pain and reported higher dissociative ability, as compared with the other two groups even after controlling for gender, motivation, medication, diagnosis, and length of hospitalization. Moreover, dissociation contributed significantly and positively to the prediction of sensation threshold. Orbach et al. explained these results as reflecting a bodily dissociation (Walsh and Rosen, 1988), rather than dissociation in general.

A lessened perception of pain during self-mutilation was also reported among inpatients with a disturbed body image exhibiting self-injurious behavior (Tameling and Sachsse, 1996). The more disturbed was the body image of the patients, the higher the frequency of self-injurious behavior (e.g., cutting the skin of the extremities, which was followed by burning the skin with cigarettes or open flames). The researchers found that the perception of pain was lessened appreciably or inactivated during the act of self-harm.

A disturbance in body image and in the experience of pain is evident in patients with eating disorders who suffer from experiences of dissociation (Vanderlinden, Spinhoven, Vandereycken, and van Dyck, 1995). Claes et al. (2006) reviewed some of the physiological mechanisms suggested to explain the high tolerance for pain in eating disorder patients: (1) It was hypothesized that the reduced pain sensitivity is mediated by the opioid system. This hypothesis was refuted by Lautenbacher et al. (1990) who found that a normalization of the increased pain thresholds could not be achieved by administering the opiate antagonist Naloxone. (2) It was suggested that the reduced pain sensitivity is caused by a subclinical malnutrition neuropathy. This hypothesis was rejected since other sensory modalities (e.g., warm, cold, and vibration sensitivity) were either not affected or showed only minor impairments (Pauls, Lautenbacher, Strian, Pirke, and Krieg, 1991). (3) It was assumed that the fasting state causes the reduced pain sensitivity and is responsible for the pain tolerance in these patients (Pirke, Pahl, Schweiger, and Warnhoff, 1985). This explanation was turned down by Lautenbacher, Barth et al. (1991) who demonstrated that pain sensitivity was not reduced in fasting healthy volunteers. (4) It was hypothesized that excessive changes in food intake (i.e., frequently shifts between reduced and excessive eating) are responsible for the increased pain threshold. This hypothesis received some support (Krieg, Roscher, Strian, Pirke, and Lautenbacher, 1993). (5) An elevated afferent vagal activation may stimulate descending pain inhibitory pathways in eating disorder patients with bingeing and purging behaviors, and might lead to an elevation in somatosensory pain thresholds in these patients (Raymond et al., 1999). It was suggested that the diminished pain sensitivity which is related to binge eating may play a role in maintaining this symptom by minimizing the physical discomfort and increasing the self-reported relief and euphoria connected with the binge/purge cycle (Faris et al., 1998 and Girdler et al., 1998). Stein et al. (2003) claimed that the tolerance for pain may be a stable trait of these patients because it persists after they recover from their binge eating. This conclusion was criticized by others who argued that it is the altered central serotonergic activity which persists after recovery from binge eating (Kaye et al., 1998) and it is that feature that is linked to the persistent decreased pain sensitivity.

The physiological mechanisms that explain why patients with eating disorders have high tolerance for pain are not clear yet. Moreover, even the role of dissociation in elevating the tolerance for pain in eating disorder patients had not been empirically proven. In a recent study (Papezová, Yamamotova, and Uher, 2005), heightened tolerance of pain in patients who suffer from eating disorders was found to exist without the contribution of what the authors referred to as "somatoform dissociation". The researchers compared thermal pain threshold latency and somatoform dissociation of 39 female patients with eating disorders (anorexia nervosa and bulimia nervosa) and of 17 healthy women. They found elevated pain threshold in patients with eating disorders, which did not depend on the level of somatoform dissociation in these patients.

In sum, although the causative link between dissociation and high tolerance for pain in eating disorder patients is not clear yet, we reviewed in this section studies that present a solid evidence that an early traumatic experience with one's body at an early age, a disturbed body image, a tendency for self-injurious behaviors, a tendency for dissociation, and high pain tolerance, are all prevalent among eating disorders patients. Specifically, we presented evidence that: (1) Women with eating disorders have a distorted body image (Pawluck and Gorey, 1998); (2) Women with eating disorders report of more dissociation than healthy controls to a degree almost comparable with patients who suffer from dissociative disorders (Vanderlinden et al., 1993). (3) A high trauma rate (especially physical abuse in childhood) was found in women with eating disorders and mainly in women with bulimia nervosa (Favaro and Santonastaso, 1995; Grave et al., 1996). (4) Many patients with borderline personality disorder, a personality disorder that is also characterized by disturbances in body image (Steiger et al., 1992), also suffer from eating disorders (Davis et al., 1997; Herzog et al., 1992); (5) Suicidal and self-injurious behaviors are common in eating disorder patients (Claes, Vandereycken, and Vertommen, 2006); (6) High tolerance for pain was evident in the abovementioned psychopathologies (Claes et al., 2006; Orbach, 1994; Orbach et al., 1997; Tameling and Sachsse, 1996). Although the relations between these factors await explanation, there is enough evidence for the role dissociation plays in the abusive stance that patients and mainly women with eating disorder take towards their body.

3. Dissociation in Women and Biological and Sociological Explanations

In this section we describe some of the social and psychological forces that may enhance women's tendency to dissociate from their body. First, we will discuss some of the non-pathological aspects of dissociation in women in general, and then we will concentrate on the relevance of these non-pathological aspects of dissociation for women with eating disorders.

Not only eating disorders but other mental problems (e.g., pelvic pain, somatization, nonepileptic seizures, self-injurious behaviors, and borderline personality disorder) link dissociation with women (Hall, 2003). However, the ability to dissociate from body sensations is not only pathological. According to Lifton (1993), dissociation is also an opportunity for personal change and a sign of resilience, as long as the person can basically rearrange in a functional and non-distressful manner. Even when forced to unbearable conditions, dissociation may be functional. Ross, Anderson, Heber, and Norton (1990) found that women who had to engage in prostitution and in exotic dancing in order to survive had increased levels of dissociation that might have protected them from pain and humiliation.

Biological explanations. Following this perceptive (Lifton, 1993; Ross et al., 1990) that regards dissociation in women as a functional coping mechanism, we suggest that dissociation may serve as an explanation for the way women adjust to various physiological changes along their youth, starting from menstruation and advancing to pregnancies and births.

Menses. During the adolescent period, young girls have to adjust to the appearance of secondary sexual signs and menses. It was found that adolescents between 11 and 15 years of age, who had been menstruating for a while, coped with these changes in their body by denying the effects of menstruation (McGrory, 1990). A study on 327 women in college found that those who had early positive menstrual experiences reported a more positive body image (McPherson and Korfine, 2004). McFarland, Ross, and DeCourville (2004) examined the relation between women's theories of menstrual distress and their recollections of physical and affective symptoms. They examined 95 women, aged 17-21 and found that the less a woman believed in the phenomenon of menstrual distress (e.g., physical pain, mood disturbance), the less she exaggerated, in recall, the negativity of her symptoms during her last period.

Based on these findings, we suggest that from the beginning of the menarche, women adjust an appeased perception of this circulatory physiological event. By concentrating on some positive aspects of the menarche, they teach themselves to ignore its unpleasant bodily aspects (e.g., pain, smell, unexpected wetness), a mechanism which restarts in each month along the women's fertility period.

Pregnancy. Pregnancy is another periodical event unique to women's physiology. A major concern that women experience during the childbearing period is about the way their pregnancy will affect their body image (Affonso, Liu-Chiang, and Mayberry, 1999). It was found that women who exercise at the beginning of their gestation (15-22 weeks) are more satisfied with their body, as compared to pregnant women who do not exercise during the same period. Exercising women seem to be more able to assimilate the bodily changes of pregnancy without a negative shift in their body image satisfaction and even to respond more favorably to changes in their bodies at early pregnancy (Boscaglia, Skouteris, and Wertheim, 2003). According to Feldmann (1977), during the second period of pregnancy, the enlarged abdomen is not perceived as a part of the woman's body, but as a child. Feldmann argues that this change in body image can be conceptualized as a mental process, which prepares the mother for the birth and for the subsequent mother-child relationship.

In line with these studies, we suggest that in both cases women partially ignore changes in their body. Women who exercise during the beginning of their pregnancy can divert their attention from unpleasant interoceptive sensations and concentrate on positive bodily aspects, such as physical fitness. At the end of their pregnancy, women depersonalize themselves from the changes that occur in their body by perceiving the abdomen part of their body (i.e., their belly) as separable.

Labor pain. Another interesting aspect of dissociation and pregnancy refers to labor pain. One of the useful techniques for pain management during child delivery is self-hypnosis which uses the ability of the patient to dissociate from her body during the process of childbirth (Oster, 1994). Smith, Collins, Cyna, and Crowther (2006) examined the effects of complementary and alternative therapies for pain management in labor on maternal and perinatal morbidity. They found that women who dissociated themselves from uneasiness through self-hypnosis had decreased requirements for pharmacological analgesia and were more satisfied with their pain management in labor compared with controls.

Menses, gestation and birth are all physiological events unique to women. We suggest that the continuous experiencing of these events may develop an ability to dissociate from disturbing, unpleasant and painful sensations. We also argue that such a dissociative ability is not necessarily a pathological mechanism, but may enable a smoother adjustment to disturbing physiological occurrences.

In the case of eating disorders, however, women use this ability to ignore painful sensations that are not caused by the patients' natural physiology, but are self initiated (e.g., self inflicted hunger or vomiting, pain which is produced by excessive physical exercise, self-injurious behaviors). Therefore, we suggest a broader perspective on dissociation in women that suffer from eating disorder. We suggest that dissociation from bodily sensations is a natural tendency in women, not a pathological one. Nevertheless, in eating disorder patients it is exaggerated and develops into a pathological pattern.

Social explanations. Several social reasons may explain the disruption in the perception of bodily sensations in women with eating disorders. First, there are the social influences, which stress the idea of the slim woman body. By concentrating on this idea, which is considered "natural" in Western societies (Bordo, 1993; Malson, 1998), women manage to dissociate from painful sensations and "succeed" in denying some of their basic physiological needs.

Conformism. In order to become convinced in the idea of the slim woman body, women have to conform to this social standard. There are studies that show that women in general are more conformist to social values and norms as compared to men (Prince-Gibson and Schwartz, 1998;. Xiao, 2000). Mason and Charney (1996) even described specific family environments that encourage consensus and achievement which according to their view may lead adolescents to adopt a more conforming personality style and thereby increase their chance to develop bulimia.

Emotional vulnerability to body image. Women are more sensitive than men to unpleasant word stimuli concerning body image (Shirao et al., 2005). In Shirao et al.'s study (2005) the researchers used functional magnetic resonance imaging to examine 13 men and 13 women during an emotional decision task. The task consisted of presenting unpleasant words concerning body image and neutral words. Whereas in women only the left amygdala was activated during the task, in men only the left medial prefrontal cortex and hippocampus were activated. The authors concluded that women processed this task more emotionally rather than cognitively, and used more intuitive processing whereas men used more rational processing. These differences may support the contention that women process information regarding their body image more sensitively than men and this is concurrent with our postulation.

In sum, we suggest biological explanations for the development of non-pathological uses of dissociation in women in general. We argue that proneness of women to use dissociation is supported by their ability to adjust to various physiological changes along their youth: (1) The power to concentrate on positive aspects of menstruation (McPherson and Korfine, 2004; McFarland et al., 2004) and gestation (Boscaglia et al., 2003); (2) The ability to create a sort of depersonalization from their changing body during the last months of their pregnancy (Feldmann, 1977); (3) The skill of using dissociation during birth, to overcome labor pains (Smith et al., 2006). Regarding the social elements that increase the use of dissociation particularly in women with eating disorders we summarize: (1) The social ideal slim body image of women that had turned into a realistic and convincing image for women (Bordo, 1993; Malson, 1998); 2) The heightened conformity of women in general (Prince-Gibson and Schwartz, 1998;. Xiao, 2000), and of women from family environments that encourage consensus and achievement in particular (Mason and Charney, 1996), enables them to comply with food restrictions even when these restrictions create unpleasant sensations; (3) The vulnerability of women to unpleasant stimuli regarding their body (i.e., their tendency to process these stimuli in an emotional way) deepens their involvement in dieting (Shirao et al., 2005).

4. Dissociation and Preventive and Therapeutic Efforts

Some of the preventive and therapeutic efforts to treat women with eating disorders concentrate on their tendency to use dissociation. Preventive efforts challenge the ideal of the slim women, and therapeutic methods use hypnosis as a mean to disrupt their pathological dissociation.

Primary and secondary prevention. Challenging the importance that women patients ascribe to becoming thin may disrupt their tendency to dissociate from unpleasant sensations in order to become thin. Piran (2005) reviewed studies on the prevention of eating disorders in pre-adolescents, high school students and young college students, and her review supports this contention. She reported on 21 studies that were published on primary prevention (i.e., the provision of knowledge in order to change attitudes and behaviors) – all methodologically well-designed studies. The prevention programs that focused on decreasing the disproportionate value of thinness were more effective in changing pathological behavioral patterns (e.g., reduced dieting or meal skipping). Although many studies reported significant changes in knowledge, most of these changes were not followed by changes in attitudes or in behavior. She also reviewed 13 studies that were done on secondary prevention of eating disorders. These studies resulted in more favorable results (i.e., attitudinal change was found in 93% of the interventions, behavioral change in 56% and maintenance of gains in 40%). Again, programs that included educational and cognitive strategies, aimed at devaluing the "normative" image of the "thin woman" were the most effective in changing the problematic behaviors. Therefore, we suggest that lessening of the persuasive potential of the idea of the "thin woman" is effective in primary and secondary prevention of eating disorders.

The use of hypnosis in tertiary prevention. Hypnosis is sometimes used as a tertiary prevention strategy in order to treat dissociation in eating disorder patients. Connection between dissociation and eating disorders was first made by Janet, who suggested to use hypnosis in order to influence the dissociated "id'e fixe" (Vanderlinden and Vandereycken, 1988). Nevertheless, according to Barabasz (2007) although there is an accumulating evidence for the efficacy of hypnotherapy in the treatment of eating disorders, the research in this field still suffers from many methodological limitations (e.g., a lack of standardized inductions, lack of control groups, procedures which cannot be replicable).

Hypnotherapy of eating disorders patients is usually combined with Cognitive behavioral methods (CBT). These methods tackle the dissociative tendencies that characterize these patients. Torem (1986, 1987) suggested that therapy with eating disorders patients should be aimed at reintegrating their dissociated ego states by hypnosis. Griffiths (1995a) in her 8-weeks therapy program offers to use positive hypnotic suggestions with a special focus on reinforcing changes in eating habits and establishing normal eating habits. She (1995b) presented positive results of a 2-year follow-up of this method. The combination of behavioral and hypnotic therapy was effective in reducing symptoms on the drive for thinness, bulimia, body dissatisfaction, ineffectiveness and interoceptive awareness, over both the short and long terms. Adding a self-hypnosis component following a behavioral treatment seemed to assist in maintaining the patients' progress in a 2-year post-treatment period. Two other studies (Griffiths, Hadzi-Pavlovic, and Channon-Little, 1994, 1996)—compared the efficacy of hypnobehavioral and CBT treatments for bulimia and demonstrated no differences between the two methods. The authors concluded that the two methods are equally effective in treating these patients. Barga and Barabasz (in press) compared the efficacy of 60-minute individual outpatient therapy sessions over 7-12 weeks of hypnotherapy and hypnotherapy with CBT. In the second session they integrated hypnosis and self-hypnosis as a means for developing relaxation, guided imagery and deepening techniques. Posthypnotic suggestions were tailored at reducing bingeing and designed to reinforce rational thoughts about body weight and shape. In this program, the hypnotic suggestions also concentrated on the urges to binge and on strengthening the participant's control and choice over these urges. In addition, participants were instructed to practice these suggestions at least once a day. The group that was treated with hypnotherapy plus CBT improved more on all measures.

Barabasz (2007) also reports on the management of anorexia with hypnotherapy. Hypnosis is introduced to the anorectic patients as a means of enhancing self-control and personal sense of power and to provide a sense of ego support. Hypnosis is also used in these patients to deal with body-image distortions. Nash and Baker (1993) reported that 76% of 36 patients that were treated by hypnosis demonstrated a remission of symptoms at 5 and 12 months after treatment, whereas only 53% of 38 women who received treatment without hypnosis demonstrated such a remission. Hornyak (1996) reported of a 20-month treatment with hypnosis in which hypnosis was used as means to control stress and initiate relaxation. Hornyak also described how to make use of spontaneous dissociative states in therapy. Barabasz (2000) reported another case study in which hypnosis was used in a case of a woman with anorexia. Most of the hypnotic suggestions in this case concentrated on body image distortions. Spiegel and Spiegel (2004) treated overweight people with hypnosis and their treatment involved reframing overeating as a poison that affects the body and eating properly as a respectful and protective way to handle the only body one would have in this life.

Dissociative tendencies during the course of psychotherapy. In order to examine whether clinical improvement in eating disorder patients is associated with decline in dissociative tendencies, Iancu et al. (2006) studied 30 eating disorder patients. The patients were active duty soldiers and 90% of them were women, 18-21 years of age. Fifteen patients suffered from bulimia nervosa, 10 from anorexia and five from eating disorder not otherwise specified. The patients met weekly for an hour and a half group therapy sessions. The therapeutic intervention took six months and included a cognitive behavioral techniques combined with a dynamic approach. This therapeutic group process was perceived by the three co-therapists of this group as a powerful mean of influencing body distortion. Several questionnaires were administered before and after the intervention and one of them was the DES (Bernstein and Putnam, 1986). No significant differences were found in the mean score of DES for the 30 patients before and after the intervention, despite a significant improvement of the eating attitudes. The authors concluded that the lack of such differences may display the complexity of the relations between eating disorders and dissociation, or that alternatively it may denote that the improvement of eating symptoms is the first and obvious sign of change, and a deeper change and emotional insight may require longer periods of treatment.

In sum, primary and secondary prevention programs focus mainly on the importance women ascribe to the idea of the "thin women". The reduction of the potential persuasion of this idea seems to be effective in changing pathological eating habits of women, habits that result from dissociation. It could be that the combination of hypnotherapy with CBT, provides better results than CBT alone because hypnosis might tackle the increased dissociative tendencies in women. Indeed, hypnotic suggestions that concentrate on the urges to binge and on strengthening the participant's control and choice over these urges are commonly used and are reported as effective.

5. Conclusions

Dissociation is common in psychiatric disturbances with a history of an abusive event at an early age (Hall, 2003). Physical or sexual abuse at an early age affects the attitude of the individual towards his/her body (Hall, 2003) and may lead to the development of psychiatric disturbances such as borderline personality disorder, post traumatic stress disorder (Jureidini, 2004), dissociative identity disorder (Gleaves, 1996) and eating disorders (Murray et al., 2008).

A history of psychological abuse at an early age in women with eating disorders had been widely reported (Allison et al., 2007). There is also solid evidence that dissociation is commonly used by patients with eating disorders (Hutchinson et al., 2007) as a mean to avoid recalling traumatic memories, and to detach from the mental and physical pain these memories evoke (Iancu et al., 2006). Dissociation in women with eating disorders can create a vicious cycle and result in problematic consequences (Iancu et al., 2006). Nevertheless, it is not yet understood how dissociation affects pain threshold in women with eating disorders (Claes et al., 2006), although it may enable the patient to starve, exercise and vomit.

Nevertheless, dissociation should not only be regarded as a pathological mechanism. It can also be considered as enabling resilience (Lifton, 1993) and even as a coping mechanism that allows better functioning, especially under stressful conditions (Ross et al, 1990). We suggest that this perspective on dissociation enables a broadened examination of this mechanism in women with eating disorders that links between dissociation and between biological and social gender differences. According to our perspective, the continuous requirement from women to adjust to continuous body changes (menstruation, gestation, birth) teaches women to dissociate from their bodies. In addition, women in general (Prince-Gibson and Schwartz, 1998; Xiao, 2000) and bulimic women in particular (Mason and Charney, 1996) are considered more conformist to social values and norms than men, and more sensitive to the social value of a thin body even on a physiological level (Mason and

Charney (1996). Certainly, in these women dissociation reaches abnormal levels and requires careful inspection.

Eating disorders are regarded as a modern western psychopathology, and as a psychiatric disturbance that can end in death. The combination of physiological differences between genders, the social pressure on women to be slim, and a personal traumatic history may all contribute to the development of dissociation from bodily sensations in these patients. Dissociation from bodily sensations and troubling memories in these patients creates and maintains pathological behaviors such as self starvation, initiated vomiting, intensive exercising, and self-injurious acts. Preventive and therapeutic efforts are effective but a continuous focus on a disruption of the pathological use of dissociation in women seems to be a promising avenue for these efforts.

REFERENCES

Affonso, D.D., Liu-Chiang, C.Y., and Mayberry, L.J. (1999). Worry: conceptual dimensions and relevance to childbearing women. *Health Care for Women International*, 20, 227-36.

Allison, K.C., Grilo, C.M., Masheb, R.M., and Stunkard, A.J. (2007). High self-reported rates of neglect and emotional abuse, by persons with binge eating disorder and night eating syndrome. *Behaviour Research and Therapy*, 45, 2874-2883.

American Psychiatric Association. Diagnostic and statistical manual of mental disorders, 4th edition (DSM-IV). Washington: American Psychiatric Association, 1994.

Axelsen, E., and Sveaass, N. (1994). Psychotherapeutic understanding of women exposed to sexual violence in political detention. Nordisk Sexlogi, 12, 1-12.

Barabasz, M. (2000). Hypnosis in the treatment of eating disorders. In L. Hornyak and J. Green (Eds.). Healing from within: Hypnosis, imagery methods and women's health care. Washington,D.C.:American Psychological Association.

Barabasz, M. (2007). Efficacy of hypnotherapy in the treatment of eating disorders. *International Journal of Clinical and Experimental Hypnosis,* 55, 318-35.

Barga, J. and Barabasz, M. (in press). Effects of hypnosis as an adjunct to Cognitive-Behavioral therapy in the treatment of Bulimia. *International Journal of Clinical and Experimental Hypnosis*.

Barry, D.T., Grilo, C.M., and Masheb, R.M. (2002). Gender differences in patients with binge eating disorder. *International Journal of Eating Disorders*, 31, 63-70.

Becker, A.E., Grinspoon S.K., Klibanski, A., and Herzog, D.B. (1999). Eating disorders. *New England Journal of Medicine,* 340, 1092-1098.

Berkman, N.D Lohr, K.N. and Bulik, C.M. (2005). Outcomes of eating disorders: a systematic review of the literature. *International Journal of Eating Disorders*, 40, 293-309.

Bernstein, E.M., and Putnam, F.W. (1986). Development, reliability and validity of a dissociation scale. *Journal of Nervous and Mental Disease*, 174, 727-735.

Bordo, S. (1993). Unbearable weight: Feminism, western culture, and the body. Berkeley, CA: University of California Press.

Boscaglia, N., Skouteris, H., and Wertheim, E.H. (2003). Changes in body image satisfaction during pregnancy: a comparison of high exercising and low exercising women. *The Australian and New Zealand Journal of Obstetrics and Gynecology*, 43, 41-45.

Braun, B. G. (1988). The BASK model of dissociation. Dissociation, 1, 4-23.

Brewerton, T.D. (2007). Eating disorders, trauma, and comorbidity: focus on PTSD. *Eating Disorders*, 15, 285-304.

Chu, J. A., and Dill, D. L. (1990). Dissociative symptoms in relation to childhood physical and sexual abuse. *American Journal of Psychiatry*, 147, 887-892.

Claes L, Vandereycken W, Vertommen H. (2001). Self-injurious behaviors in eating-disordered patients. *Eating Behavior*, 2, 263-72.

Claes, L., Vandereycken, W., and Vertommen, H. (2006). Pain experience related to self-injury in eating disorder patients. *Eating Behaviors*, 7, 204-213.

Claridge, G., Davisb, C., Bellhouse, M., and Kapteinb, S. (1998). Borderline personality, nightmares, and adverse life events in the risk for eating disorders. *Personality and Individual Differences*, 25, 339-351.

Davis, C., Claridge, G., and Cerullo, D. (1997). Personality factors predisposing to weight preoccupation: a continuum approach to the association between eating disorders and personality disorders. *Journal of Psychiatric Research*, 31, 467-480.

Demitrack, M. A., Putnam, F. W., Brewerton, T. D., Brandt, H. A., and . Gold, P. W. (1990). Relation of clinical variables to dissociative phenomena in eating disorders. *American Journal of Psychiatry*, 147, 1184–1188.

Diekstra, R.F. (1993). The epidemiology of suicide and parasuicide. Acta Psychiatrica Scandinavica, 371, 9-20.

Eddy KT, Keel PK, Dorer DJ, et al. Longitudinal comparison of anorexia nervosa subtypes. *International Journal of Eating Disorders,* 31, 191–201.

Everill, J., Waller, G., and Macdonald, W. (1995). Dissociation in bulimic and non-eating-disordered women. *International Journal of Eating Disorders*, 17, 127-34.

Fairburn, C. G. and Harrison, P. J. (2003) Eating disorders. Lancet, 361, 407-416.

Faris, P. L., Kim, S. W., Meller, W. H., Goodale, R. L., Hofbauer, R. D., Oakman, S. A., et al. (1998). Effect of ondansetron, a 5-HT3 receptor antagonist, on the dynamic association between bulimic behaviors and pain thresholds. *Pain*, 77, 297– 303.

Favaro, A., and Santonastaso, P. (1995). Dissociative experiences, trauma and eating disorders in a female college sample. *European Eating Disorders Review*, 3, 136–200.

Feldmann, H. (1977). Body image in pregnancy. *Zeitschrift für Psychosomatische Medizin und Psychoanalyse*, 23, 310-28.

Girdler, S. S., Koo-Loeb, J., Pedersen, C. A., Brown, H. J., and Maixner, W. (1998). Blood pressure-related hypoalgesia in bulimia nervosa. Psychosomatic Medicine, 60, 736–743.

Gleaves, D.H. (1996). The sociocognitive model of dissociative identity disorder: a reexamination of the evidence. *Psychological Bulletin*, 120, 42-59.

Grave, R. D., Oliosi, M., Todisco, P., and Vanderlinden, J. (1997). Self-reported traumatic experiences and dissociative symptoms in obese women with and without being-eating disorder. Eating Disorders: *Journal of Treatment and Prevention,* 5, 105–109.

Grave, R. D., Rigamonti, R., Todisco, P., and Oliosi, E. (1998). Dissociation and traumatic experiences in eating disorders. *European Eating Disorders Review*, 4, 232–240.

Griffiths, R. A., Hadzi-Pavlovic, D. and Channon-Little, L. (1994). A controlled evaluation of hypnobehavioral treatment for bulimia nervosa: Immediate pre-post treatment effects. *European Eating Disorders Review*, 2, 202-220.

Griffiths, R. (1995a) Hypnobehavioral treatment for bulimia nervosa: A treatment manual. *Australian Journal of Clinical and Experimental Hypnosis* 21, 25-40.

Griffiths, R. A. (1995b) Two-year follow-up findings of hypnobehavioural treatment for bulimia nervosa. *Australian Journal of Clinical and Experimental Hypnosis*, 23, 135-144.

Griffiths, R. A., Hadzi-Pavlovic, D. and Channon-Little, L. (1996) The short-term follow-up effects of hypnobehavioural and cognitive behavioural treatment for bulimia nervosa. *European Eating Disorders Review*, 4, 12-31.

Hall, J.M. (2003). Dissociative Experiences of Women Child Abuse Survivors: A Selective Constructivist Review. Trauma Violence Abuse, 4, 283-308.

Herzog, D.B., Hopkins, J.D., and Burns, C.D. (1993). A follow-up study of 33 subdiagnostic eating disordered women. *International Journal of Eating Disorders*, 14, 261–67.

Hornyak, L.M. (Lynn, S. J., Kirsch, I. and Rhue, J. W. eds.) (1996) Hypnosis in the treatment of anorexia nervosa. Casebook of Clinical Hypnosis pp. 51-73. American Psychological Association , Washington, DC.

Hutchinson, Gow, and Jamieson (2007). Hypnotizability, Eating Behaviors, Attitudes, and Concerns: A Literature Survey. *Journal of Clinical and Experimental Hypnosis*, 55, 84–113.

Iancu, I., Cohen, E., Yehuda, Y.B., and Kotler, M. (2006). Treatment of eating disorders improves eating symptoms but not alexithymia and dissociation proneness. *Comprehensive Psychiatry*, 47, 189–193.

Jureidini, J. (2004). Does dissociation offer a useful explanation for psychopathology? *Psychopathology*, 37, 259-265.

Kaye, W. H., Greeno, C. G., Moss, H., Fernstrom, J., Fernstrom, M., Lilenfeld, L. R., et al. (1998). Alterations in serotonin activity and psychiatric symptoms after recovery from bulimia nervosa. *Archives of General Psychiatry*, 55, 927– 935.

Kluft RP: Dissociative identity disorder; in Michelson LK, Ray WJ (eds): Handbook of Dissociation. New York, Plenum Press, 1996, pp. 337-366.

Krieg, J.C., Roscher, S., Strian, F., Pirke, K.M., and Lautenbacher, S. (1993). Pain sensitivity in recovered anorexics, restrained and unrestrained eaters. *Journal of Psychosomatic Research*, 37, 595-601.

Lautenbacher, S., Barth, K., Friess, E., Strian, F., Pirke, K.M., and Krieg, J.C. (1991). Dieting and pain sensitivity: a validation of clinical findings. *Physiological Behavior*, 50, 629-31.

Lautenbacher, S., Pauls, A.M., Strian, F., Pirke, K.M., and Krieg, J.C. (1990). Pain perception in patients with eating disorders. *Psychosomatic Medicine,* 52, 673-82.

Lifton, R. J. (1993). The protean self: Human resilience in an age of fragmentation. New York: Basic Books.

Lucas, A.R., Beard, C.M., O'Fallon, W.M., and Kurland, L.T. (1991). 50-year trends in the incidence of anorexia nervosa in Rochester, Minn.: A population-based study. *American Journal of Psychiatry,* 148, 917-922.

Lucas, A.R., Crowson, C.S., O'Fallon, W.M., and Melton LJ. (1999). The ups and downs of anorexia nervosa. *International Journal of Eating Disorders*, 26, 397-405.

Lynn, S. J. and Kirsch, I. (2006) Essentials of clinical hypnosis: An evidence-based approach. American Psychological Association , Washington, DC.

Malson, H. (1998). The Thin Woman. London: Routledge.

Mason, N. S. and Chaney, J. M. (1996). Bulimia nervosa in undergraduate women: Factors associated with internalization of the sociocultural standard of thinness. *Applied and Preventive Psychology*, 5, 249-259.

McFarland, C., Ross, M., and DeCourville, N. (2004). Women's theories of menstruation and biases in recall of menstrual symptoms. *Journal of Personality and Social Psychology*, 57, 522-31.

McGrory, A. (1990). Menarche: responses of early adolescent females. Adolescence, 25, 265-70.

McPherson, M.E, and Korfine, L. (2004). Menstruation across time: menarche, menstrual attitudes, experiences, and behaviors. Womens Health Issues, 14, 193-200.

Miller, D.A., McCluskey-Fawcett, K., and Irving, L.M. (1993). The relationship between childhood sexual abuse and subsequent onset of bulimia nervosa. *Child Abuse and Neglect,* 17, 305-14.

Mitchell, J.E., Hatsukami, D., Pyle, R.L., Eckert, E.D., and Boutacoff, L.I. (1987).

Metabolic acidosis as a marker for laxative abuse in patients with bulimia. *International Journal of Eating Disorders,* 6, 557–560.

Murray, C.D., Macdonald, S., and Fox J. (2008). Body satisfaction, eating disorders and suicide ideation in an Internet sample of self-harmers reporting and not reporting childhood sexual abuse. *Psychology, Health and Medicine*, 13, 29-42.

Nagata, T., Kiriike, N., Iketani, T., Kawarada, Y., and Tanaka, H. (1999). History of childhood sexual or physical abuse in Japanese patients with eating disorders: relationship with dissociation and impulsive behaviors. *Psychological Medicine* 29, 935-942.

Nash, M.R. and Baker, E.L. (Rhue, J. W., Lynn, S. J. and Kirsch, I. eds.) (1993). Hypnosis in the treatment of anorexia nervosa. Handbook of clinical hypnosis pp. 383-394. American Psychological Association , Washington, DC

Nielsen S. (2001). Epidemiology and mortality of eating disorders. The Psychiatric Clinics of North America, 24, 201–14.

Nock, M.K., Prinstein, M.J. (2004). A functional approach to the assessment of self-mutilative behavior. *Journal of Consulting and Clinical Psychology,* 72, 885-890.of fragmentation. New York: Basic Books.

Orbach, I. (1994). Dissociation, physical pain, and suicide: A hypothesis. Suicide and Life-Threatening Behavior, 24, 68-79.

Orbach, I., Mikulincer, M., King, R., Cohen, D., and Stein, D. (1997). Thresholds and tolerance of physical pain in suicidal and nonsuicidal adolescents, *Journal of Consulting and Clinical Psychology*, 65, 646-652.

Oster, M.I. (1994). Psychological preparation for labor and delivery using hypnosis. *American Journal of Clinical Hypnosis,* 37, 12-21.

Palmer, R. (2004). Bulimia nervosa: *25 years on. British Journal of Psychiatry*, 185, 447-448.

Papezová, H., Yamamotová, A., and Uher, R. (2005). Elevated pain threshold in eating disorders: physiological and psychological factors. *Journal of Psychiatric Research*, 39, 431-8.

Paul, T., Schroeter, K., Dahme, B., and Nutzinger, D.O. (2002). Self-injurious behavior in women with eating disorders. *American Journal of Psychiatry*, 159, 408-411.

Pauls, A.M., Lautenbacher, S., Strian, F., Pirke, K.M., and Krieg, J.C. (1991). Assessment of somatosensory indicators of polyneuropathy in patients with eating disorders. *European Archives of Psychiatry and Clinical Neuroscience* 241, 8-12.

Pawluck, D.E., and Gorey, K.M.(1998). Secular trends in the incidence of anorexia nervosa: integrative review of population-based studies. *International Journal of Eating Disorders*, 23, 347–352.

Piran, N. (2005). Prevention of Eating Disorders: A Review of Outcome Evaluation Research. *Israeli Journal of Psychiatry and Related Sciences*, 42, 172–177.

Pirke, K.M., Pahl. J., Schweiger, U., Warnhoff, M. (1985). Metabolic and endocrine indices of starvation in bulimia: a comparison with anorexia nervosa. *Psychiatry Research*, 15, 33-39.

Prince-Gibson, Eetta, and Shalom H. Schwartz. 1998. Value priorities and gender. Social Psychology Quarterly, 61,49-67.

Putnam F.W. (1993). Dissociative phenomena; in Spiegel D (ed): Dissociative Disorders. A Clinical Review. Lutherville, Sidran Press, pp 1-16.

Putnam, F. W., Carlson, E. B., Ross, C. A., Anderson, G., Clark, P., Torem, M., et al. (1996). Patterns of dissociation in clinical and nonclinical samples. *Journal of Nervous and Mental Disorders*, 184, 673-679.

Rastam, M., Gillberg, C., and Garton, M. (1989). Anorexia nervosa in a Swedish urban region: a population-based study. *British Journal of Psychiatry*, 155, 642–46.

Raymond, N.C., Eckert, E.D., Hamalainen, M., Evanson, D., Thuras, P.D., Hartman, B.K., and Faris, P.L. (1999). A preliminary report on pain thresholds in bulimia nervosa during a bulimic episode. *Comprehensive Psychiatry*, 40, 229-33.

Ricca V, Mannucci E, Mezzani B, et al. Psychopathological and clinical features of outpatients with an eating disorder not otherwise specified. *Eating and Weight Disorders*, 6, 157–65.

Riley, K. C. (1988). Measurement of dissociation. *Journal of Nervous and Mental Disease*, 176, 449–450.

Robinson, A.D., Duffy, J.C. (1989). A comparison of self-injury and self-poisoning from the Regional Poisoning Treatment Centre, Edinburgh. *Acta Psychiatrica Scandinavica*, 80, 272-279.

Rodin, J., Silberstein, L., and Striegel-Moore, R. (1984). Women and weight: A normative discontent. In: *Sonderegger T*, editor. Psychology and Gender. Lincoln, NE: University of Nebraska, pp. 267-307.

Rosen, J.C., Leitenberg, H., Fisher, C., and Khazam, C. (1986). Binge-eating episodes in bulimia nervosa: the amount and type of food consumed. *International Journal of Eating Disorders,* 5, 255–267.

Ross, C. A., Anderson, G., Heber, S.,andNorton, G. R. (1990). Dissociation and abuse among multiple personality patients, prostitutes, and exotic dancers. *Hospital and Community Psychiatry*, 41, 328-330.

Schumaker, J. F., Warren, W. G., Schreiber, G. S., and Jackson, C. C. (1994). Dissociation in anorexia nervosa and bulimia nervosa. *Social Behavior and Personality*, 22, 385–393.

Shirao, N., Okamoto, Y., Mantani, T., Okamoto, Y., and Yamawaki, S. (2005). Gender differences in brain activity generated by unpleasant word stimuli concerning body image: an fMRI study. *British Journal of Psychiatry*, 186, 48-53.

Smith, C.A., Collins, C.T., Cyna, A.M., and Crowther, C.A. (2006). Complementary and alternative therapies for pain management in labour. Cochrane Database Syst Rev. 18, CD003521. Review.

Steiger, H., Leung, F.Y., and Houle, L. (1992). Relationships among borderline features, body dissatisfaction and bulimic symptoms in nonclinical females. *Addictive Behavior*, 17, 397-406.

Stein, D., Kaye, W.H., Matsunaga, H., Myers, D., Orbach, I., Har-Even, D., Frank, G., and Rao R. (2003). Pain perception in recovered bulimia nervosa patients. *The International Journal of Eating Disorders*, 34, 331-6.

Tameling, A., and Sachsse, U. (1996). Symptom complex, prevalence of trauma and body image of psychiatric patients with self-injury behavior. Psychotherapie, Psychosomatik, *Medizinische Psychologie*, 46, 61-67.

Tobin, D.L., Molteni, A.L., and Elin, M.R. (1995). Early trauma, dissociation, and late onset in the eating disorders. *International Journal of Eating Disorders*, 17, 305-8.

Torem, M. S. (1986). Dissociative states presenting as an eating disorder. *American Journal of Clinical Hypnosis*, 29, 137–142.

Torem, M. S. (1987). Ego-state therapy for eating disorders. *American Journal of Clinical Hypnosis*, 30, 94–103.

Vanderlinden, J., Spinhoven, P., Vandereycken, W., and Van Dyck, R. (1995). Dissociative and hypnotic experiences in eating disorder patients: An exploratory study. *American Journal of Clinical Hypnosis*, 38, 97–108.

Vanderlinden, J., Van Dyck, R., Vandereycken, W. Vertommen, H. and Verkes, R. J. (1993). The Dissociation Questionnaire: Development and characteristics of a new self-report questionnaire. *Clinical Psychology and Psychotherapy*, 1, 21–27.

Vanderlinden, J., Vandereycken, W. (1988). Perception of changes in eating disorder patients during group treatment. *Psychotherapy and Psychosomatic,* 49, 160-163.

Waller, G. (1994). Childhood sexual abuse and borderline personality disorder in the eating disorders. Child Abuse and Neglect, 18, 97-101.

Walsh, B. W., and Rosen, P. M. (1988). Self-mutilation: Theory, research, and treatment. New York: Guilford Press.

Welch, S.L., and Fairburn, C.G. (1996). Impulsivity or comorbidity in bulimia nervosa. A controlled study of deliberate self-harm and alcohol and drug misuse in a community sample. *British Journal of Psychiatry*, 169, 451-458.

Xiao, H. (2000). Class, Gender, and Parental Values in the 1990. Gender and Society, 14, 785-803.

Yates, T.M. (2004). The developmental psychopathology of self-injurious behavior: compensatory regulation in posttraumatic adaptation. *Clinical Psychology Review*, 24, 35-74.

Zlotnick, C., Zakriski, A. L., Shea, M. T., Costello, E., Begin, A., Pearlstein, T., et al. (1996). The long-term sequelae of sexual abuse: Support for a complex post-traumatic stress disorder. *Journal of Traumatic Stress*, 9, 195-205.

In: Eating Disorders in Adult Women
Editor: Julian N. Fuchs

ISBN 978-1-60456-673-4

Chapter 7

THE EXPERIENCE OF MEXICAN EATING DISORDERED PATIENTS: AN APPROACH FROM A GENDER PERSPECTIVE

Claudia Unikel Santoncini*[*], *Martha Patricia Romero Mendoza and Ietza Bojorquez Chapela

Epidemiological and Psychosocial Research at the Ramón de la Fuente Muñiz National Institute of Psychiatry
Secretaría de Salud, Mexico

ABSTRACT

This paper reviewed the gender perspective approach to eating disorders and analyzed certain socio-cultural and psychological aspects related to the development of the latter, such as the relationship of food and emotions, control and identity, the acceptance of the feminine body and, the mother-daughter relationship. The study belongs within the field of the study of clinical psychology and uses a qualitative approach. In-depth interviews were conducted with patients with eating disorders currently receiving specialized treatment at the Ramón de la Fuente Muñiz National Institute of Psychiatry. The testimonies were audiotaped, transcribed and subsequently analyzed using meaning condensation and categorization. Certain themes were selected to be discussed in light of the gender perspective and were illustrated using the interviewees' testimonies. The paper ends with a discussion of the importance of a qualitative approach in the study of these pathologies.

Keywords: *Eating disorders, gender studies, qualitative research, anorexia nervosa, bulimia nervosa, Mexico.*

[*] Correspondence address: Dra. Claudia Unikel, Dirección de Investigaciones Epidemiológicas y Psicosociales, Instituto Nacional de Psiquiatría, Calz. México-Xochimilco 101, Col. San Lorenzo Huipulco, México D.F. 14370, Tel. 56 55 28 11 Ext. 185, Fax: 55 13 34 46, Email: unikels@imp.edu.mx.

> It is the fear of letting go, of loosening the reins that tie you to the prison, a prison constructed to survive life's ups and downs, a prison that has been so sturdily built that it is almost impossible to destroy it, particularly because you feel that once it has been destroyed, there will be nothing left. The need for protection chooses a way out, getting rid of everything. It builds a vacuum because it does not feel that it is worthy of receiving or capable of living. You can devote your life to abandoning yourself and pleasing others, with the false conviction that it is your life. It is the fear of being seen, the terrible fear that others will notice the desire, the need, the fragility and the sensitivity reflected in the inability to inhabit one's own body. And above all, it is the fear of something that is virtually unknown, the possibility of feeling good.
>
> *Claudia Unikel*

Eating disorders are not a fully developed field of knowledge in Mexico. Although the studies carried out to date have contributed valuable data that has shed light on the nature of these diseases in certain sectors of the Mexican population, several issues have yet to be resolved, such as research aimed at detecting risk factors, the development of prevention programs, and early, appropriate referral for treatment of persons that are either at risk or are already suffering from the disease.

Since eating disorders are a novel theme in Mexico, explanations of their root causes have tended to be based on research carried out in other socio-cultural contexts, which are not necessarily relevant to Mexican culture. There is therefore a need for studies to be carried out in Mexico that will reveal the characteristics that are crucial to the development of these disorders in the Mexican socio-cultural context and will permit the design of screening tests, preventive strategies and appropriate treatment.

The multi-causal origin of eating disorders includes areas of human experience that are difficult to understand using quantitative methodologies, for example sexual abuse, substance use and depression, as shown by studies carried out previously in Mexico (Romero, Rodríguez, Durand-Smith, Aguilera, 2003; Unikel, Villatoro, Medina-Mora, Fleiz, Alcántar and Navarro, 2001). It is a fact that people with eating disorders need to be listened to, understood, interpreted, accompanied, empowered and actually taken by the hand to discover the possibility of pleasure. Hsu, Crisp and Callender (1992) found that for patients, being understood was crucial to their recovery.

Some researchers have noted how the expression of the particular experiences of women as women is rarely listened to, particularly when these experiences differ from those of men. Women often silence what they think and feel when they try to describe their lives in terms of prevailing concepts and conceptions. Consequently, in order to listen to women's perspective, one should learn to hear both the dominant and the silenced discourse, in order to understand the relationship that exists between them (Anderson and Jack, 1991).

Approaching eating disorders from a qualitative research perspective responds to the need to listen to the language of patients, since it involves a high-risk psychosomatic pathology, in which the body is compromised in its actual dimensions. It is a scenario in which conflicts arise that cannot be expressed any other way, that do not emerge in the subject's discourse but intervene in their bodies, and in this respect, it involves a pathology of action: a person does what she cannot say, "We are with subjects who speak through their bodies" (Tubert, 2000). It is therefore essential to incorporate techniques such as in-depth interviews, to take advantage of the benefits of "face-to-face" situations into research, as well as the possibility of constructing knowledge together with the interviewee during the course of the research, taking up issues that have scarcely been explored and including those that were not initially contemplated. This technique will also make it easier to establish a more favorable atmosphere for the interview that will reduce bias and create a more comfortable atmosphere for the informant. The interaction between the interviewee and the interviewer creates the possibility of going beyond conventional life stories, to reveal experience in a less culturally biased manner. Just as in psychoanalysis, it is a clinic of listening, in which the person is given the opportunity to talk, since her subjectivity will only be able to emerge in her speech, insofar as she manages to put her symptoms into words (Tubert, 2000). Qualitative research seeks to consider the ways in which people experience their lives and use them to interpret and construct the world that surrounds them, in other words, the way they can lend meaning to their world.

The methodology used in qualitative research is characterized by an approach that attempts to describe and analyze the culture and behavior of human beings and groups from the point of view of those that are being studied. This methodology places particular emphasis on the holistic understanding of the social contexts in which research is conducted. Beyond the search for generalizations, qualitative research attempts to delve into the essence of a particular phenomenon. One of the most important contributions of the interpretative and feminist developments of sociological research (Owen, 1995) has been the insistence on the researcher's position within the research process as a social agent, affected by and affecting all the stages of the research process. The reformulation of the "act of researching" is posited as a dynamic social process rather than as a controlled experimental event.

In qualitative research, interviewees' lives are filtered by researchers and the stories filtered by researchers are present (whether or not we admit this) in their writings. It is better to acknowledge and analyze this than to attribute it to the false notion of objectivity or to collapse and confuse the experiences of our informants with our own (Cotterill and Letherby, quoted in Owen, 1995). This approach opens up new perspectives in the study of eating disorders insofar as it goes beyond the first level at which only the symptoms are dealt with, as a response to the anguish the illness causes the researcher. An attempt is made to understand the essence of the illness in such a way that, together with the interviewee, the researcher, in constant interaction with the interviewer, as an interlocutor who creates the space for discourse to emerge, helps reconstruct the origin of the flaw in the resolution of the teenage crisis, by approaching the personal experience and the way of interpreting, constructing, and lending meaning and significance to the world that surrounds them.

Throughout this process, researchers are unable to avoid being affected. They are also moved from their original position and, as in any therapeutic process, their task is to deal with the anguish and to process the resistance that the interviewee causes them. Thus, the working material is not only derived from the discourse of the other, but also from the researcher's own reflection on the difficulties or ease generated within the exchange, which makes qualitative research an extremely enriching tool for understanding women's discontent.

Etiology of Eating Disorders

Although various models are used to explain eating disorders, each of which clarifies specific aspects of the disease, none of them offers a complete explanation. This is why several researchers tend to regard anorexia and bulimia nervosa as the result of the complex interaction of underlying, precipitating and perpetuating factors. This complaint is the result of a series of influences that vary with each patient but which interact in a way that makes it difficult to distinguish cause and effect (Garfinkel and Garner, 1982).

Vandereycken and van Deth (1994) note that anorexia nervosa has attracted researchers' attention for over a century, giving rise to a series of hypotheses and speculations about its causes and meanings. Several theories attempt to provide an explanation and promote their corresponding line of therapy. From a biological point of view, anorexic patients display an astounding range of hormonal and metabolic disorders. It is as yet unclear, however, whether they are the cause or effect of the disease. The psychodynamic approach posits that anorexics fear sexual maturation and female growth as was stated in Freud's first studies (Freud, 1981). Emaciation hampers development, with the aim of maintaining an asexual, infantilized life both physically and mentally. However, researchers lack information on the origin of this fear and the way these hypotheses can be proved. The same is true of the learning theory (Kleifield, Wagner and Halmi, 1996), which postulates that anorexia constitutes a phobia about getting fat, which is rewarded in two ways. By losing weight, a young woman reduces her fear of getting fat while attracting attention from others, particularly her parents. The psychodynamic point of view is linked to the systems theory (Selvini-Palazolli, 1974), in which anorexia nervosa is regarded as a sign of the presence of distorted structures and interactions within the family. Nevertheless, researchers still do not know whether this distorted familial system is the cause or effect of self-starvation, or why the disorder occurs in a particular way or in a particular family member. Finally, the increase of anorexia nervosa in women in Western countries has led to the development of socio-cultural theories often inspired by feminist ideas based on the premise that anorexia nervosa is a sign of women's subjection to an ideal of thinness in a patriarchal society surrounded by abundance. According to Orbach (1986), dieting and fasting are an expression of this oppression.

Mara Selvini Palazolli took a definitive step towards the cultural explanation of anorexia nervosa. She attributed the increase in anorexia after the Second World War to the emergence of an opulent society oriented towards consumerism, with middle-class families who focused on their children and with women who were experiencing a contradictory situation caused by growing pressure for them to become emancipated (Toro, 1996). During the war, women in large number could experience the benefits of emancipation, working in the public sphere and having access to higher education, but still being restrained in the private sphere. In the body terrain this translates into the accomplishment of contradictory roles: the nurturing and caring mother; the soft, sexy and giving wife; and the sexually independent, competitive, and ambitious career woman. The current body ideal embodies all of these qualities, conveying through the body the contradictions women face in their lives today. These contradictions raise conflicts for girls in the context of our current body ideal; girls often try to generate self-esteem by loosing weight, a strategy that is reinforced by the body-development double bind (Brown and Jasper, 1993).

On the basis of this, it is important to contribute knowledge on the explanation of the origin of eating disorders, focusing in this particular case on the clinical population, i.e. women diagnosed with an eating disorder who have sought psychiatric treatment, through the use of qualitative research methodology.

Gender Perspective

This study regards gender as a constituent element of the reality that operates within the framework of social relations. As a relationship, the gender perspective refers, as other social relations do, to human coexistence and to the actions that this coexistence creates and recreates, based on solidly built asymmetries. These asymmetries are constructed on the basis of a set of guidelines. The understanding of these asymmetries is influenced by the view that they will never be able to be considered mere derivations of the differences between persons of different sexes but rather as elements that create social inequalities, in other words, as culturally instituted norms (Salles, 1997).

Nowadays, social standards for thinness in women are both widespread and largely unachievable for the average person, as a result of which thinness has acquired a higher value in society while obesity has been denigrated, meaning that being obese is a genuine social stigma (Rand and Kuldau, 1986; Rodin, Silberstein, and Striegel-Moore, 1985). Habits and customs form a subtle network of which we all form part, which consists of rejecting anyone who fails to observe the rules of the bodily aesthetic currently in force (Toro, 1996). Female obesity is the subject of public passion and women feel guilty about it, because it is implicitly acknowledged that within the myth, our bodies do not belong to us but rather to society and that thinness is not a private aesthetic, while hunger is a concession granted by the community (Wolf, 1994).

According to feminist theories, an important aspect of women's social learning is the equivalence between physical attractiveness and self-esteem (Franks, 1986, Nagel and Jones, 1992). Several authors note that women usually over-identify with their bodies and that their sense of self-esteem is intimately linked to current standards of thinness and physical attraction (Bergner, Remer and Whetsell, 1985; Striegel-Moore and Marcus, 1995). Likewise, women are socialized to place more emphasis on interpersonal relations than men. In other words, female identity is organized around the value, search, maintenance and nourishment of social relations, in addition to the fact that women are taught to assume responsibility for the success of their interpersonal relations.

The question some authors ask is what eating disorders say about women's position in a world ruled by men. From a feminist perspective, women with eating disorders are desperately trying to fit into a stereotyped female role (imposed by a sexist society) which is reflected both in the search for a thin body and in a passive, despairing attitude towards life. Turner (1984), however, suggests that it is a more complex phenomenon, involving a symbolic struggle against forms of authority and the attempt to resolve the contradictions of the female self. Eating disorders regarded as a form of addiction (Van Der Bergh, 1991) have been explained by the relationship that exists between the conditions of isolation and oppression exercised by patriarchal cultures. Growing up in an atmosphere in which one has to exercise power over others to be successful and where success is measured by external factors rather than by innate qualities may create feelings of inadequacy, lack of power, despair and loss. An addiction provides the illusory sensation of omnipotence and control. However, it also consumes psychic energy, which is necessary for nutrition and growth, meaning that if it is not stopped in time, it can cause a person even more severe problems.

Brown and Jasper (1993) explain eating disorders from a gender perspective through the control of one's body, which is used by women to gain self-esteem and a sense of power and control over their lives. The sensations of lack of power and dissatisfaction can be replaced by self-satisfaction, social approval and a sense of achievement obtained by controlling one's shape and body weight. Women's bodies become the space in which discontent and protest are expressed and focusing on "improving" their bodies to feel better about themselves becomes a distracter from the true sources of discontent.

Steiner-Adair (1990) uses the development model to suggest that when men and women reach adolescence, they undergo different processes, insofar as for men, acquiring muscles and height, as well as a deep voice, are characteristics that meet social expectations, in that they are associated with power, effectiveness and authority. However, women are expected to be assertive, independent and self-controlled, characteristics that do not fit the increase in the amount of body fat necessary for menstruation, since fat is a symbol of lack of power, ineffectiveness and lack of control. A woman who has control over her life, but is fat, will feel that this characteristic contradicts her effectiveness and control, which in turn will lead her to think that being overweight makes her possible flaws more obvious to others.

From a metaphorical point of view, a woman who eats emotionally is aware that she needs something, but does not know what. She is usually capable of nourishing others, but receives little in return. The anorexic tends to minimize her needs and has difficulty inserting anything into herself. Since she experiences relationships as intrusive, she focuses on self-sufficiency and absolute self-control. Conversely, the bulimic woman may experience elements of both, since she can insert certain things into herself, yet finds it difficult to retain the goodness of nutrients within herself. She realizes that she has needs, although she does not feel happy about them and feels generally guilty about her needs and feeding herself. Anorexia and bulimia do not revolve around weight or eating. Instead, they are an attempt to combat the psychological discontent in women's lives. When a young woman concentrates on her weight and food, other more important aspects are overlooked.

As several authors have already mentioned (Chernin, 1985; Friedman, 1985; Orbach, 1986), anorexia is something that women do for themselves. It is a fruitless attempt to achieve strength and well being, and a paradox of control, since insofar as the anorexic has a greater need to control her body, she is increasingly removed from the latter. The anorexic is communicating with herself and others that there is something very wrong and that she is very unhappy. Her body and her behavior are proof of her frustration and she may perceive them as the only way of expressing feelings in such a way that it will not affect others.

Table 1. Demographic Data and Diagnosis

Informant	A	B	C	D	E	F	G	H	I
Age	20	28	24	32	22	20	26	28	20
Marital status	Single	Single	Single	Married	Single	Single	Single	Single	Single
Occupation	Gastronomy student	Human science student	Psychology student	Shopkeeper	Food engineering student	Business student	Graphic design student	Accountant	Communication sciences student
Socio-Economic Level	Middle	Middle	Upper middle	Upper middle	Upper middle	Lower	Lower	Middle	Middle
Place of birth and residence	Puebla, Puebla	MEXICO CITY	MEXICO CITY	MEXICO CITY	MEXICO CITY	Pénjamo, Guanajuato	Mexico State	MEXICO CITY	Mexico State
Person she lives with	Father, mother, brother and sister	Father, mother and brothers	Father, mother and brother	Husband	Father, mother and brothers	Mother, aunts and sister	Mother and brother	Father, mother and brothers	Father, mother and sister
Father's occupation	School teacher	Shopkeeper	Employee at private firm	Shopkeeper	Employee	School teacher	Deceased	Own business	Housewife
Mother's occupation	Retiree	Housewife	Housewife	Shopkeeper	Housewife	Shopkeeper	Housewife	Housewife	Retiree
Diagnosis	ANP	EDNOS	ANR	ANR	BNP	ANR	BNP	BNP	ANP

ANR= Anorexia nervosa restrictive type

ANP =Anorexia nervosa purging type

BNP = Bulimia nervosa purging type

EDNOS= Eating disorder not otherwise specified

METHOD

The study was carried out by interviewing 9 women with an eating disorder defined on the basis of DSM-IV diagnostic criteria (APA, 1994), who were currently receiving treatment at the eating disorder clinic of the Ramón de la Fuente Muñiz National Institute of Psychiatry (INP). Informants were distributed in terms of diagnosis as follows: anorexia nervosa restrictive type (3 cases), anorexia nervosa purging type (2 cases), bulimia nervosa purging type (3 cases), eating disorder not otherwise specified (one case). The demographic data of the informants are described in Table 1. Six out of nine informants were born and lived in Mexico City, the other three were born and lived outside MC, one at a 2 hour drive, one at a four hour drive and the other at an hour drive.

They're ages ranged from 20 to 32 years, and all but one was single. All but two were college students and the others were working. Two were from low socioeconomic status, 5 from middle and two from middle-high socioeconomic status. Six out of nine informants came from a nuclear family, two from a monoparental family and one lived with her husband. Mother's of interviewees worked in only three out of nine cases, five were housewives and two were retirees. Regarding fathers working status, seven of them worked, one was deceased and one was a housewife.

The criteria for inclusion in the study were 1) having received treatment regularly for a minimum of three months; 2) being in a suitable physical and emotional condition to be able to participate in the research, according to the doctor responsible for their treatment and 3) agreeing to participate in the study. El estudio fue aprobado por el comité de ética del INP. The interviewees were informed of the confidentiality and privacy nature, the possible risks and benefits of the research. They were asked to give their consent to be audio-taped and they were informed that their participation was voluntary and would in no way affect their ability to go to the institution for consultations and that they could stop participating whenever they wished to do so. The interviews were carried out by the first author of this paper, who has an ample experience on clinical work with eating disorder patients and on research practice with adolescents.

In-depth interviews[1] were conducted individually on the Institute's premises, using the number of sessions required to be able to compile all the experiences to complete the interview guide, which was sub-divided into three areas with the following themes. Interviews length ranged from one single session to 9 sessions, with a taping time of one to 16 hours. In six out of nine cases, all the previewed themes were completed, but in three cases the interviewees declined before finishing. In-depth interviews were selected as the preferable method of interviewing because the aim of the study was to acquire knowledge regarding specific issues related to eating disorders previously signaled by the literature, although as it was mentioned above, any new issues mentioned during the interviews were welcome, which is one of the advantages of qualitative research.

---

[1] In contrast with more exploratory interviews, intensively investigate a particular topic. The purpose of an in-depth, or focused interview is to gain as complete and detailed an understanding as possible of the topic at hand. In-depth interviews involve semi-structured interview guides, and assume enough prior exploration of the topic to know what the relevant questions are that relate to the topic to be investigated (Hudelson, 1994).

Socio-cultural aspects	Psychosocial aspects	Individual aspects
Demographic data Domestic routine and family activities. Relations with parents, siblings and other close relatives. Peer groups. Personal and social values regarding their bodies. Professional choice	Self-esteem Body image. Depression. Personality traits. Family history of eating disorders and other mental disorders. Attempts to seek help and treatment. Identity. Sexuality.	Eating behavior. History of body weight. Academic life. Relations with boyfriend/partner. Experiences of rejection related to the body. Domestic violence.

The taped material was transcribed verbatim and the information in it subsequently analyzed using meaning condensation and categorization (Kvale, 1996).

RESULTS

Interviews yielded information on a wide range of issues related to the areas acknowledged. Some of them are father's alcohol use, mother's depression, experience of sexual abuse, criticism about body features by relatives, peers, teachers and other persons; comorbidity of abnormal eating behaviors with affective disorders, suicidal ideation and suicide intent, anxiety, impulsivity and drug use. Overweight or obesity was common characteristics during infancy, as well as body image distortion and dissatisfaction. Features such as low self esteem, perfectionism, maturity fears, shame feelings and interpersonal relationships with relatives and men in general, were found among interviewees. Social pressure to be thin was seen in certain beliefs about the importance a thin figure has to be a successful person.

In the present paper results are presented divided in four areas in which some of the issues mentioned above are included, these were named: food and emotions, identity and control, acceptance of the female body and the mother-daughter relationship. Below is an analysis of the material, followed by testimonies drawn from the interviews conducted, each text can be identified according to the initial letter, same one shown at the top of table 1.

FOOD AND EMOTIONS

Food is always linked to emotional needs. "Emotional eaters" use food as an attempt to fill the emptiness they feel inside, or as a form of distraction from feelings of dissatisfaction and unhappiness. Compulsive eating is a way of providing comfort and food, whereas diets are experienced as a means of physiological and emotional deprivation, while purging can be experienced as a way of relieving emotional tension, particularly anger.

Eating disorders, or the deterioration of the eating function are the way some people attempt to solve or camouflage problems in their life which they feel are insoluble (Bruch, 1973) or as Orbach notes (1978) weight control is used by many women as a substitute for controlling their real problems over which they lack control. Eating disorders can be understood as the most open, global and symptomatic expression of women's inability to control their lives and offset its traumatic effects. The cultural over-valuation of the body (and eating) becomes a means of expressing aggression, sexuality and desire as well as simultaneously acquiring power and comfort (Zerbe, 1996).

The female body often serves as an amplifier of the discontent and psychic conflicts that are not conscious and cannot be verbally expressed, which is reflected in the fact that nearly all typically female psychopathological forms have somatic expressions. At the same time, only the somatic aspects of the processes related to female physiology (contraception, abortion, pregnancy, childbirth and menopause) are dealt with, whereas all the psychosocial factors that accompany or generate them are ignored (González de Chávez, 1993).

> (G, 26 years old)"That's actually what used to happen to me when I had a problem, when I felt depressed or that I was a failure, when I felt people looked down on me, when I felt my family didn't love me. I used to think about eating, so there was always a reason why I used to feel bad and eating was a way of getting over it…"
>
> "I used to feel anguished, perhaps about being lonely, and that no-one loved me, and above all, that I was no good, because nobody loved me, or I used to feel that no-one would love me because I was fat, or because I was stupid, or because I had never had a boyfriend and those thoughts were very painful. And because I felt that I was like that, that was my situation, and the only nice thing I could have was to eat whatever I wanted, in other words, with no limits. It was sort of my only pleasure."
>
> (I, 20 years old) "For example, the last time was when I had a really bad fight with my boyfriend. We broke up and he started going out with someone else and instead of saying, 'You know what? You really hurt me,' instead of saying it to his face or paying someone to beat him up, like lots of people do, I was punishing myself. I said, 'It's all my fault,' and whereas before I used to have a cup of cereal, after that I started to have less. When I tried to commit suicide, it was because he had hurt me and I knew it was my fault because I was tired of struggling between wanting to eat and on the other hand, having something inside me say, 'No, you shouldn't eat, you mustn't eat.' And during that time, I had a car crash and instead of expressing it another way or shouting or telling him to his face or doing something else, I hurt myself."

As one can see from the testimonies presented, there is a link between emotional states and the way a person eats. The inability to exteriorize emotions is turned against oneself into self-destructive acts such as stopping eating or overeating and vomiting, among other things. Thus, eating behavior is a way of relieving unpleasant sensations such as depression, failure, inadequacy, lack of love, anguish, loneliness and pain, caused by stressful situations.

Identity and Control

Eating disorders are an extreme, distorted expression of social expectations of women that have emerged since the 20th century. In a relatively short space of time, young women have been forced to deal with a series of new demands, with a strong orientation towards success, competition and independence, and a series of values that conflict with the traditional female role. At times of numerous opportunities but also of enormous pressure, many women have found it difficult to find a viable identity, which is why they have a feeling of fragmentation, confusion and doubt about themselves (Gordon, 1990).

Women's relationship with food is also partly shaped by her role as a provider of food. Women learn through feeding others that food is a form of giving and looking after others. At the same time, women are fundamentally identified with their bodies, which is how they obtain power in society. The body is a socially accepted means of expression, yet it is also a depository of fear, hatred and distrust. According to Zimberg (1993), this contradictory message forces women to take control of their bodies and acknowledge that their bodies are their source of power.

In eating disorders, control is synonymous with identity. It is the core symptom which a person must hold on to for two reasons; first, because the rewards obtained from it are the very center of the disease and second, because letting go of this symptom may mean losing everything, including one's identity. Identity is based on the need to have everything under control and the loss of the latter involves subjecting oneself to the most heartrending sensation of vulnerability, weakness and death.

For Schilling (1993), bodies have become crucial to giving people a sense of identity in modern times. An increasing number of people are interested in health, and the shape and appearance of their own bodies as expressions of individual identity, particularly among the middle classes, although in recent years, this phenomenon has extended beyond these limited confines. Among its many effects, modernity has led to an increase in the degree of control that nations in general and the medical professions in particular have exerted over their citizens' bodies. People's relationships with their bodies can be understood as one of the ways of defining modernity.

Nowadays, women express the conflicts in their lives through their bodies and food for two main reasons: the spread and internalization of the aesthetic thin ideal and the conflictive relationship that women in Western societies have with food and their bodies. The experiences of violence and sexual abuse add another conflict and appear to increase the tendency in women to worry about their weight and to develop eating disorders as a result of trying to achieve a greater sense of control and self-esteem by regulating the consumption of food and the shape of their bodies. During this contradictory, unsafe stage in the history of women, eating disorders have become a viable response (Brown and Jaspers, 1993).

In the West, there is a tendency to see the body as an entity that is undergoing a process of development, that it is a project that must be worked on and perfected as part of the individual's identity. Thus, the appearance, size, shape and contents of the body can be reconstructed, which makes individuals both aware and worried about the handling and maintenance of the appearance of their bodies. This involves recognizing the body as a social symbol and source of resources that provide messages about a person's identity. It entails investing in the body and giving people a means of self-expression and a potential way of feeling good and increasing the degree of control they have over themselves.

Tubert (2000) notes that "the search for thinness, identified with perfection, also has other aspects; it serves as a defense against the anguish caused by bodily disorders, associated in both the social imagination and the family and women's subjectivity primarily with the female body, punishment, the search for an identity that restores lost stability. What is usually created is a pseudo-identity, in that it is based on an over-adaptation to the experiences of others. In general terms, it affects girls who have been excessively responsible, perfectionist, and submissive. During adolescence, they are also subjected to ideal cultural models, which they interpret "literally", yet exaggerate, taking them to their ultimate consequences, in a parody which, as such, reveals a suppressed hostility that involves self-destruction, and an aborted rebelliousness."

The body, as the anthropologist Mary Douglas notes, is a powerful symbolic form, an area in which the central rules, hierarchies and even the metaphysical commitments of a culture are inscribed and reinforced. Female bodies are docile bodies, bodies whose energy is accustomed to regulation, subjection, transformation and "improvement." Through the discipline of diet, make-up and clothes, women are oriented more towards self-modification and less towards the social. Taken to an extreme, the practices of femininity can lead to demoralization, weakness and even death (Bordo, 1999).

> (C-24 years old) "A little while ago, I had a little spotting which lasted two days and I told the doctor and all and he said, 'Great!' but I was a bit hesitant about telling my mother. I thought it would be like when I was 11 years old again, and I thought, 'Should I or shouldn't I tell her?' and I finally decided to tell her. I said, 'Guess what, Mum, I've had a period again,' and she actually had a party and hugged and kissed me and so on. And I remembered a friend whose mum had made a real fuss and I said, 'You should have had a party when I had my first period,' and I thought about all that and I said, 'Oh!' and then I felt bad because I said, 'Damn! I've failed, I'm not doing what I want to do, I haven't managed to get the better of my body, why did it have to happen to me?' I thought. I handle my body and I decide when to lose weight and get really skinny and when to put on weight, I'm responsible for my body, so when I started to get my period, I thought, 'I didn't want it to be like this, I didn't want to have my period yet,' I felt like a real failure, my body got the better of me, because that's what my Mum wanted!"
>
> "...I don't want to see them again, that is, when we leave the faculty, I don't want to see them, because they'll see that I've put on weight again. They'll say, 'Serves her right for being so cocksure of herself,' because I used to say, 'I went on a very strict diet and did exercise,' I was very orderly and so on and because of that, I felt really proud to have lost so much weight, so when they see me looking fat again, they'll say, 'The perfect girl isn't so perfect after all, her diet wasn't that great after all.' I wanted to keep up an image with them, of being the perfect girl because they always thought I was perfect, and that everything was going great for me, and that I controlled everything, so if they see me looking fat again, I don't want them to see me, they'll say, 'Isn't she fat?' or at least they'll think it."
>
> "When I was very thin, I felt comfortable with my body, I used to say that everything fitted me, that I could wear anything, everything that I had always dreamt of wearing, everything fitted me perfectly. Then I'd go into the changing rooms in shops and try on trousers and blouses, you know, those really tight trousers, but they'd still be loose on me, and I'd say, 'Drat, they're loose on me," but then I'd say, 'That's great, and I felt really good."
>
> "I find that the opposite is true. For me, being an anorexic is a source of pride, because being anorexic gives me control over my life, over food, I do what I want, whatever I feel like whereas being bulimic is just the opposite. Being bulimic gives you a poor sort of control, you don't really know what's going on, it's really imperfect. But being anorexic is perfect, it's almost perfect, because during my anorexic phase, I used to come in and do the dishes, my room was always impeccable, and I used to put everything away. There wasn't a single dish left drying in the dish rack because I used to wash the dishes, then dry them and put them away. I used to leave the table perfectly clean, but not any more. I don't leave my clothes all over the place in my room, but there are one or two. I don't wash the dishes any more, I just leave them there to drain. Before I used to brush my teeth as soon as I had finished eating, because they felt dirty, but now I can wait for an hour or so and then brush them. For me,

being bulimic is like being a slob, being fat but anorexia is something you can admire, don't you think?"

(A, 20 years old) "Yes, I definitely want to get ahead or find myself again, I want to have my own life, I need to be alone, I need to be able to survive on my own and I need to stop feeling anxious, because I feel that it is preventing me from doing lots of things, and I need to be independent of my mother and not depend on her so much any more."

(H, 28 years old) "When I'm fat I lose everything, I've thought about my vanity, but I know that when you have a good figure, people automatically think you're a professional."

(G, 26 years old) "I always thought that thin people, in other words, those that have always been accepted or are the most accepted…or that thinness is the only way of finding success…and that they are perfect people…"

These testimonies reflect the fragile identities of the women identified, by pointing out the places in which it is located: beauty and the search for the perfect body, understood as thinness, and the control of bodily functions such as menstruation, which provides a sense of belonging, achievement and strength. It is sometimes confused with the search for "male" characteristics, since the latter contain qualities that could make up for what is missing in femininity, such as freedom, respect and autonomy. The body "project" can be modified in such as way that it will reflect a certain identity, yet at the same time, the latter is exposed to any change, and therefore ends up being extremely vulnerable.

Acceptance of the Female Body

Historically, women's social value has never been separate from her body. Her social role has been identified with and expressed through her body: in feeding her children, in satisfying men's sexual needs and in looking after the emotional and physical needs of male children and adults. The "ideal" image of the female body has been transformed in relation to the social roles they have played. The most significant of these transformation has been the change from the round, female forms that predominated when women's role as caretaker was more important (Beller, 1977, Bruch, 1973) to the thin, muscular body of today. The emphasis on woman's fertility declined after the industrialization of Western societies and insofar as women experienced progress in economic, political and social life, thinness became a symbol of wealth, independence and freedom, and a thin body that emphasized sexuality that was unrelated to reproduction began to be valued.

Thinness has also constituted a form of anti-patriarchal rebellion. A thin bodily image expresses freedom through its connotation of mobility, independence, sexuality and freedom. However, it also expresses woman's continuous oppression and despite its muscular expression, it also signifies smallness, dependence and vulnerability, through woman's delicacy and small size.

Since the 1960s, diets and thinness have acquired the status of a cultural obsession, the main protagonists of which have been women. This is due to the importance of physical appearance and sexual attraction as conditions for women's self-esteem and social success (Gordon, 1990). Turner (1984) notes that in contemporary Western society, self-starvation is a form of self-affirmation of female beauty or sexual attraction as well as the negation of sexuality, and above all, fertility. As Orbach (quoted in Bordo, 1993) points out, women's current situation is one in which the constellation of social, economic and psychological factors combines to produce a generation of women who feel profoundly imperfect, ashamed of their needs and not entitled to exist unless they are transformed into creatures with new values (in other words, without needs, desires or bodies).

From the perspective of Susie Orbach, the message is clear: "a woman's body does not belong to her" (Bordo, 1993). The cultural emphasis is placed on "how feminine a woman is" while at the same time pointing out that enjoyment is bad. You can make people desire you, but never admit far less realize your desire, because pleasure is prohibited. Bodily needs must be controlled as much as possible, because otherwise, they would lead women to satisfy their desires. How else can one understand the level of self-aggression expressed in an eating disorder? In the words of Susan Bordo, "Culture scorns and suppresses female hunger. It makes women ashamed of their appetites and needs and requires women to strive constantly to transform their bodies" (Bordo, 1993).

According to modern Christian discourse, femininity has a negative value derived from the association of femininity with nature, otherness, being a threat to human nature and cultural matters, an obscure force (unknowable, enigmatic) a symbol of evil and an alliance with negative powers that drag man into perdition. Woman is basically body, sexuality, impurity, temptation and sin. Her redemption depends on her being able to deny her intrinsic nature and accepting the subjection she owes man because of his greater proximity to God. Women's personal fulfillment and salvation depend on living a life for others (Alfie, Rueda and Serret, 1994).

Food has become an area of conflict for women, since she is expected to provide physical sustenance and food for others, while denying herself this same possibility. Passionate, unrestricted eating is regarded as unattractive and unfeminine, while diets and asceticism are accepted and even encouraged. It is hardly surprising then, that bulimia is associated with a feeling of spiritual weakness, whereas anorexia is associated with force. This allows one to understand anorexia as an attempt to escape from the same voracity to which the bulimic surrenders.

> (B, 28 years old) "I've got big hips and a small waist and I've always had a complex about that, so to hide that, I always used to tie sweaters round my waist, and I went through high school like that."
>
> "I think I was a bit confused about relations between men and women because I think my dad didn't really like women. If Mum got dressed up to go out, all hell would be let loose, so it was better not to look like a woman, it was better to be either a little girl forever or something neutral, in other words, without...just a person, without...because my father thought sex was awful and disgusting."
>
> "...When I was a little girl, I used to say, 'I don't want to grow up, it was as though I didn't want to grow up, I didn't want to become a woman, I always played at being a man, in other words, I wanted to be like my dad, not like my mum, never like my mum, I wanted to be a man, because I felt that men were...freer, they were more respected, in other words, they had more auton...it was as though men were more valuable, in other words, they could do more things, and as a woman, you had to act lifeless, and you were weak, in other words, women were weak and I didn't want to be weak, I wanted to be strong. I didn't even want my bust to grow...but when I knew I was going to get my period, and all that...I rejected it, I didn't want to be a woman...and my mum wanted me to wear stockings and a skirt and to be really flirty and I thought that was silly because she never got dressed up like that, so why did she want me to get dressed up like her? She didn't set an example for me, she felt guilty about

putting make-up on or when she wore skirts above the knee, she felt she was the most immoral woman in the world…."

(E, 22 years old)"There came a time when I couldn't stand it any more, and I said, 'I'm not interested. I prefer to stay shut up at home. I won't be able to study for a degree, have a boyfriend or be happy until I lose weight."

"Because I was scared that, even if I changed physically, and had a period, I would never be able to attract anyone. I wanted to get used to the idea that as long as I was like that, without a period or breasts or anything, people would go on saying things to me, and I would go on being unhappy, so I didn't want to grow or have responsibilities, I didn't want to mature or get on in life."

(I, 20 years old) "…I was about 15, about 5 years ago, when I realized that everyone used to compare me with my sister because I really was fat, I wasn't at all attractive and my friends attracted boys because they were thin and very sure of themselves, and from the moment I realized that I didn't have the figure to make people realize that I existed, that's when the problem started.

(C, 24 years old) "I get very embarrassed when I'm eating without control, I start thinking, 'If anyone could see me now, I must look really disgusting,' I don't know, I eat things without enjoying them, without chewing them or anything, Sometimes I think, I really disgust myself, yuck, and then of course I feel guilty, and think that I wasn't that hungry after all, I didn't need to eat those things. For example, yesterday, I ate three bags of gumdrops and they didn't agree with me, I felt awful, I wondered why on earth I had eaten so many, when I didn't need to at all, I'm disgusting, and then when I saw my mother, I was really embarrassed, so I think I find it really difficult to accept the fact that I'm bulimic, we haven't talked about it directly in our family when we are alone, like, 'What's all this about your bulimia?' we haven't talked about it. They say, 'As an anorexic, you must…' I mean they accept that I'm an anorexic, but they never say that I'm bulimic.'

The constant struggle to achieve an "ideal" figure according to current socio-cultural standards of thinness reflects the negation of the subject as a person with desires. This is reflected in the words of the women interviewed, who mention their fear of being seen, of being a magnet for the opposite sex or admitting their physiological or affective needs.

Standing at the center of this hostile crossroads, teenage girls apparently have the power to dominate their own bodies, and thereby exercise power. For some, perfection means having absolute control of their bodies (being the perfect dieter) whereas for others, power is exercised by playing two opposing roles in the public and private sphere. The woman who is perfect in public, i.e. the best worker, daughter, mother, sister and student, is the most disgusting, repugnant and impulsive person in private (a bulimic) yet still maintains control, albeit in secret. Nevertheless, this "ability to control makes her feel powerful and worthy of admiration in the "world" from which, deep down, she actually feels excluded and devalued."

The Mother-Daughter Relationship

On the basis of the material compiled, we noticed that discontent (Burin)[2] is expressed in a person's failure to recognize her own desires, which are usually confused with the mother's

2 The term "discontent" includes all those who complain of something, even though they do not fit into psychiatric diagnostic categories. Researchers in the area of eating disorders have attempted to do this by calling undifferentiated forms of disorders partial or sub-clinical syndromes although they end up being

wishes. This creates a sensation of total impotence and hostility that is concealed by self-aggression (eating disorders, guilt, lack of self-esteem and a permanent need for recognition). Mabel Burín and cols. (1990) mention the fact that the inhibition of hostility together with the centrality of the maternal gender role imposes ideals for the constitution of women as subjects, which often seem unattainable, cause frustration and are therefore a major depressant factor.

It is interesting to note that most mothers of anorexic and bulimic daughters also suffer from similar disorders that are usually not recognized as such. The mother's role is ambivalent because she must not only take care not to overfeed, but also to maintain her daughter's health. What mothers fail to do is to teach their daughters to feed themselves emotionally, in other words, to provide the tools to achieve sufficient autonomy, self-esteem and independence. As Susie Orbach points out (1980) women's energy is channeled into looking after others. If the maternal role is what gives women their identity, the loss of this role is devastating when the daughter is faced with the decision to become independent, which in turn, signifies the rejection of her own mother.

> (C, 24 years old) "The thing is that she's not anorexic or bulimic or anything of the sort, but she is always worried about her weight, always, always, she says, 'Oh no, I've put on weight, I've put on two kilos and now I weigh 51 kilos and I should weigh 48 and she's always going on about her 48, 48, 48 kilos."
>
> (F, 20 years old) "My mum's like that too. Mum's got this idea into her head that she should never have supper, and that she wants to wear our clothes even though she's a bit fatter and I say, 'That doesn't look good on you,' and she says, 'But I'm thin,' but she's not thin and then she criticizes people who eat or put on weight."
>
> (B, 28 years old) "My mum says, 'That's why I'm healthy and thin. I eat a little bit of everything. I find it really annoying when she says that. 'That's why I'm thin. As though being thin was the best thing in the world.'

Mothers of bulimic women have been described as emotionally distant, critical and unaccepting (Root, Fallon and Friedrich, 1986). They find it difficult to tolerate and moderate emotions and tend to deny painful emotions. When the father or mother is physically present yet emotionally absent or abusive, the situation becomes extremely confusing for the child, because there is no obvious reason for her to feel bad. Within this atmosphere, a child's emotional needs are not met, meaning that she fails to internalize the capacity to affirm, console and cheer herself up. With a profound sense of shame, combined with trust in disassociation as a form of defense, and a deficit in the structure of her ego, and the ability to regulate herself, she does not learn to connect with her own experiences. She therefore runs the risk of rejecting herself and losing control because she lacks the ability to regulate her physical and emotional states (Reindl, 2001).

Women with anorexia nervosa experience difficulty in relating to others, a difficulty that is based on the need for a close relationship that is not one of fusion, coupled with the need for separation that is not synonymous with distancing. Commitment becomes confused with

---

operationalized and therefore exclusive. This shifts the focus from the mind in the search for the illness as suffering (in the health-illness dichotomy) towards the search for experience, which is not static, nor can it be cured nor given a prescription for, since it travels through time, has close and distant antecedents and is complicated because it is anchored in the most basic features of identity and because it is intertwined with the researcher's subjectivity.

being trapped and connection is feared because it represents the loss of the sense of autonomy of the ego. In extreme cases, she fears that being connected means becoming lost in a malevolent, overwhelming presence, while admitting the need for connection with others means exposing herself to danger in a dependent, destructive position. Attempting to separate herself from this would imply the destruction of others and of herself, as well as incurring tremendous wrath (Steiner-Adair, 1991).

(A, 20 years old) "…I think that these things are too intimate for her to be telling me, so I felt a bit uncomfortable and thought, they are too delicate for her to be able to talk about with her daughter, and then I thought, well, at least she trusts me…"

"…When she cries, it is nearly always because she'd like to have her mother with her, to give her advice. She says she cries because she can't ask her mother for advice any more. The other day, I was talking to her and I said, 'You're going to cry!' and she said, 'You're the only person I feel I can talk to. When she says that, I feel awful, and even worse, because I want to tell her that I want to leave home. Imagine how I feel when she says I'm the only person she feels she can talk to. That's when I say, 'I can't leave home. I'll have to stay with them!"

"I felt I had to be sad, because if she didn't enjoy life, then how could I? It was as though I felt I didn't have the right to be happy, if she wasn't happy, I didn't have the right to feel happy, I got it into my head that I had to be in the same mood as she was."

(C, 24 years old) "…if she doesn't like me being fat, then why does she buy me bread? As I said to my therapist, why is she sabotaging me like that? What does she want? For me to be fat or thin?" "I feel really rejected by my mother, which is why I am always doing things to please her."

(E, 22 years old) "The thing about my mother is that she was proud of me when I lost weight, she said, 'Just look at my daughter.' So that's when things started to go wrong. In other words, I was accepted if I lost weight, and if I put on weight, I had to go on a diet. So it's difficult, it's been really hard for me and it got to the point where I used to cry at the thought that I was going to put on a kilo."

(D, 32 years old) "My mum decides a lot of the things in my life. But I can't tell her because she really did it because she wanted the best for me, you can't really blame her. When I decided to finish high school in the English system, classes had already started there, so when I arrived, I was already enrolled at the Maddox and my mother said, 'Guess what? I've enrolled you. So I said, 'Alright, I'll study English for a year,' and she said, 'If you don't like it, you can change to the university of your choice. I wanted to study design, and she said, 'You can study wherever you like,' and then I stayed there because my friends were there and then I went on to do a degree. It's not something I would have chosen to do, but I stayed there because of my friends. So what do you do? And it's a degree course, a four-year degree, like any other degree, so I feel that with lots of things, I always end up doing what she wants, to please her."

(B, 28 years old) "…I don't know why she used to get depressed, sometimes I used to think that it was because of me, when I started having problems with food, I thought it was because of me, because I didn't have a boyfriend or because I was fat or whatever, or because I didn't turn out the way she expected me to…"

"…apparently she's busy getting lunch ready, but suddenly she says, 'Don't do that! In other words, she's keeping an eye on me. Or she used to look at me when I was eating, or she'd say, 'You've already had a lot of rice!" or when I was getting ready to go out, she'd say, 'That doesn't look good on you!' So whenever I came out of my room, my mother would always inspect me…"

(C, 24 years old)"…if my mother says that I look slim, my face lights up, and my eyes sparkle and I feel proud of myself, and that makes me feel good in other words happy, you know, if my mother says so, then I'm alright then, aren't I?

"…one of the things they suggested we should do in our habit modifying therapy was that we should plan our menus every day. I did that, and I'd put my food in the fridge, and then when my mother was getting lunch ready, she'd say, 'So that's what you want to eat, is it? So she'd fix lunch. Until recently, I couldn't be bothered to prepare my menu but then I thought, I'll stop letting her have so much control over me. For breakfast, I'm going to have whatever I like, I'm going to plan my menu in my head, so mum won't know. So she'd come up and ask me and I'd say, 'I don't know, I haven't thought about it, and then she'd say, 'What are you having for breakfast?' And I'd say, 'I don't know, I have no idea,' so she'd say, 'Make it yourself, then," and I'd think, 'That's exactly what I want.' So I'd gradually start to have control over my life again. Before I'd go around the city in peseros (collective taxis) and then my mum started coming everywhere with me."

The testimonies show that the maternal relationship is experienced by the interviewees in an extremely close way, with the mothers involving their daughters in intimate aspects of their own lives, supervising their activities or making decisions on such personal matters as their professional careers. Conversely, the relationship is sometimes so distant that it is experienced as rejection. In both cases, however, the daughter experiences the same sensation, of not being good enough to be valued, loved or accepted by her mother. The lack of connection with her daughter makes the mother re-live her feelings of inadequacy (when needs are not acknowledged), and she will make every effort to please her, without managing to change the feeling of being incapable of pleasing her, and of never being good enough to deserve her love (Jordan, 1989; Murray, Waller and Legg, 2000).

Discussion

Along this chapter, we have presented the testimonies of women diagnosed with an ED, exploring the relationship of gender-related factors with their illness. Subject themes proposed by the literature where approached during in-depth interviews, and the resulting conversations show that they mirror the experience of these women. In their accounts, the relation of food with emotions is clear-cut, the confusion about identity, the feminine aspects of the body are experienced as enemies, and the enmeshment of mothers and daughters desires appears as a source of confusion and emotional pain.

It is interesting to note that, for the interviewees, dietary restriction was consciously aimed at loosing weight. They did not, as the Chinese women reported by Lee (Lee, Lee, Ngai, Lee and Wing), explain their food avoidance in terms of digestive discomfort, and neither did they restrict their intake of food without a clear reason, as in the case stories from India presented by Khandelwal et al (Khandelwal, Sharan and Saxena, 1995). Their alimentary practices were thus inscribed in the western context of the pursuit of thinness, which places them in what we could call the mainstream of eating disorders. Food restriction can be an expression of emotional (and gendered) conflict, for which the individual can give a variety of culturally modelled conscious explanations (Lee, 1995), and we can see how these women from a Latin American country, discursively situated their behaviour within the mainstream rationale.

Going back to the subject of the gender dimension and its relation to ED, the experience of being a woman for the interviewees was probably also "typical", in the sense of living through the double exigencies of the superwoman ideal: career and family, being seductive and yet caste, asserting oneself and at the same time yielding to others. If these conflicts are at the root of the bodily discontent expressed through anorexia and bulimia nervosa, interventions addressed at improving women's self acceptance are urgently needed, but in the clinical and the general, preventive, context.

Since the seminal work by Bruch (1962) on the genesis of anorexia nervosa, it has been more or less accepted that some problem with identity is at the core of the eating disorders. According to that author, a lack of acceptance of children's self expression results in a deficiency in the formation of personality, where the child is incapable to recognize her own needs and desires, and accepts her parents (usually her mother's) as her own. Although this situation can be seen in the interviewees' accounts of their relations with their mothers, a gender perspective must consider those aspects of identity formation which are determined by the sex-gender system.

Identity is generally understood as a person's self-account, the sense of being a unit. This sense is inseparable of the bodily sensations, and in fact, according to Freud, the perception of the body is the basis for the formation of the identity. However, this perception is not a natural, simple one. Diverse parts of the body, and the body as a whole, are invested with meaning, and the sense of identity is a reflection of this (Gras, 1994). In the case of the eating-disordered women, the lack of recognition of their own bodily sensations results in an impaired sense of identity. The practices oriented towards the control of the body weight allow for a sort of recovering of that sense. Paradoxically, even while the person feels affirmed through the control exerted over her body, she is actually responding to the social mandate for women to be slim, contained, small and fragile. The feeling of control is, then, the result of its opposite, a stereotyped response in accord with what society expects (Bordo, 1993).

Another aspect of the dynamics of identity in the eating disorders is worth examining. If we consider that identity is not a fixed situation, but a construction that has to be maintained, and amenable to constant transformation in response to the exigencies and experiences of the life course, we must accept that being a patient is also a form of identity. The women whose accounts we have analyzed here are all "eating disorders patients", recognized as such by themselves and others. How this position modifies their perceptions of their bodies and their eating practices would be interesting to explore. It is also important to remember that, at the time they were interviewed, all the participants had already been diagnosed, and must have had some idea of the core psychopathology they were supposed to have. Their accounts, then, can be read as an affirmation of a subject position they have adopted, the position of a woman with an eating disorder. The further exploration of this might shed light on the process of moving from a position where the controlling of food is the only identity available, to a situation where the possibility of exploring a diversity of identities is possible.

Being anorexic or bulimic constitutes a response to the answer about one's own identity, an existential problem, which causes a great deal of anguish in adolescence, which explains the tenacity with which patients appear to cling to these diagnostic labels. However as Tubert (2000) signals, these labels only serve to confirm a false identity, which is why it is necessary to go beyond the symptom in both the diagnostic and the therapeutic process.

Objectification theory specifies that women in particular tend to reflect and evaluate their bodies in relation to cultural standards. The female body is accepted only under determined circumstances. Invariably the image of women shown by the media is young, thin and white. Animal functions are symbolically removed in such a way that the body is presented as attractive. The objectification of female sexuality has a symbolic function as it divorces women from their animal nature, being up to cultural standards, becomes a protection, as it transforms "natural women" into beauty and desire objects (Roberts and Goldenberg, 2007). As we could observe from the interviewees, they showed their struggle when growing into a woman's body, hiding body parts, desiring to stay with a girl's body to deal with interpersonal relationships with men, comparing themselves to idealize others to achieve happiness and to be capable of attracting boys. From testimonies it could be observed the disgust interviewees expressed with themselves because of the way they eat and because their not able to control their eating, as among eating disorder patients anorexia is catalogued as higher in the hierarchy of eating disorders because its closer to perfection and control.

The body is that part of us that is immediately observable to others, and even though we may think ourselves as rational beings, our existence can only be held at an embodied self. Our body often operates outside our control, it grows, gets old, changes its functions, gets sick or impeded and eventually it will die. Sickness, to loose control over our bodily functions, our abilities or mind, can be a source of shame as we need to be cared for, here the attitudes from the ones surrounding us are enormously important. And the way we get sick can also be a source of stigma, we can hate our bodies or harmonize with them (Gilbert, 2002).

Women with eating disorders are more prone to feel bad with themselves in particular in relation to their bodies than with their behaviors. Fodor (1996) suggests that a woman with an eating disorder can feel ashamed about her desire for food, when she perceives herself ineffective, when she doesn't meet the expectancies from others or because of her use of compensatory behaviors to maintain herself slim. According to the author, this feeling of shame forms part of the core sense of self of the anorexic.

It is possible that the feelings of shame and guilt related to the appetites experimented by eating disordered patients develop within the context of familial relationships which have been described by some authors as enmeshed or not empathic (Bruch, 1973; Minuchin, 1978). Such familial bounds lack of an empathic care, and even though there appears to be an apparent intense closeness, only the parent's needs are met by the child, the child is not recognized as an individual and can have difficulty acknowledging the unmet needs in the context of such enmeshment. For some young girls, guilt and shame in relation to food, hunger and appetite, can symbolize the guilt they feel as a consequence of their need to be fed. The enmeshment that characterizes these families can be exacerbated when the daughter develops an eating disorder, as her symptoms provoke an inappropriate intrusiveness to the people surrounding her, as a part of a vicious cycle; this exacerbation provokes more guilt and shame feelings (Frank, 1991).

Body shame is a relatively recent concept in psychology. It can be defined as severe perception of having body attributes that others find not attractive and that cause rejection and attack. Body shame involves a conscious and shame state evoked when the others observe that someone's body does not reach the standards of the social ideal representation of men and women (Skårderud, 2007). As Rosen (1992) states, women with eating disorders often process the information related to self worth in terms of body shape and size, and impersonal issues as directly related to the self. This is how they erase the difference between physical appearance, self worth and eating problems, which are distortions consistent with shame proneness.

Eating disorders, highlighting anorexia and bulimia, are clear examples of specific gender psychopathology. Along the revised testimonies in the present work, the ambivalence and the internal fights of women in relation with themselves and to the relationship with their mother are highlighted: "I control or I let others control me", "I eat or I don't eat", "I self-harm or I feel pleasure", "Being anorexic is a source of pride", "I need to be independent…I don't want to depend so much on her", "To grow up or not to".

According to some psychoanalysts like Lawrence (2001) and Beattie (2006) women's vulnerability to such disorders derives at least at some point from the nature of female psychosexual development. The early process of individuation-separation from the pre-aedipical almighty mothers is enormously more difficult for girls than for boys, because girls simultaneously carry out a process of individuation and identification with their main carer of the same sex. The hostile-dependent conflicts and the ambivalent fights to acquire independence from the mother can persist for their whole life and are very easily acted by the abnormal control of feeding and body image.

Two essential experiences in girls that were studied separately by Chasseguet-Smirgel (1970) are distancing from mother and to acquire autonomy. The first one is ample and normal while the second is extremely pathologic, even fatal, not symbolic and profoundly narcissistic. The second experience (the pathological way) has been called "escaping from the mother through eating disorders". The daughter seeks "autarky", a narcissistic self efficiency. The separatedness from the maternal body is crucial for identity development.

Chasseguet-Smirgel (1970) sets the hypothesis that eating disorders begin during adolescence because the daughter's body acquires secondary sexual characters that turn her body similar to that of her mother; and this increases the state of not differentiation from the mother. The daughter then, fears to emerge as her adult body blurs the differences between them.

Anorexia and bulimia are desperate essays to differentiate the body, from the mother's body; (in contrast, the male adolescent acquires secondary sexual characteristics tan differentiate him profoundly from his mother). Eating disorders are a cartoon of autonomy, a desperate way out of an irresoluble conflict.

The ample and normal phenomena that seek the mothers distancing is the penis envy. Chasseguet-Smirgel (1970) mentioned long ago that the main function of the penis besides its sexual function is that it is a sign of the difference from the mother. When the child is driven by the desire to be autonomous, the normal way to get distanced from the mother is to become an individual through the identification with his father (in normal development boys and girls identify themselves with both parents). To become autonomous is to be able to replace the mother and all the need for her, by the possibility of doing for oneself what she is supposed to do.

In view of these remarks, one thing remains to be said about the research carried out for this study. Academic training in psychology and research at a psychiatric institution forces one to take a number of factors into account, such as diagnostic criteria, symptomatology and the causes and consequences of the illness. As a result, the interview guide was drawn up on the basis of the information compiled from an extensive review of the literature. In other words, the subjects included were influenced by previous readings and by my experience of dealing with people with eating disorders. Although my position as a researcher in relation to the interviewee was not neutral, since I had a predetermined interest in obtaining information on certain issues, the situation within the interview enabled me to deal with unforeseen issues and forms, for example, when the interviewee directed the interview towards aspects that were apparently not included in the interview guide, certain personality traits of the interviewees that altered the interaction, which either enabled the conversation to flow freely or limited it, since it was an impediment at the counter-transferal level, aspects that could have prevented the conclusion of some of the interviewees. This was offset by the gratification I obtained from finding out from the interviewees that they had found the experience beneficial, since it either enabled them to discuss important issues or ones they had never talked about, or allowed them to find out about themselves by being listened to or served as a guide enabling them to continue. It was also very interesting to watch the intense process of reflection that some of them engaged in during the period when they were interviewed.

Finally, the main implication of carrying out qualitative research within an institution is that it involves an alternative proposal for constructing knowledge, using a holistic approach in which context and meanings are considered, whose main implication lies in the search and proposal for an improvement in the detection of cases and the care of the persons affected, as well as constructing theories more in keeping with the reality of a given socio-cultural context; dealing with issues that cannot be researched in depth with other kinds of methodology; and approaching aspects involving the researcher's subjectivity such as intolerance towards a particular type of mental pathology and increasing the quantity and quality of professionals in the area.

ACKNOWLEDGEMENTS

I am extremely grateful to all those who allowed me to find out about their lives, without whose help this research could never have been completed. I am also grateful to the final year psychology students at the Universidad Autónoma Metropolitana-Xochimilco who collaborated in the transcription and analysis of the information: Fabiola Barrera Beltrán, Mireya Barreiro Esquivel, Adriana Cruz Ortega, Martha Cavazos Milanés, Rocío Gómez Mendoza, Cecilia Monroy Vallejo, Cecilia Quiroz Cerón, Araceli Martínez Espinosa, Rosario Martínez Martínez and Lorena Loza López. I would also like to thank the Interdisciplinary Program of Women's Studies at El Colegio de México for financing this project.

REFERENCES

American Psychiatric Association. (1994). *Diagnostic and Statistical Manual of Mental Disorders*. 4ª ed. American Psychiatric Association, Washington.

Alfie, M., Rueda, M.T. and Serret, E. (1994). *Identidad femenina y religión*. México:Departamento de Sociología, UAM-A.

Anderson, K. and Jack, D.C. (1991). Learning to listen: Interview techniques and analyses. In Berger Gluck, S., and Patai, D. (Eds.) *Women's Words. The feminist practice of oral history.* New York: Routlegde.

Beattie, H. (2006). Eating disorders and the mother-daughter relationship. *International Journal of eating disorders*, 7, 452-460.

Beller, A. (1977). *Fat and thin: a natural history of obesity.* New York:Farrar Starus and Giroux.

Bergner, M., Remer, P., and Whetsell, C. 1985: Transforming women's body image: a feminist counseling approach. *Women and Therapy*, 4, 25-38.

Bordo, S.R. (1993). *Unbearable weight. Feminism, western culture, and the body.* Berkeley:University of California Press.

Bordo, S.R. (1999). The body and the reproduction of femininity: a feminist appropriation of Foucault In A.M., Jaggar, and S.R., Bordo (Eds.). *Gender/Body/Knowledge: Feminist reconstructions of being and knowing*. New Jersey:Rutgers University Press.

Brown, C. and Jasper, K. (1993). Why weight? Why women? Why now?. In C., Brown, and K., Jasper (Eds.). *Consuming Passions. Feminist approaches to weight preoccupation and eating disorders* (pp. 16-35). Toronto:Second Story Press.

Bruch, H. (1962). Perceptual and conceptual disturbances in anorexia nervosa. *Psychosomatic Medicine*, 24, 187-194.

Bruch, H. (1973). *Eating disorders: obesity, anorexia nervosa and the person within.* London:Routledge and Kegan Paul.

Burín, M., Moncarz, E. and Velásquez, S. (1990). *El malestar de las mujeres. La tranquilidad recetada.* Argentina:Paidós.

Chasseguet-Smirgel, J. (1970). *Female sexuality: new psychoanalytic view.* Ed. Ann Arbor. University of Michigan Press.

Chernin, K. (1985). *The hungry self: women, eating and identity*. Toronto:Randon House.

Cotterill, P., and Letherby, G. (1993). "Weaving stories: personal auto/biography in feminist research". *Sociology* 27, 67-79.

Fodor, I.E. (1996). A woman and her body: the cycles of pride and shame In: R.G. Lee and G. Wheeler (Eds.) *The voice of shame: silence and connection in psychotherapy.* San Francisco:Jossey-Bass.

Foucault, M. (1980). *Discipline and punish.* New York:Vintage.

Frank, E.S. (1991). Shame and guilt in eating disorders. *American Journal of Orthopsychiatry*, 61, 303-306.

Franks, V. (1986). Sex stereotyping and diagnosis of psychopathology. *Women and Therapy*, 5, 219-232.

Freud, S. (1981). *Obras completas*. Madrid:Biblioteca Nueva.

Friedman, M. (1985). Bulimia. *Women and Therapy*, 4/2 (Summer), 63-69.

Garfinkel, P.E., and Garner, D.M. (1982). *Anorexia nervosa: A multidimentional perspective.* New York:Brunner/Mazel.

Gilbert, P. (2002). Body shame In: *Body shame. Conceptualisation, research and treatment.* P. Gilbert and J. Miles (Eds.). New Cork: Brunner-Routlegde.

González de Chávez, M.A. (1993). Sistema Sanitario, concepción de la salud y condición de las mujeres In: González de Chávez, M.A. (Compilator). *Cuerpo y Subjetividad Femenina.* España:Siglo XXI editores.

Gordon, R.A. (1990). *Anorexia and bulimia. Anatomy of a social epidemic*. Cambridge:Basil Blackwell.

Gras, E. (1994). *Volatile bodies. Toward a corporeal feminism*. Bloomington: Indiana University Press.

Hsu, L.K.G., Crisp, A.H., and Callender, J.S. (1992). Recovery in anorexia nervosa: the patient's perspective. *International Journal of Eating Disorders*, 11, 341-350.

Hudelson, P.M. (1994). *Qualitative research for health programmes*. Division of Mental Health World Health Organization. Geneva.

Jordan, J.V. (1989). Relational development: Therapeutic implications of empathy and shame. Work in progress, N° 39. Wellesley MA:The Stone Center.

Khandelwal, S., Sharan, P., and Saxena, S. (1995). Eating Disorders: An Indian Perspective. *International Journal of Social Psychiatry,* 41, 132-146.

Kleifield, E.I., Wagner, S. and Halmi, K.A. (1996). Cognitive-behavioral treatment of anorexia nervosa. *The Psychiatric Clinics of North America*, 19, 715-737.

Kvale, S. (1996). *Interviews. An introduction to qualitative research interviewing*. Thousand Oaks: Sage Publications.

Lawrence, M. (2001). Loving them to death: the anorexic and her objects. *International Journal of Psychoanalisis*, 82, 43-55.

Lee, S. (1995). Self-Starvation in Context: Towards a Culturally Sensitive Understanding of Anorexia Nervosa. *Social Science and Medicine*, 41, 25-36.

Lee, S., Lee, A., Ngai, E., Lee, D.T.S., and Wing, Y.K. (2001). Rationales for food refusal in Chinese patients with anorexia nervosa. *International Journal of Eating Disorders*, 29, 224-229.

Minuchin, S., Rosman, B., and Baker, L. (1978). *Psychosomatic families*. Cambridge:Harvard University Press.

Murray, C., Waller, G. and Legg, C. (2000). Family function and bulimic psychopathology: The mediating role of shame. *International Journal of Eating Disorders*, 28, 84-89.

Nagel, K.L., and Jones, K.H. (1992). Sociocultural factors in the development of eating disorders. *Adolescence*, 27, 107-113.

Orbach, S. (1978). *Fat is a feminist issue: A self-help guide for compulsive eaters*. Berkeley:Berkeley Books.

Orbach, S. (1980). La obesidad, una perspectiva feminista. In: D., Cardacci, and L., Alvarez, (compilators). *Mujeres y medicina. De cómo fuimos perdiendo nuestros cuerpos*. México:UAM-X.

Orbach, S. (1986). *Hunger strike. The anorectic struggle as a metaphor of our age*. New York:W.W. Norton.

Owen, J.M. (1995). Women-talk and men-talk: Defining and resisting victim status. In R.E., Dobash, R.P., Dobash, and L. Noaks, (Eds.). *Gender and crime*. Cardiff: University of Wales Press.

Rand, C.S.W., and Kuldau, J.M. (1986). Eating patterns in normal weight individuals: bulimia, restrained eating, and the night eating syndrome. *International Journal of Eating Disorders*, 5, 75-84.

Reed, K. (2006). Mothers and daughters. *Journal of the American Psychoanalytic Association* www.apsa.org/portals/1/docs/japa/544/reed-1245a.pdf.

Reindl, S. (2001). *Sensing the self*. Cambridge: Harvard University Press.

Roberts, T.A. and Goldenberg, J.L. (2007). Wrestling with nature: an existential perspective on the body and gender in self-conscious emotions In J.L., Tracy, R.W. Robins, and J.P. Tangney (Eds.). *The self-conscious emotions*. New York:The Guilford Press.

Rodin, J., Silberstein, L.R., and Striegel-Moore, R.H. (1985). Women and weight: a normative discontent. In T.B. Sonderegger (Ed.). Nebraska Symposium on motivation: Vol. 32. Psychology and gender (pp. 267-307). Lincoln:University of Nebraska Press.

Romero, M., Rodríguez, E.M., Durand-Smith, A., and Aguilera, R.M. (2003). Veinticinco años de investigación cualitativa en Salud Mental y Adicciones con poblaciones ocultas. Primera parte. *Salud Mental*, 26, 76-83.

Root, M.P., Fallon, P., and Friedrich, W. (1986). *Bulimia: A systems approach to treatment*. New York:Norton.

Rosen, J.C. (1992). Bodu-image disorder: Definition, development, and contribution to eating disorders. In J.H. Crowther, D.L. Tennenbaum, S.E. Hobfoll, and M.A.P. Stephens (Eds.). *The etiology of bulimia: The individual and familial context*. Washington, D.C.:Hemisphere Publishing Corporation.

Salles, V. (1997). *EL género: ¿Una perspectiva útil para la elaboración de indicadores?* México:Centro de Estudios Sociológicos de El Colegio de México.

Schilling, C. (1993). *The body and social theory*. London:Sage.

Selvini-Palazzolli, M. (1974). *Self-starvation*. London:Chaucer.

Skårderud, F. (2007). Shame and prime in anorexia nervosa: a qualitative study. *European Eating Disorders Review*, 15, 81-97.

Steiner-Adair, C. (1990). Paper presented on a panel called "The psychology of women and the treatment of eating disorders", at the International Conference on Eating Disorders, New York.

Steiner-Adair, C. (1991). New maps of development, new models of therapy: the psychology of women and the treatment of eating disorders. In C.L. Johnson (Ed.) *Psychodinamic treatment of anorexia nervosa and bulimia*. New York:The Guilford Press.

Striegel-Moore, R., and Marcus, M. (1995). Eating disorders in women: current issues and debates. In Stanton, A. and Gallant, S., (Eds.). *Psychology of women's health: progress and challenges in research and application*. Washington DC: American Psychological Association.

Surrey, J.L. (1985). Self-in-relation: A theory of women's development. Work in progress, N° 13. Wellesley MA:The Stone Center.

Toro, J. (1996). *El cuerpo como delito. Anorexia, bulimia, cultura y sociedad.* Barcelona:Editorial Ariel.

Tubert, S. (2000). Anorexia: una perspectiva psicoanalítica. *Debate Feminista*, 11, 257-290.

Turner, B.S. (1984). *El cuerpo y la sociedad. Exploraciones en teoría social*. México:Fondo de Cultura Económica.

Unikel, C., Villatoro, J., Medina-Mora, M.E., Fleiz, C., Alcántar, E.N., and Navarro, C. (2001). Validación de una escala para medir conductas alimentarias de riesgo en adolescentes mexicanas. Paper presented at the IX Congreso Mexicano de Psicología. Aplicación de la investigación científica a la práctica profesional del psicólogo en la década de la conducta.

Van Den Bergh, N. (1991). Having bitten the apple: A feminist perspective on Addictions. In *Feminist Perspectives on Addictions*. New York :Springer Publishing Company.

Vandereycken, W., and van Deth, R. (1994). *From the fasting saints to anorexic girls. The history of self starvation*. New York:New York University Press.

Wolf, N. 1994: Hunger. In P., Fallon, M., Katzman, and S., Wooley (Eds.). *Feminist Perspectives on Eating Disorders*. New York:The Guilford Press.

Zerbe, K.J. (1996). Feminist psychodinamic psychotherapy of eating disorders. Theoretic integration informing clinical practice. *The Psychiatric Clinics of North America*, 19, 811-827.

Zimberg, R. (1993). Food, needs and entitlement: women's experience of emotional eating. Brown, C. and Jasper, K., (Eds.). *Consuming Passions. Feminist approaches to weight preoccupation and eating disorders*. (pp. 16-35). Toronto:Second Story Press.

In: Eating Disorders in Adult Women
Editor: Julian N. Fuchs

ISBN 978-1-60456-673-4

Chapter 8

THE IMPACT OF MEDIA INFLUENCES ON DISORDERED EATING BEHAVIOR

Daniel J. Munoz
University of Indianapolis, USA

ABSTRACT

While global prevalence rates of eating disorders have been increasing, there still exists a wide disparity in rates between westernized countries and the rest of the world. In fact, eating disorders are often referred to as "culture bound" syndromes due to the near exclusivity of the disorders in westernized countries. One explanation for this disparity is the "thin ideal" represented in the media in countries with elevated rates of eating disorders. This proposed book chapter will explore the research on the relationship between eating disorders and media exposure. In particular the specific images and messages that are disseminated in the media and the influence that may have on body image, and in turn risk factor for eating disorders. Topics to be discussed include current research on media influences on body image, the relationship between media exposure and eating disorder symptomatology and intervention and prevention programs that have been developed to minimize the risk of such exposure.

INTRODUCTION

Eating disorders, while found across the world, are predominantly a Westernized disorder. It is this finding that may explain why eating disorders are more likely to occur in societies where food is abundantly available, but also where the idealized body shape for women is slender, despite the dichotomy of the vast majority of the populace in these food abundant societies not matching such a thin-ideal. The idealization of thinness (and corresponding derogation of fatness) has become increasingly pronounced for females over the last few decades (Polivy and Herman, 2004).

While not diagnostic criteria prescribed by the DSM-IV-TR for a diagnosis of an eating disorder, impact of media and socio-cultural influences on the development and maintenance of anorexia nervosa and bulimia nervosa are highlighted as significant contributory factors (APA, 1994 REF). Body image disturbance, a hallmark of eating disorders, is a subjective evaluation that leads to profound distress (Thompson and Stice, 2001). This distress is not exclusive to eating disorders among women and is also a contributory factor to comborbid disorders such as depression and anxiety (Thompson and Stice, 2001).

The "sociocultural model" attempts to account for the relationship between the media thin-ideal and disordered eating behavior in women. First, women feel bad about themselves due to what they regard as their own shortcomings of the presupposed idealized feminine body resulting in body dissatisfaction. This has been substantiated in research supporting an increase in depression and decrease in reported self-esteem following exposure to media thin ideal images (Pinhas, Toner, Ali, Garfinkel, and Stuckless ,1999). Secondly this body dissatisfaction compels women to engage in various methods of dietary restraint eating patterns that easily and often deteriorate into eating disorders (Polivy and Herman, 2004).

Certainly the vast majority of women who watch television and read fashion magazines do not suffer from an eating disorder. However, while the impact for most women in a westernized media culture does not approach the level of a severe illness such as anorexia or bulimia- evidence does support that there is an overall impact on other attitudes and behaviors that in the face of other factors may lead to disordered eating. Far more women who have been exposed to the thin media ideal demonstrate increases in body dissatisfaction, social comparison and even increased desire in cosmetic procedures such as liposuction and breast enlargement (Harrison, 2003). In fact, some research has found no demonstrable differences on body dissatisfaction between women with and without current anorectic behaviors after exposure to thin models (Ogden and Mundray, 1996). Thus for a minority of these women, this general unhappiness of not living up to the thin ideal promoted by the media, may potentiate the impact of other vulnerabilities that lead to disordered eating behaviors.

This present chapter will examine the body of research on media, body image and eating disorders. First, an overview of the thin ideal as promoted in the media will be presented. Second, the mechanisms by which exposure to the media affect cognitive and affective processes. Finally, innovative programs at the primary, secondary and tertiary level to minimize the impact of media on negative body image will be discussed.

The Media and the Thin-Ideal

The thin-ideal exists in the media because of the perception it sells merchandise. This has been substantiated by industry insiders such as a spokesperson for a top modeling agency whom stated in an interview, "If you stick a beautiful, skinny girl on the cover of a magazine, you will sell more copies…this is a business and the fact is that these models sell the products" (Gillian, 2000). While the accuracy of that statement is not confirmed, what is fact is the fashion industry is enormous. In the United States alone, $368 billion dollars was spent in the last year on apparel (Standard and Poor's, 2008). As the industry has exponentially grown, the size of models over time has decreased.

A forty-year examination of cover models for Glamour, Vogue, Cosmopolitan and Mademoiselle reveals the steady and dramatic convergence to a thin-ideal promoted in the media. Sypeck and colleagues (2004) examined 1,920 magazine covers over the past four decades and matched the size of the model to a standardized set of body shape silhouettes. In addition they calculated the amount of body displayed on each cover. On the first question regarding body size, all magazines except for Glamour indicated a significant decrease over time in the size of the models. Secondly for all magazines there was an exponential increase in full body displays of the models. Whereas cover models from the 1960's and 1970's were more likely presented as facial or upper-torso shots, covers from the 1980's and 1990's moved almost exclusively to full body shots of the models. Thus the most popular women magazines have indicated a demonstrable emphasis on smaller models and increased attention to full body portrayals.

The genesis of the socialization of women to a thin ideal by the media may be traced back to a multibillion dollar icon- the Barbie Doll. Barbie, first launched by the Mattel toy corporation in 1959 has since sold over one billion dolls in over 150 countries worldwide (Sutton-Smith 1986). It is this global worldwide popularity that has long troubled the eating disorder community as it examines the grossly unrealistic body shape (large chest, thin waist and hips) that the doll represents. A fascinating study out of Australia examined the anthropometric relationships of fourteen dimensions of body parts among the figure of a Barbie doll extrapolated to an adult woman size then compared that to a sample of anorexics, models and the mean body shape of women in Australia (Norton, Olds, Olive, and Dank, 1996). The findings revealed that the Barbie was significantly smaller on all dimensions compared to the reference group of average women. Even more shocking was Barbie was smaller than anorexics on all dimensions with the exception of chest. While one can argue there may be methodological problems with the determination of Barbie's "adult woman" measurements, the "models" group, determined by a sample of models commonly seen on television and in magazines, were also all significantly smaller than the reference group and were found to be no different with anorexics on nine of the metrics.

Even when magazines attempt to discuss the dangers of eating disorders they may inadvertently reinforce the thin ideal that is such an extant risk factor. Schulze and Gray (1990) had female college students read a textbook article on bulimia and one excerpted from a fashion magazine. The participants who read the magazine profile were more likely to describe the subject of the article as attractive, minimize the severity of her disorder and thought her eating behavior was better controlled compared to the textbook profile. A related qualitative analysis of a fashion magazine portrayal of a young female with anorexia versus a textbook profile suggest that the magazine in fact may minimize the health consequences associated with eating disorders (Bishop, 2001). Inch and Muralli (2006) further analyzed the content of 43 fashion and young woman-oriented magazine articles on eating disorders and found that anorexia was the most commonly discussed disorder (a disorder more consistent with a thin ideal compared to bulimia) and furthermore there was a significant discrepancy between the degree the article discussed the weight loss achievements of the profiled female and discussion of the physical and health consequences. In other words, the magazine profiles may have covertly promoted the radical steps anorexics use to achieve a desired weight at the expense of describing the severe medical consequences and possible lethality of the disorder (Inch and Muralli, 2006).

The Influence of the Thin-Ideal on Disordered Eating

In the past few decades, an inverse correlation between prevalence of eating disorders and the decrease in the average body weight of women portrayed in the media has emerged (Wiseman, Gray, Mosimann, and Ahrens, 1992). Multiple pathways by which media exposure is related to body distress among women have been proposed. One line of research proposes the stable personality characteristic of body dissatisfaction moderates the vulnerability to media exposure, suggesting that in absence of such preexisting concerns, the media-thin ideal yields a negligible effect (Posavac, Posavac, and Posavac, 1998). There is support for this model, as research has consistently found women with higher degrees of pre-existing body dissatisfaction are more likely to be affected by presentation to thin models (e.g. Trampe, Stapel, and Siero, 2007). There is also evidence that body dissatisfied females interpret thin celebrities to be smaller in size than in reality (Willinge, Touyz, and Charles, 2006). Exposure to a feminine media thin ideal on men also impacts women. Research has suggested that men who have viewed thin models on television and in magazines were more likely to view those sizes as normative and furthermore desire their girlfriends to attain those sizes (Hargreaves and Tiggeman, 2003).

However, the argument that media exposure only affects those prone to body dissatisfaction is spurious, as the prevalence of body dissatisfaction is so prevalent among women and adolescent girls that it has been referred to as "normative discontent" (Rodin, Silberstein, and Streigel-Moore, 1985). Thus it is not "comforting" to extrapolate the media thin-ideal only negatively impacts those with body dissatisfaction, since that represents the plurality of women in our society. In other words, the continuum is not necessarily ranging from dissatisfied to satisfied; rather it appears to predominantly cover varying degrees of the magnitude of dissatisfaction.

Three potential mechanisms that potentially account for the translation of media content to body dissatisfaction are social comparison, internalization of the thin ideal and investment in the appearance for self-evaluation (Tiggeman, 2002). The latter two, however presume a developmental process that requires ongoing exposure to idealized images and thus would not account for the robust experimental findings demonstrating singular, isolated exposure to media images produces demonstrable decreases in body dissatisfaction.

Social comparison may be the critically important construct that accounts for the more proximal impact of media images on body dissatisfaction. When women compare themselves to images presented of actresses or fashion models, this is almost invariably an upward social comparison process thus leading to immediate experiences of negative self-evaluation centered on appearance. This idea has been tested directly with women who affirm statements such as "I often compare myself to the models in *Vogue, Cosmopolitan and Glamour*" report higher degrees of body dissatisfaction (Heinberg and Thompson, 1995). Furthermore social comparison effects seem to be unique to media images as exposure to thin peers does not appear to elicit similar degrees of negative affect and thin-ideal internalization (Krones, Stice, Batres, and Orjada, 2005)

An example of research supporting the direct effects of social comparison resulting from media exposure can be found in a sample of 126 Australian women (Tiggeman and McGill, 2004). Within the sample, participants on average read four fashion and beauty magazines a month and watched on average ten hours of television a week. Results indicate that brief exposure, consisting of viewing eleven images over the course of ten minutes was enough to result in increased self reported body dissatisfaction. Furthermore, the finding remained stable even controlling for individual differences related to pre-morbid body image or eating disordered related behaviors. In addition, presentation of only specific body parts elicited as much body distress as full pictures of models. Finally, support was lent to the social comparison hypothesis with results indicating elevated self reporting of social comparison after presentation of models and body parts compared to controlled image presentations. Support has also been found for a mediating effect of social comparison. Bessenoff (2006) found that in a sample of college women, the degree of social comparison mediated the effects of media thin-ideal exposure on body dissatisfaction and disordered eating attitudes and behaviors. These findings have been replicated in other research with adult women (e.g. Englen-Maddox, 2005; Lin and Kulik, 2002, Dittmar and Howard, 2004; Groesz, Levine, and Murnen, 2002)

The pressure to be thin and degree of body dissatisfaction has been found to be fairly consistent across ethnic groups (Shaw, Ramirez, Trost, Randall, and Stice, 2004). The long-term effects of exposure to media images of a thin-ideal have been also been demonstrated cross-culturally. Haregreaves and Tiggeman (2003) followed 80 Australian adolescents over two years and found that body dissatisfaction after viewing body-image related commercials at time one predicted greater body dissatisfaction at time two. In other words, in this sample of Australian adolescent females, a cumulative effect of media exposure evidenced greater body distress two years later. Similar research in New Zealand indicated that while media consumption equally predicted awareness of a thin ideal among male and female college students, only the females showed a clear decrease in body satisfaction as a function of media consumption (Miller and Halberstadt, 2005).

Even non-Westernized cultures report the effects of media influences on body dissatisfaction. Bilushka and Utermohlen (2002) examined the impact of Western media culture on 616 women in the Ukraine. There was a clear and convincing relationship demonstrating the more exposure to American television (via satellite television) and magazines, the higher reported rates of body dissatisfaction and dieting attempts. Eddy and colleagues (2007) found similar results in a sample of 213 young adult females in the East African nation of Tanzania. The authors found a positive association between those women in the sample who endorsed eating disorder pathology and their exposure to Westernized media (Eddy, Hennessey, and Thompson-Brenner, 2007).

The above research suggests that the relationship between the media thin-ideal and disordered eating is the function of mediated and moderated interactions among an array of other factors such as gender-role endorsement, body dissatisfaction and self-esteem. However some research has indicated media exposure independently predicts eating disorder symptomatology. Stice and colleagues (Stice, Schupak-Neuberg, Shaw, and Stein, 1994) conducted structured equation modeling on data collected from 238 women. The analyses of pathways found that, while other associated factors accounted for variance on outcome measures of disordered eating symptomatology, the strongest predictor was the linear relationship with media exposure .

PREVENTION AND INTERVENTION

Empirically supported treatments for eating disorders (i.e. Cognitive Behavioral Therapy) traditionally feature components to challenge distorted beliefs about the viability and importance of attaining the thin ideal as presented in the media. Techniques such as behavioral experiments like assessing the true base rate of the body sizes purported in the media to that of those in the vicinity of the patient and identifying and reframing beliefs about normative sizes and the veracity of media images are integral components in treatment. While the therapeutic components of an integrated challenge to the media thin-ideal are established, it should be noted these are interventions that are provided at the tertiary level. That is, these are interventions provided to patients once they are in the throes of a diagnosable eating disorder. Thus only a small minority of females will be exposed to those treatment factors, despite the fact far more women are exposed to media images of the thin ideal and engage in behaviors that may not reach the threshold of a diagnosable eating disorder that would provide them access to treatment. Therefore it may be more necessary to examine larger scale community and more focused targeted primary and secondary interventions that can attenuate the likelihood of development of a full-blown diagnosable disorder.

Dissonance-based intervention programs have emerged recently as a promising means of altering the impact of a societal promoted thin ideal. The proposed mechanism by which these types of interventions are based on is the theory of cognitive dissonance (Aronson, 1969). Cognitive dissonance, a theory derived from the field of social psychology, describes the uncomfortable tension that may result from having conflicting cognitions, while at the same time or engaging in behavior that conflicts with one's beliefs. More broadly, it also refers to attempts to reduce the discomfort of conflicting thoughts, beliefs and actions (Aronson, 1969). With regards to interventions designed to alter attitudes and behaviors impacted by exposure to messages about the thin ideal, cognitive dissonance theory would predict that tension would arise when participants have to argue against thin ideal standards and in order to reduce such tension, participants would then engage in behaviors (i.e. developing and adhering to more realistic body standards) that are more commensurate with such arguments (Stice, Mazotti, Weibel, and Agras, 2000).

A recent study comparing the effectiveness of eating disorder prevention programs for adolescent and young adult females illuminated the importance of challenging society's thin ideal. Stice and colleagues (Stice, Presnelll, Gau, and Shaw, 2007) randomized 335 females ages 14-19 to one of three conditions- a group where healthy eating was discussed, an expressive writing control group and the primary group of interest, a dissonance intervention whereby participants were encouraged to participate in activities that encouraged development of a skeptical attitude towards a thin ideal. Examples of a dissonance based activity included having the participants engage in a role-play whereby they attempted to dissuade facilitators from pursuing a thin ideal. The results indicated that compared to the other interventions, the dissonance-based group realized significantly greater reductions in endorsement of a thin ideal and body dissatisfaction. Furthermore, participation in the dissonance-based intervention mediated the impact of outcome on measures of dietary restraint and bulimic symptoms. Thus, challenging the societal thin ideal appears to be an effective pathway to reduce the likelihood of disordered eating symptomatology. Other studies have confirmed that the success of dissonance-based interventions are mediated by the reduction of adherence to a thin-ideal which in turn significantly reduces outcomes related to eating disorders such as negative affect, dietary restraint, body dissatisfaction and bulimic symptomatology (Stice, Presnell, Gau, and Shaw, (2007).

CONCLUSION

The rates of eating disorders, while relatively low in the general population increase exponentially when the most at-risk groups- adolescent and young adult females, are examined. This increased prevalence within that group also correlates with those most likely to be exposed to fashion magazines, television shows and music videos exalting the thin-ideal. Thus while one cannot extrapolate that media exposure to a thin ideal leads to eating disorders, there undeniably is a relationship between the two.

It is clear the motivation for the portrayal of a thin ideal in the media is because it is presumed to be an effective marketing tool. It is foolish to think the goal of television and magazines is to induce an eating disorder, rather the prominence of unrealistically thin models is due to the belief they are best at motivating viewers to purchase their products. Experimental research such as Halliwell and Dittmar's (2004) challenge that notion. Their sample of 202 women found that while presentation of thin models activated body dissatisfaction, they in fact did not increase advertising effectiveness. In other words, compared to an average sized model, participants were as likely to like the product being sold. The only demonstrable effect of having a thin model compared to an average-sized model was the induction of body anxiety.

Another promising development is a movement by several fashion houses to bar unhealthy appearing models from the runway. For example, public outcry over the death of Uruguayan model Luisel Ramos due to anorexia resulted in a global agreement among fashion houses and the Italian government to ban size zero models (Hodgson, 2006). Additionally popular fashion-oriented television shows such as "America's Next Top Model" and "Project Runway" have made concerted efforts to deemphasize gratuitously thin models and promote healthier sizes on their programs.

These are all small, positive steps in the right direction. As encouraging as previously mentioned interventions are in attenuating the effects of a media thin ideal on body dissatisfaction and disordered eating sequelae, true impact can only come from a societal level. While some impact can be made at a public policy level, issues of freedom of speech and restraint of trade would certainly pose a problem. That however has not stopped Spain's ministry of health from launching an initiative to encourage fashion retailers to make available larger sizes and deemphasize the use of thin models to sell their fashions (Tremlett, 2006).

Ultimately it will be consumers whom can decide to not patronize corporations that promote unhealthy body images, parents whom can monitor their children's access to media content and schools to deliver consistent messages about healthy body attitudes.

References

American Psychiatric Association (1994). The Diagnostic and Statistical Manual of Mental Disorders-IV. Washington D.C.

Aronson, E. (1969). The theory of cognitive dissonance: A current perspective. In L. Berkowitz (Ed.). Advances in Experimental Social Psychology, Volume 4, pp1-34. New York: Academic Press

Bessenoff, G. (2006). Can the media affect us? Social comparison, self-discrepancy the thin ideal. *Psychology of Women Quarterly, 30,* 239-251.

Biluksha, O., and Utermohlen, V. (2002). Internalization of Western standards of appearance, body dissatisfaction and dieting in urban educated Ukrainian females. *European Eating Disorders Review, 10(2),* 120-137

Bishop, R. (2001). The pursuit of perfection: A narrative analysis of how women's magazines cover eating disorders. *The Howard Journal of Communications, 12,* 221–240.

Dittmar, H.,and Howard, S., (2004). Thin-ideal internalization and social comparison tendencies as moderators of media models' impact on women's body-focused anxiety. *Journal of Social and Clinical Psychology, 23(6).*768-791

Eddy, K., Hennessey, M., and Thompson-Brenner, H. (2007). Eating pathology in East African women: The role of media exposure. *Journal of Nervous and Mental Disease, 95(3),* 196-202.

Englen-Maddox, R. (2005). Cognitive responses to idealized media images of women: The relationship of social comparison and critical processing to body image disturbances in college women. *Journal of Social and Clinical Psychology, 24(8).* 1114-1138

Gillian, A. (2000, May 31). Skinny models 'send unhealthy message'. *Guardian* (p. 7). London: Guardian Newspapers Ltd

Groesz, L., Levine, M., and Murnen, S. (2002). The effect of experimental presentation of thin media images on body satisfaction: A meta-analytic review. *International Journal of Eating Disorders, 31,* 1-16.

Halliwell, E. and Dittmar, H. (2004). Does size matter? The impact of model's body size on women's body-focused anxiety and advertising effectiveness. *Journal of Social and Clinical Psychology, 23(1),* 104-122

Hargreaves D, Tiggemann M. (2003) Female ''thin ideal'' media images and boys' attitudes towards girls. *Sex Roles* 49:539–544.

Hargreaves, D and Tiggeman, M (2003) Longer-term implications of responsiveness to "thin-deal" television: support for a cumulative hypothesis of body image disturbances. *European Eating Disorders Review, 11(6),* 465-477

Harrison, K. Television viewers' ideal body proportions: The case of the curvaceously thin woman. *Sex Roles, 48(5),* 255-264.

Heinberg, L. J., and Thompson, J. K. (1995). Body image and televised images of thinness and attractiveness: A controlled laboratory investigation. *Journal of Social and Clinical Psychology, 14,* 325–338.

Hodgson, M. (December 3, 2006). Fashion industry publishes charter to ban size-zero models. Retrieved February 10, 2008 via the internet at http://findarticles. com/p/ articles/mi_qn4159/is_20061217/ai_n16899862/pg_1

Inch, R., and Merali, N. (2006). A content analysis of popular magazine articles on eating disorders. *Eating Disorders, 14,* 109-120.

Krones, P., Stice, E., Batres, C., and Orjada, K. (2005). In vivo social comparison to a thin-ideal peer promotes body dissatisfaction: A randomized experiment. *International Journal of Eating Disorders, 38,* 134-142.

Lin, L., and Kulik, J. (2002). Social comparison and women's body satisfaction. *Basic and Applied Social Psychology, 24*(2), 115-123.

Miller, E., and Halberstadt, J. (2005). Media consumption, body image and thin ideals in New Zealand Males and Females. *New Zealand Journal of Psychology 34(3),* 189-197.

Ogden, J. and Mundray, K. (1996). The effect of the media on body satisfaction: the Role of gender and size. *European Eating Disorders Review, 4(3),* 171-182.

Pinhas, L., Toner, B., Ali, A., Garfinkel, P. and Stuckless, N. (1999). The effects of the ideal of female beauty on mood and body satisfaction. *International Journal of Eating Disorders, 25,* 223-226.

Polivy, J., and Herman, P. (2004). Sociocultural idealization of female body shapes: An introduction to the special issue on body image and eating disorders. *Journal of Social and Clinical Psychology, 23(1),* 1-6

Posavac, H., Posavac, S., and Posavac, E. (1998). Exposure to media images of female attractiveness and concern with body weight among young women. *Sex Roles, 38 (3/4),* 187-201

Schulze, E. A., and Gray, J. J. (1990). The effects of popular and textbook presentations of bulimia nervosa on attitudes toward bulimia nervosa and individuals with bulimia nervosa. *British Review of Bulimia and Anorexia Nervosa, 4,* 83–91.

Shaw, H., Ramirez, L., Trost, A., Randall, P., and Stice, E. (2004). Body image and eating disturbances across ethnic groups: More similarities than differences. *Psychology of Addictive Behaviors, 18(1),* 12-18.

Sypeck, M., Gray, J., and Ahrens, A. (2004). No longer just a pretty face: Fashion magazines' depictions of ideal female beauty from 1959 to 1999. *International Journal of Eating Disorders, 36,* 342-347.

Standard and Poor's (2008) Industry Profile: Apparel and Footwear. Accessed via the internet on February 9, 2008 at http://kml.uindy.edu:2074/NASApp /NetAdvantage/ showIndustrySurvey.do?code=apf

Stice, E., Mazotti, L., Weibel, D., and Agras, W. S. (2000). Dissonance prevention program decreases thin-ideal internalization, body dissatisfaction, dieting, negative affect, and bulimic symptoms: A preliminary experiment. *International Journal of Eating Disorders, 27,* 206–217.

Stice, E., Presnell, K., Gau, J., and Shaw, H. (2007). Testing mediators of intervention effects in randomized controlled trials: An evaluation of two eating disorder prevention programs. *Journal of Consulting and Clinical Psychology, 75,* 20-32.

Stice, E., Schupak-Neuberg, E., Shaw, H., and Stein, R., (1994). Relation of media exposure to eating disordered symptomatology: An examination of mediating mechanisms. *Journal of Abnormal Psychology, 103,* 836-840.

Sutton-Smith, B. (1986). *Toys as Culture*. New York: Gardner Press

Thompson, J., and Stice, E. (2001). Thin-ideal internalization: Mounting evidence for a new risk factor for body-image disturbance and eating pathology. *Current Directions in Psychological Science, 10(5),* 181-183.

Tiggemann, M. (2002). Media influences on body image development. In T.F. Cash and T. Pruzinsky (Eds.), Body image: A handbook of theory, research and clinical practice. New York: Guilford.

Tiggemann, M., and McGill, B. (2004). The role of social comparison in the effect of magazine advertisements on women's mood and body dissatisfaction. *Journal of Social and Clinical Psychology, 23(1),* 23-44.

Trampe, D., Stapel, D., and Siero, F. (2007). On models and vases: Body dissatisfaction and proneness to comparison effects. *Journal of Personality and Social Psychology, 92(1),* 106-118.

Tremlett, G. (April 21, 2006). Spain to size up fashion industry. Retrieved via the internet on February 10, 2008 at http://www.guardian.co.uk/ spain/article/ 0,,1758202, 00.html?gusrc=rss

Willinge, A., Touyz, S., and Charles, M. (2006). How do body dissatisfied and body-satisfied males and females judge the size of thin female celebrities. *International Journal of Eating Disorders, 39(7),* 576-582.

Wiseman, C.V., Gray, J.J., Mosimann, J.H., and Ahrens, A.H. (1992). Cultural expectations of thinness in women: An update. *International Journal of Eating Disorders, 11(1),* 85-89.

In: Eating Disorders in Adult Women
Editor: Julian N. Fuchs

ISBN 978-1-60456-673-4

Chapter 9

SOCIAL PHYSIQUE ANXIETY ACROSS PHYSICAL ACTIVITY CONTEXTS: A META-ANALYTIC REVIEW

Diane E. Mack*[1], *Philip M. Wilson, Lindsay Waddell, and Jennifer Gasparotto
Brock University
Department of Physical Education and Kinesiology, Canada

ABSTRACT

The purpose of this investigation was to review the empirical evidence specific to the relationship between physical activity contexts and social physique anxiety (SPA). English language studies were located from computer and manual literature searches. Studies included in the meta-analysis presented at least one empirical effect for SPA between physical activity participants (i.e., athletes or exercisers) and non-physical activity participants. The final sample included sixteen studies with a total sample size of 3595. Studies were coded for mean SPA between physical activity participants and non-physical activity participants with type of physical activity participation serving as a moderator variable. Using Hunter and Schmidt's (2004) protocol, statistical artifacts were corrected. Results indicated that, practically speaking, those who were physically active reported lower levels of SPA than the comparison group (dcorr = -0.15; SDcorr. = 0.21). Moderator analysis generally reiterated this trend, although concerns over generalizability were noted. Results offer support for the potential bi-directionality of the relationship between physical activity and SPA; however, the direction of causality warrants additional investigation. Future consideration of the dose-response effects of physical activity on SPA, as well as the nature of exercise behavior and sport classification may help elucidate the role of physical activity contexts on SPA.

[1] Address for reprint requests and correspondence: Diane E. Mack Department of Physical Education and Kinesiology Brock University 500 Glenridge Ave St. Catharines, ON CANADA L2S 3A1 Tel: (905) 688-5550 (4360) E-mail: dmack@brocku.ca.

Social physique anxiety across physical activity contexts: A meta-analytic review Eating disorders (EDs) reflect a significant public health concern with population health data estimating lifetime prevalence of EDs ranging from 0.6 - 4.5% (Hudson, Hiripi, Pope, and Kessler, 2007). Although typically associated with adolescent girls and young adult women, eating disorders span across gender, age, race/ethnicity and socioeconomic status (Hudson et al., 2007; Striegel-Moore and Bulik, 2007). Three classifications of EDs have been identified: 1) anorexia nervosa, 2) bulimia nervosa, and 3) eating disorders not otherwise specified (EDNOS) a broadly defined heterogeneous category *(Diagnostic and Statistical Manual*; *DSM-IV*; American Psychiatric Association, 1994). Classification into ED categories is based on diagnostic criteria including body image disturbance, and extreme behaviors to control weight or shape (e.g., over- or under-control of eating behavior, excessive exercise) which often result in impaired physical health and psychosocial functioning (American Psychiatric Association, 1994; Fairburn and Harrison, 2003).

A diverse array of variables have been linked with EDs in the literature (Becker, Keel, Anderson-Fye, and Thomas, 2004; Fassino, Amianto, Gramaglia, Facchini, and Abbate Daga, 2004; Yanovski, 1993). One variable pertinent to this investigation is the association between EDs and anxiety disorders (see Swinbourne and Touyz, 2007, for a review) with social forms of anxiety identified as a central psychopathology linked to the development of EDs (Black Becker, DeViva, and Zayfert, 2004; Hinrichson, Wright, Waller, and Meyer, 2003; Kaye et al., 2004). *Social anxiety* has been identified as a marked and persistent fear of one or more situations that vary in social (e.g., meeting new people) and/or performance (e.g., public speaking, sport performance) expectations imposed on the self (American Psychiatric Association, 1994). Population health estimates identify between 24.80% and 41.30% of those with social anxiety also self-reporting an ED (Hudson et al., 2007).

Given the consistent link established between social forms of anxiety and EDs, it is hardly surprising that a number of approaches for understanding social anxiety have been advanced. Most approaches emphasize one of three antecedents: biological mechanisms; cognitions associated with how a person think about themselves and his/her social world; and interpersonal processes (Leitenberg, 1990). Self-presentational frameworks envelop both cognitive and interpersonal processes as mechanisms accounting for social anxiety by proposing that people may experience social anxiety when they are motivated to make a desired impression on others, but doubt their ability to do so (Leary and Kowalski, 1995a, 1995b; Schlenker and Leary, 1982). Social physique anxiety (SPA) represents one subtype of social anxiety embedded within self-presentational perspectives which results from the prospect or presence of negative interpersonal evaluation involving one's physique (Hart, Leary, and Rejeski, 1989).

Correlates of SPA identified have often demonstrated patterns of association with EDs. SPA has been linked to varied demographic (Berry and Howe, 2004; Mack, Strong, Kowalski, and Crocker, 2007a; Russell, 2002; Russell and Cox, 2003) and anthropometric characteristics (Greenleaf, 2004; Hausenblas and Fallon, 2002; Russell, 2002; Russell and Cox, 2003). Cognitive and perceptual correlates of SPA include (but are not limited to): body dissatisfaction and drive for thinness (Krane, Stiles-Shipley, Waldron, and Michalenok, 2001; Thompson and Chad, 2002), motivational processes including social anxiety, fear of negative evaluation and public self-consciousness (Martin and Leary, 2001; Carron and Prapavessis, 1997), maladaptive or neurotic perfectionism (Haase, Prapavessis, and Owens, 2002; Krane et al., 2001), and social comparison (Thornton and Maurice, 1997). Behavioral variables have also been associated with SPA including body checking behaviours (e.g., examining one's reflection in glass; Haase, Mountford, and Waller, 2007), orthorexia (Eriksson, Biagi, Marklund and Lindgren, 2007) and eating behaviors (Cox, Lantz, and Mayhew, 1997). While rarely examined in those diagnosed with EDs, SPA has been found to differentiate females currently in-treatment for EDs to those not in-treatment, with higher scores for the former found on the measure of SPA (Mack, Strong, Kowalski, and Crocker, 2007b).

Physical Activity and EDs

The biological and psychological benefits conferred by physical activity for many chronic and acute health conditions are well documented (Bouchard, Blair, and Haskell, 2007). Nevertheless, physical activity has been implicated in the development and maintenance of EDs with prevalence estimates of excessive exercise ranging from 20.2% - 54.5% depending on ED classification (Shroff et al., 2006). Athletes report more (albeit a weak effect) eating disordered symptoms than non-athletes (Hausenblas and Carron, 1999) with the physique salient nature of the sport moderating this relationship as those involved in non-physique salient sports (e.g., ball sports) reported lower levels of ED symptoms than non-athletes. While research has demonstrated the beneficial effects of exercise in terms of possible treatment for EDs (Pendleton, Goodrick, Poston, Reeves, and Foreyt, 2002; Sundgot-Borgen, Rosenvinge, Bahr, and Schneider, 2002), current recommendations do not include physical activity an adjunctive ED treatment strategy (Hausenblas, Cook, and Chittester, 2008).

Narrative reviews and empirical evidence have implicated sport and exercise as contexts which emphasize physical salience for social and performance outcomes (Crocker, Sabiston, Forrester, Kowalski, and McDonough, 2003; Crocker, Synder, Kowalski, and Hoar, 2000; Hausenblas, Brewer, and Van Raalte, 2004; Gammage, Martin Ginis, and Hall, 2004). Therefore, it is possible that athletes/exercisers may report higher levels of SPA than individuals not involved in physical activity contexts due to the increased emphasis on the physique for performance outcomes embedded within these contexts. With this in mind, the influence of physical activity contexts on SPA has been investigated with inconsistent findings (e.g., Berry and Howe, 2004; Cox, Lantz, and Mayhew, 1997; Haase and Prapavessis, 2001; Hausenblas and Mack, 1999; Martin Ginis, Prapavessis, and Lindwall, 2007) that offer little clarification as to the role of variation in physical activity contexts on SPA. Consequently, the relative impact of physical activity contexts on SPA remains a topic for continued investigation to determine the underlying factors contributing to variation in anxiety associated with the physique.

The present investigation contributes to existing literature through its use of meta-analytic techniques to address the influence of physical activity contexts on SPA. Inconsistent and often contradictory findings as to whether participation in sport or physical activity leads to elevated levels of SPA impedes theory development and delays the advancement of knowledge. Meta-analyses refer to "…the statistical analysis of a large collection of analysis results from individual studies for the purpose of integrating the findings" (Glass, 1976, p.3). Although criticisms of this approach to reviewing evidence have been identified (Davies and Crombie, 2003), meta-analyses can provide a more precise estimate of treatment effects, may explain heterogeneity between the results of individual studies, increase statistical power, and offers one avenue towards resolving uncertainty (Egger and Davey Smith, 1997).

The main purpose of the present study was to synthesize the evidence attesting to the role played by physical activity contexts in the tendency to report variation in SPA. Given the current conceptualization of SPA as a trait, it was hypothesized that no differences in SPA across physical activity and more general contexts would be found. A secondary aim was to examine the influence of the type of physical activity participation (i.e., sport and exercise) as a moderator of SPA between those participating in physical activity and those not identified as participants.[2] Given inconsistent conclusions derived from existing reviews (Hausenblas et al., 2004; Martin Ginis et al., 2007), no *a priori* hypotheses were advanced.

METHOD

Selection of the Data

Literature searches were completed to identify studies that recorded the use of the Social Physique Anxiety Scale (SPAS; Hart et al., 1989) in various groups and situations. The SPAS is a multi-item inventory assessing an individuals' dispositional tendency to experience elevated anxiety when they perceive their physique to be evaluated by others in social contexts. Respondents rate the extent to which each item is characteristics of them across a 5-point Likert response scale with higher scores reflective of greater anxiety associated with physique evaluation in social contexts. While controversy exists regarding the psychometric properties of SPAS scores (Eklund, 1998; Martin et al., 1997; Haggar et al., 2007), the SPAS remains the instrument of choice among sport and exercise psychology researchers interested in examining SPA. Literature searches did not extend prior to the publication date (i.e., 1989) of the SPAS and were obtained through two processes--computer and manual searches. Computer searches included exhaustive examination of the following databases: Academic Search Premier, MEDLINE, PsychLIT, PsychInfo, SPORTDISCUS, and ERIC. Keywords entered for the computer searches were social physique anxiety, SPA, SPAS, social anxiety, appearance anxiety, impression management, and self-presentation.

Manual searches involved obtaining articles from reference lists contained in empirical studies and narrative reviews identified through the computer search. In addition, a hand search of select journals (those where a significant number of relevant articles were found) was conducted. Finally, supplement volumes of published abstracts from relevant professional meetings since 1989 (e.g., North American Society for the Psychology of Physical Activity and Sport) were reviewed for relevant content. Six authors were contacted where information was missing for the calculation of effect sizes, three of whom provided the requested data.

---

[2] Although other demographic, design, and measurement moderator variables were originally hypothesized to influence SPA in different physical activity settings, their influence was not tested.

Data Coding

Each study obtained was coded for study characteristics and potential moderators. Clear and detailed coding rules were generated based on recommendations advocated by Hunter and Schmidt (2004) to limit concerns over ambiguity and reliability during the process of coding the data. Two reviewers with expertise in meta-analytic investigations and knowledge of the self-presentation literature in sport and exercise reviewed the coding form for clarity and comprehensiveness. Based on their recommendations, modifications to the coding form (e.g., wording) were made.[3] Two trained coders (neither of the reviewers) independently coded all studies selected for inclusion with discrepancies discussed and consensus reached after deliberation.

From the original search, 150 articles that included the use of the SPAS were independently coded. The final database included 16 studies ($N = 3595$) of the initial search that directly addressed the primary research question. To be included, studies had to incorporate participants that were physically active as well as a comparison group. Individual studies with multiple effect sizes were averaged such that each study that met inclusion criteria contributed one ES to the overall meta-analysis (Hunter and Schmidt, 2004).

Data Analysis

Calculating effect sizes. Data were analyzed employing the Hunter and Schmidt (2000; 2004) meta-analytic method. Consistent with this approach, a random effects model was adopted which corrects *ES* estimates for the attenuating effect of errors (e.g., unreliability) and provides an estimate of the amount of *ES* variance due to artifacts such as sampling error. As recommended by Hunter and Schmidt (2004), when the internal consistency reliability of test scores from the SPAS was not reported, the internal consistency estimate from the oringial development and item validation study was used.[4]

Standardized mean difference (Cohen's d). For between-subjects designs, athletes/exercisers were compared to a comparison group. Mean values and pooled standard deviations (SD_{pooled}) were used to calculate *ES*s resulting in a Cohen's *d* statistic (Cohen, 1977). For a within subjects design, the measure of variability was based on the standard deviation of the difference score rather than the SD_{pooled}. For within-subject designs, the following within-subjects *ES*s were calculated: pre-post athlete/exerciser, pre-post comparison, pre-athlete/exerciser vs. pre-comparison and post-athlete/exerciser vs. post-comparison. For mixed methods study designs, both within and between subjects *ES*s were calculated and the average entered to maintain statistical independence (Hunter and Schmidt,

---

[3] The coding sheet is available from the first author upon request.

[4] Internal consistency reliability estimates vary based on several characteristics and coefficient α (Cronbach, 1951) is sensitive to the number of items (Crocker and Algina, 1980). Research adopting the SPAS remains ambiguous with regards to the number of items to be included in the instrument (Hart et al., 1989; Martin et al., 1997; Haggar et al., 2007). Consistent with Hunter and Schmidt (2004), when estimates of internal consistency reliability were not reported in the primary source, imputation of estimates from the initial validation study are recommended. As such, where coefficient α was not reported in the primary sources, the alpha coefficient associated with the validation study based on the number of items was inserted (e.g., Hart et al., 1989; 12-item SPAS $\alpha = .90$).

2004). Consistent with Cohen (1969, 1992), *ES* (*d*) values of 0.20, 0.50, and 0.80 were interpreted as "small", "medium", and "large" respectively.

Bias in effect size. The effect size is subject to a statistical phenomenon known as bias which reflects the discrepancy between the average sample effect size and the population effect size (Hunter and Schmidt, 2004). For sample sizes greater than 20, the bias is trivial in magnitude (Hunter and Schmidt, 2004), however given criticisms levelled against meta-analyses, the correction for small sample size was employed.

Confidence and credibility intervals. As part of the analysis, 95% confidence intervals and 80% credibility intervals were computed. A confidence interval gives an estimated bandwidth of potential population values that are reasonable given the observed value. The confidence interval examines the extent to which a finding may be due to sampling error, with wider intervals which span zero indicating definitive conclusions cannot be derived. A confidence interval that includes zero reflects that the corrected *ES* was not significantly different from zero (i.e., the null). A confidence interval that does not include zero indicates that the mean corrected *ES* was significantly different from zero.

Credibility intervals are independent of sampling error and represent an index that the true relationship generalizes across samples and situations. If the lower 80% credibility value is greater than zero, confidence that a relationship generalizes across situations examined in the study can be concluded. However, if the credibility interval includes zero, another variable is believed to moderate the effect (Whitener, 1990), especially when the corrected *SD* (SD_{corr}) is large relative to the corrected *d* (d_{corr}).

Moderator analysis. Appropriate *ES* subgroups (i.e., athletes or exercisers *vs* non-physical activity participants) were tested as a portion of the analysis in this study. Moderators were explored by examining differences between d_{corr} values and changes in the SD_{corr} across moderator subgroupings (Hunter and Schmidt, 2004). One indication of the possible presence of a moderator is the difference in mean effect size estimates between subsets. A second indicator is based on a reduction in the variance in SD_{corr} compared to the overall SD_{corr}. The reduction in SD_{corr} was afforded more attention when the number of studies and sample size was relatively equal across subsets. When unequal, attention to the difference in mean effect sizes was undertaken (Hunter and Schmidt, 2004). Finally, the 80% CrI values were used to determine the likelihood that the effect generalized across situations, or to suggest the presence of additional unexamined moderators.

File drawer. A file drawer analysis provides a measure of certainty that the *ES* was not caused by publication bias. This calculation identified the number of unreported studies with null findings there would have to be such that the mean effect size was not significantly different from zero. The formula employed was based on recommendations by Orwin (1983).

Meta-analyses. The following statistics were computed: total sample size (*N*), number of *ES*s (*K*), mean sample-size weighted observed (d_{obs}), d_{obs} 95% confidence interval (95% CI), mean sample-size weighted corrected *ES* (d_{corr}), corrected standard deviation (SD_{corr}), residual standard deviation (SD_{res}), percent of d_{obs} variance due to sampling error (%*VARe*), 80% credibility interval (80% CrI), and d_{corr} fail-safe *N* (d_{fs}). The d_{corr} fail-safe *N* estimates the number of unlocated *ES*s with null results needed to reduce d_{corr} to the lowest critical *ES* considered practically or theoretically important (Hunter and Schmidt, 2004). However, when the d_{corr} was less than an *ES* deemed theoretically important (i.e., $ES < 0.20$), then the fail-safe *N* was calculated to examine the number of unlocated *ES*s with a d_{corr} of 0.40 to increase the current *ES* up to 0.20. The critical *ES* was set at 0.2, the value typically associated with a small effect. The d_{corr} and SD_{corr} were interpreted as best estimates of the population parameters.

RESULTS

Primary Sources: Study Characteristics

Data were collected from studies ($N = 16$) identified using our inclusion/exclusion criteria ranged from 1996 and 2007. Age was reported in 87.50% (n = 14) of the included studies with a mean age of 21.18 years (SD = 4.10). Gender was reported in 93.75% (n = 15) studies, where male participants comprised 12.50% (n = 2), female participants 43.75% (n = 7), and studies that included both male and female participants 37.50% (n = 6). BMI was reported in 31.25% (n = 5) of the studies (M = 23.23kg/m^2; SD = 3.60 kg/m^2). Race/ethnicity was reported in 18.75% (n = 3) of studies, and in all cases participants were of 'mixed' origin. Publication type was identified with 93.75% (n = 15) of primary sources appearing in peer-reviewed journals, and 6.25% (n = 1) included as an unpublished thesis. Study design was considered with 62.50% (n = 10) classified as non-experimental, 31.25% (n = 5) quasi-experimental, and 6.25% (n = 1) adopting a randomized experimental design.[5] Non-probability based sampling techniques were employed in all studies, with convenience 56.20% (n = 9) and purposive 43.80% (n = 7) techniques recorded in the studies included for review. Of the studies examining athletes, sport classification was identified with 33.30% (n = 2) of the participants competing in a physique-salient sport, and 66.70% (n = 4) represented heterogeneous sporting classifications. In terms of the exercisers, 31.25% (n = 5) of the studies reported the exercise setting in which they were engaged (all public contexts), 18.80% (n = 3) reported the gender composition [66.70% (n = 2) same-gender and 33.30% (n = 1) mixed-gender], and 25.00% (n = 4) reported the public *vs.* private nature of the setting (all group setting). Frequency of exercise with respect to number of sessions engaged in per week was reported in 18.75% (n = 3) studies. With regards to the SPAS, 50.00% (n = 5) used the 12-item scale, 31.25% (n = 5) used the 9-item, and 18.75% (n = 3) used a version other than the 12- or 9-item SPAS.

Overall Meta-Analytic Results

An examination of descriptive statistics revealed that participants, regardless of physical activity classification, reported moderate levels of SPA. Across the 5-point Likert response scale those classified as physically active reported a mean score of 2.84 (SD = 0.75; Range = 2.32 to 3.27). Those in the comparison group reported on average SPA scores of 3.05 (SD = 0.78; Range = 2.59 to 3.51). Results of the overall analysis showed that differences between physical activity participants and the comparison group were quite small ($d_{corr} = -0.15$; $SD_{corr} = 0.21$; see Table 1) indicative of a 0.15 SD difference in SPA between those who were physically active compared to those in the comparison group.

---

[5] The classification of designs was based on the work of Trochim (2001) along with Pedhauzer and Pedhauzer Schmelkin (1991).

Table 1. Overall meta-analysis of effect and moderator analysis for physical activity participation on social physique anxiety

Analysis	N	K	d_{obs}	95% CI	d_{corr}	SD_{corr}	SD_{res}	%Var$_e$	80% CrI	d_{fs}
Overall	3595	16	-.136	-.430 to .158	-.148	.214	.143	44.85	-.351 to .055	4.0
Moderator*										
Type of PA										
Sport	1113	6	-.228	-.553 to -.097	-.242	.236	.157	44.20	-.468 to -.017	1.0
Exercise	2609	12	-.086	-.360 to .188	-.095	.149	.209	48.97	-.286 to .096	10.0

Note: N, total sample size; K, number of ESs; d_{obs}, mean sample-size weighted observed ES; 95% CI, d_{obs} 95% confidence interval; d_{corr}, mean sample-size weighted corrected ES; SD_{corr}, sample-size weighted corrected standard deviation; SD_{res}, residual standard deviation; %Var$_e$, percent of d_{obs} variance due to sampling and measurement error; 80% CrI, 80% credibility interval; d_{fs}, d_{corr} fail-safe N with $d_{critical}$ = .20, [$d_{unlocated}$ = .00 for d_{corr} values above .20 and $d_{unlocated}$ = .40 for d_{corr} values below .20]. Boldface entries are best estimates of the population mean ES. *The reporting of sample sizes differ between the overall and moderator analysis as two primary sources included athletes *vs* non-physical activity participants and exercisers *vs*.non-physical activity participants. As such, the comparison groups (i.e., non physical activity participants) were included twice in the moderator analysis.

The 95% CI spanned zero (-0.35 to 0.06). The large SD_{corr} and %VAR$_e$ below 75% (Hunter and Schmidt, 2004) suggested the presence of potential moderators. The 80% CrI included zero, which suggests that the effects of physical activity context on SPA may not generalize. The calculated fail-safe N of 4.0 does not imply a particularly strong tolerance to availability bias as four additional studies with a d_{corr} of 0.40 would have to be found and included in the present investigation to increase d_{corr} values to 0.20.

Moderator Analysis

Type of physical activity. The type of physical activity (i.e., athletes *vs*. exercisers) was investigated as a plausible moderator of the influence of physical activity on SPA. Descriptive statistics demonstrated slightly higher mean SPA values for athletes (M = 2.90; SD = 0.59) compared to exercisers (M = 2.82; SD = 0.80). Athletes reported lower levels of SPA than their comparison group (d_{corr} = -0.24, SD_{corr} = 0.24) as did exercisers with their respective comparison group (d_{corr} = -0.10, SD_{corr} = 0.15). Interpretation of the 95% CI demonstrated statistically significant findings for the athletes and the 80% CrI did not cross zero suggestive of a relationship that would generalize to similar situations. The magnitude of difference between exercisers and their comparison group was not statistically significant (i.e., the upper and lower bound of the 95% CI assumed 0). For exercisers, the 80% CrI crossed zero suggesting that additional (untested) moderators may influence this effect (Whitener, 1990). Fail-safe N values were not suggestive of good tolerance of availability bias for the athlete subsample as one study with a $d_{corr} = 0.00$ would be necessary to lower the reported value to $d_{corr} = 0.20$. Ten studies comparing exercisers to non-physically active samples with $d_{corr} = 0.40$ would need to be added to increase the reported d_{corr} value to the critical value of 0.20

DISCUSSION

EDs represent a meaningful public health concern (Hudson et al., 2007) independent of their deleterious effect on physical and psychiatric health (Chavez and Insel, 2007). Developing an enriched understanding of ED etiology, in conjunction with known effective treatments represent meaningful avenues for applied health research. Physical activity has been linked with condition onset and maintenance (Schroff et al., 2006) and excessive exercise following treatment release has been implicated in condition relapse (Carter, Blackmore, Sutandar-Pinnick, and Woodside, 2004). The contribution of the present investigation to the available literature was to synthesize the role afforded physical activity contexts in the prevalence of body-related anxiety reported in conjunction with EDs and associated symptomology (Erikkson et al., 2007; Mack et al., 2007b). SPA represents an important sub-type of social anxiety specific to the body that co-exists with EDs (Swinbourne and Touyze, 2007).

Results of this investigation suggest that, in general, those who were physically active reported lower levels of SPA than the comparison group. This observation is consistent with existing literature (Berry and Howe, 2004; Hausenblas and Mack, 1999) and corroborates previous findings on adolescent samples that physical activity is not strongly endorsed as a strategy to cope with SPA (Kowalski, Mack, Crocker, Niefer, and Fleming, 2006; Sabiston, Sedgwick, Crocker, Kowalski, and Mack, 2007). Interpretation of the 95% CI suggest that the actual influence of physical activity contexts on SPA spans zero suggestive that the true effect of physical activity context may result in decreased, increased, or no influence on SPA compared to non-physical activity contexts. The overall effect should be interpreted with caution as the overall *ES* was based on sixteen primary studies, suggestive of the possibility of second-order sampling error emanating from variation in effect sizes across primary sources that demonstrate particular influence on the deviation surrounding the *ES* (Hunter and Schmidt, 2004). The results do offer some support for the bi-directionality of the relationship between physical activity and SPA; however, a causal interpretation cannot be imposed on these findings and the motivational significance of SPA remains open for further scrutiny as an architectural element of behavioral change.

The amount of variance accounted for within meta-analytic investigations reflects one interpretation of its importance (Hunter and Schmidt, 2004). However, small effects (as noted in the present study) may have important implications in a practical context, and may be quite important theoretically (Bland and Altman, 1995; Prentice and Miller, 1992). As such, continued exploration into the role of the physical activity contexts on SPA is encouraged to elucidate the self-presentational mechanisms contributing to SPA. One direction for further inquiry concerns the nature of research designs and the type of data collected in studies examining the influence of physical activity contexts on SPA. Few studies have embraced rigorous designs (e.g., randomized vs. cross-sectional/non-experimental) or explored the potential for qualitative approaches in this area (e.g., Sabiston et al., 2007) to tease out the causal influence of physical activity contexts on SPA. Finally, the measurement of SPA may present a limiting factor as interpretation of the $\%VAR_e$ suggests that over 44% of the variance d_{obs} was due to sampling and measurement error. Although primarily linked to sampling error (Koslowsky and Sagie, 1994), the measurement error implications cannot be ignored. The instrument designed to assess SPA has undergone considerable scrutiny (Martin et al., 1997; Motl and Conroy, 2000; Haggar et al., 2007) and is still not without controversy (Eklund, 1998).

The manner in which SPA was experienced and the criteria used to classify participants in the primary sources warrants further consideration to explain the findings of the present investigation. The distributional properties of scores derived from the SPAS regardless of physical activity classification, suggest low- to- moderate levels of SPA which may explain the small differences between groups. Decisions applied to the classification of participants as non-physically active have proven to be vexing issues in health psychology (Bennett, Winter-Stone, Nail, and Scherer, 2006; Welk, 2002) and may also have influenced results. The present investigation relied on classification terms (i.e., exerciser vs. non-exerciser) identified in the primary source, however concerns may be raised over classification strategies employed (e.g., Bowden, Rust, Dunsmore, and Briggs, 2005). Future investigations should give careful consideration to the criteria used to categorize individuals into active or inactive groups to reduce further inconsistency that can obfuscate important theoretical and applied developments (Forscher, 1966).

Physical activity participation was dichotomized into sport or exercise to test for the moderating effects of context with differences noted. While both athletes and exercisers report lower levels of SPA than their comparison groups, the magnitude, and strength of conclusions emanating from these findings differed. The lower *ES* value reported for the exercise moderator analysis may have been influenced by the conceptualization of an "exerciser" in the primary source. Participants were classified as exercisers regardless of the mode of physical activity engaged in, how long, or how often exercise was undertaken. Conversely, those comprising the athlete sub-sample competed at relatively high levels suggestive of greater physical activity behavior overall. Exercise behavior, based on the above considerations, may be a factor in explaining difference in mean *ES* values between physical activity participants classified as exercise or athletes and their respective comparison groups. The difference in magnitude of the reported *ES*s may be somewhat misleading as consideration of descriptive statistics demonstrates that those classified as exercisers reported lower SPA mean scores (albeit greater dispersion surrounding the mean) than those classified as athletes. As such, reported differences in *ES* values may be a function of the differences in dispersion noted, or from descriptive statistics on the measure of SPA derived from the comparison group as opposed to the physical activity context group.

The results of this investigation speak to the restricted nature of the studies that have been conducted investigating SPA in different physical activity contexts and the resultant need for more research. Future research should attempt to determine in which situations the overall context-SPA effect would re-occur, and whether this effect is apparent in other physically active populations (i.e., diverse age groups, participants with a BMI level outside of the 'normal' range, etc). Additional longitudinal research examining the bi-directionality of causal flow between SPA and physical activity would clarify if lower levels of SPA lead individuals' to engage in (or avoid) physical activity participation. Efforts in this regard have been limited, with Crocker, Sabiston, Kowalski, McDonough, and Kowalski (2007) providing preliminary evidence to demonstrate the physical activity was generally independent from SPA across three years in a sample of adolescent females. The relative variability of SPA may also be of interest as Crocker et al. (2007) demonstrated considerable stability in test scores derived from the SPAS. Given the conceptualization of SPA as a trait, meaningful changes to anxiety associated with physique evaluation may demonstrate considerable resistance to varied personal (e.g., changes in physical self-perceptions) and environmental (e.g., engaging in physical activity behavior) factors which deserve further study. Finally, the dose-response effects of physical activity on the experience of SPA are minimally understood. For example, does more intense physical activity provide different results from lower intensity exercise? Or does SPA differ commensurate with those who engage in physical activity at levels commensurate with public health guidelines in comparison to those who do not?

Results of cross-sectional (Sundgot-Borgen et al., 2002) and randomized designs (Pendleton et al., 2002) have demonstrated the beneficial effect of physical activity interventions, in isolation and in combination, with more recognized forms of treatment (e.g., cognitive behavior therapy for EDs). Further research should consider the complementary nature of physical activity with established strategies to reduce the influence of social forms of anxiety associated with EDs. Health practitioners will need to decide whether the promotion of physical activity can be offered and monitored without compromising core aspects of treatment and sequenced such that exercise interventions can be targeted to relevant personal and treatment goals. Finally, it is important to remember that exercise has a wide variety of health benefits outside the realm of EDs (Bouchard et al., 2007) which may be of benefit to more broadly defined physical and mental health goals.

Despite the limitations presented earlier, a meta-analysis based on a conceptual framework can provide useful insights such as global estimates of effect and the illustration of moderators using procedures that overcome traditional problems associated with narrative reviews (Hunter and Schmidt, 2004). Overall, results indicate that those who are physically active do report lower levels of SPA than the comparison group; however, the magnitude of the ES is small. Furthermore although in the same direction, the effects of SPA in physical activity settings seem to be more substantial when physical activity is introduced through sport-based as opposed to an exercise-based movement. However future research is deemed necessary to confirm the robustness of meta-analytic findings.

AUTHORS' NOTE

The first and second authors were supported by grants from the Social Sciences and Humanities Research Council of Canada during the preparation of this manuscript. This manuscript represents a portion of a Master of Arts thesis conducted by the third author while under direction of the primary investigator. The fourth author was a graduate student during data collection and was trained in meta-analytic techniques.

ACKNOWLEDGEMENTS

The authors would like to extend their appreciation to A. V. Carron and S. M. Burke for their thoughtful review of the coding sheet used in the present investigation.

REFERENCES

American Psychiatric Association (1994). *Diagnostic and statistical manual of mental disorders* (4th ed.). Washington, DC: Author.

¥Bartlewski, P. P., Van Raalte, J. L., and Brewer, B. W. (1996). Effects of aerobic exercise on the social physique anxiety and body esteem of female college students. *Women in Sport and Physical Activity Journal, 5*, 49-62.

Becker A. E., Keel, P., Anderson-Fye, E. P., and Thomas, J. J. (2004). Genes and/or jeans?: Genetic and socio-cultural contributions to risk for eating disorders. *Journal of Addictive Disorders, 23*, 81-103.

Bennett, J. A., Winter-Stone, K., Nail, L., and Scherer, J. (2006). Definitions of sedentary in physical activity intervention trials: A summary of the literature. *Journal of Aging and Physical Activity, 14*, 456-477.

¥Berry, T. R. and Howe, B. L. (2004). Effects of health-based and appearance-based exercise advertising on exercise attitudes, social physique anxiety and self-presentation in an exercise setting. *Social Behavior and Personality, 32*, 1-12.

Black Becker, C., DeViva, J., and Zayfert, C. (2004). Eating disorder symptoms among female anxiety disorder patients in clinical practice: The importance of co-morbidity assessment. *Journal of Anxiety Disorders, 18*, 255-275.

Bland, D. G., and Altman, J. M., (1995). Absence of evidence is not evidence of absence. *British Medical Journal, 311,* 485.

Bouchard C., Blair, S. N., and Haskell, W. L. (2007). *Physical activity and health.* Champaign, IL: Human Kinetics.

¥Bowden, R. G., Rust, D. M., Dunsmore, S., and Briggs, J. (2005). Changes in social physique anxiety during 16-week physical activity courses. *Psychological Reports, 96,* 690-692.

¥Burke, S. M., Carron, A. V., and Eys, M. A. (2006). Physical activity context: Preferences of university students. *Psychology of Sport and Exercise, 7,* 1-13.

Bulik, C. M. (2003). Anxiety, depression and eating disorders. In J. Treasure, U. Schmidt, and E. van Furth (Eds.), *Handbook of eating disorders* (pp. 193-198). Chichester, UK: Wiley.

Carron, A. V., and Prapavessis, H. (1997). Self-presentation and group influence. *Small Group Research, 28,* 500-516.

Carter, J. C., Blackmore, E., Sutandar-Pinnok, K., and Woodside, D. B. (2004). Relapse in anorexia nervosa: A survival analysis. *Psychological Medicine, 34*, 671-679.

Chavez, M., and Insel, T. R. (2007). Eating disorders: National Institute of Mental Health's Perspective. *American Psychologist, 62,* 159-166.

Cohen, J. (1992). Quantitative methods in psychology: A power primer. *Psychological Bulletin, 112*, 155-159.

Cohen, J. (1977). *Statistical power analysis for the behavioral sciences* (Rev.ed.). New York: Academic Press

Cohen, J. (1969). *Statistical power analysis for the behavioural sciences*. New York: Academic Press.

¥Cox, L. M., Lantz, C. D., and Mayhew, J. L. (1997). The role of social physique anxiety and other variables in predicting eating behaviors in college students. *International Journal of Sport Nutrition, 7*, 310-317.

Crocker, L., and Algina, J. (1986). *Introduction to classical and modern test theory.* New York: Harcourt Brace Jovanovich College Publishers.

Cronbach, L. J. (1951). Coefficient alpha and the internal structure of tests. *Psychometrika. 16*, 297-334.

Crocker, P. R. E., Sabiston, C. M., Kowalski, K. C., McDonough, M. H., and Kowalski, N. C. (2007). Longitudinal assessment of the relationship between physical self-concept and health related behavior and emotion in adolescent girls. *Journal of Applied Sport Psychology, 18*, 185-200.

Crocker, P. R. E., Sabiston, C., Forrester, S., Kowalski, N. C. Kowalski, K. C., and McDonough, M. (2003). Predicting change in physical activity, dietary restraint, and physique anxiety in adolescent girls: Examining covariance in physical self-perceptions. *Canadian Journal of Public Health, 94*, 332-337.

Crocker, P. R. E. and Synder, J., Kowalski, K. C., and Hoar, S. (2000). Don't let me be fat or physically incompetent! The relationship between physical self-concept and social physique anxiety in Canadian high performance female adolescent athletes. *AVANTE, 6*, 1-8.

Davies, H. T. O., and Crombie, I. K. (2003). *What is a meta-analysis?* Newmarket: Hayward Medical Communications.

Egger, M., and Davey Smith G. (1997). Meta-analysis: Potentials and promise. *British Medical Journal, 315*, 1371-1374.

Eklund, R. C. (1998). With regard to the Social Physique Anxiety Scale (Conceptually Speaking). *Journal of Sport and Exercise Psychology, 20*, 225-227.

¥Erikkson, L., Baigl, A., Marklund, B., and Lindgren, E. C. (2007). Social physique anxiety and sociocultural attitudes toward appearance impact on orthorexia test in fitness participants. *Scandinavian Journal of Medicine and Science in Sports*. Available on-line at doi:10.1111/j.1600-0838.2007.00723.x

Fairburn, C. G., and Harrison, P. J. (2003). Eating disorders. *The Lancet, 36,* 407-416.Fassino, S., Amianto, F., Gramaglia, C., Faccini, F., and Abbate Daga, G. (2004). Temperament and character in eating disorders: ten years of studies. *European Journal of Eating Disorders, 9*, 81-90.

¥Finkenberg, M. E., DiNucci, J. M., McCune, S. L., Chenette, T., and McCoy, P. (1998). Commitment to physical activity and anxiety about physique among college women. *Perceptual and Motor Skills, 87,* 1393-1394.

Forscher, B. K. (1966). Chaos in the brickyard. *Science, 142*, 3590.

Gammage, K. L., Martin Ginis, K. A., and Hall, C. R. (2004). Self-presentational efficacy expectancy: Its influence on anxiety in an exercise context. *Journal of Sport and Exercise Psychology, 26*, 179-190.

Glass, G. V. (1976). Primary, secondary and meta-analysis of research. *Educational Researcher, 5*, 3-8.

Godart, N., Falment, M., Curt, F., Perdereau, F., Lang, F., Venisse, J. L., Halfon, O., Bizaouard, P., Loas, G., Corcos M., Jeammet, P., and Fermanian, J. (2003). Anxiety disorders in subjects seeking treatment for eating disorders: A DSM-IV controlled study. *Psychiatric Research, 117*, 245-258.

Greenleaf, C. (2004). Weight pressures and social physique anxiety among collegiate synchronized skaters. *Journal of Sport Behavior, 27*, 260-277.

¥Grise, S. M. (1997). *The relationship between perceived sport competence, body attractiveness, physical self-worth, and social physique anxiety to girls' physical activity participation.* Unpublished Master of Arts thesis, McGill University.

Haase, A., Mountford, V., and Waller G. (2007). Understanding the link between body checking cognitions and behaviors: The role of social physique anxiety. *International Journal of Eating Disorders, 40,* 241-246.Haase, A. M., Prapavessis, H., and Owens, R. G. (2002). Perfectionism, social physique anxiety and disordered eating: a comparison of male and female elite athletes. *Psychology of Sport and Exercise, 3,* 209-222.¥Haase A. M., and Prapavessis H. (2001). Social physique anxiety and eating attitudes in female athletic and non-athletic groups. *Journal of Medicine and Science in Sport, 4*, 396-405.Hagger, M. S., Aşçı, F. H., Lindwall, M., Hein, V., Mülazımoğlu-Ballı, O., Tarrant, M., Ruiz, Y. P., and Sell, V. (2007). Cross-cultural validity and measurement invariance of the social physique anxiety scale in five European nations. *Scandianavian Journal of Medicine and Science in Sports*, 17, 709-719.

Hart, E. A., Leary, M. R., and Rejeski, W. J. (1989). The measurement of social physique anxiety. *Journal of Sport and Exercise Psychology, 11,* 94-104.

Hausenblas, H. A., Cook, B. J., and Chittester, N. I. (2008). Can exercise treat eating disorders? *Exercise and Sport Science Reviews, 36*, 43-47.

Hausenblas, H. A., Brewer, B. W., and Van Raalte, J. L. (2004). Self-presentation and exercise. *Journal of Applied Sport Psychology, 16,* 3-18.

Hausenblas, H. A., and Carron, A. V. (1999). Eating disorder indices and athletes: An integration. *Journal of Sport and Exercise Psychology, 21*, 230-258.

Hausenblas, H. A., and Fallon, E. A. (2002). Relationship among body image, exercise behavior, and exercise dependence symptoms. *International Journal of Eating Disorders, 32*, 179-185.

¥Hausenblas, H. A. and Mack, D. E. (1999). Social physique anxiety and eating disorder correlates among female athletic and nonathletic populations. *Journal of Sport Behavior, 22*, 502-514.

Hinrichson, H., Wright, F., Waller, G., and Meyer, C. (2003). Social anxiety and coping strategies in eating disorders. *Eating Behaviors, 4,* 117-126.

Hudson, J. I., Hiripi, E., Pope, H. G., and Kessler, R. C. (2007). The prevalence and correlates of eating disorders in the National Comorbidity Survey Replication. *Biological Psychiatry, 61*, 348-358.

Hunter, J. E., and Schmidt, F. L. (2004). *Methods of meta-analysis: Correcting error and bias in research findings: 2nd Edition.* Newbury Park: Sage Publications.

Hunter, J. E., and Schmidt, F. L. (2000). Fixed effects vs. random effects meta analysis models: Implications for cumulative knowledge in Psychology. *International Journal of Selection and Assessment, 8*, 275-292.

Kaye, W., Bulik, C., Thorton, L., Barbarich. N., Masers, K., and the Price Foundation Collaborative Group (2004). Co-morbidity of anxiety disorders with Anorexia and Bulimia Nervosa. *The American Journal of Psychiatry, 161*, 2215-2221.

Kowlowsky, M., and Sagie, A. (1994). Component of artifactual variance in meta-analytic research. *Personnel Psychology, 47*, 561-574.

Krane, V., Stiles-Shipley, J. A., Waldron, J., Michalenok, J. (2001). Relationships among body satisfaction, social physique anxiety, and eating behaviors in female athletes and exercisers. *Journal of Sport Behavior, 24,* 247-264.

Kowalski, K. C., Mack, D. E., Crocker, P. R. E., Niefer, C. B., and Fleming, T. L. (2006). Coping with social physique anxiety in adolescence. *Journal of Adolescent Health, 39*, 275.e9-275.e16.

Leary, M. R., and Kowalski, R. M. (1995a). *Social anxiety.* New York: Guilford.

Leary, M. R., and Kowalski, R. M. (1995b). The self-presentational model of social phobia.In R. G. Heimberg, M. R. Liebowitz, D. A. Hope, and F. R. Schneier (Eds.), *Social phobia: Diagnosis, assessment, and treatment.* New York: Guilford.

Leary, M. R. (1992). Self-presentational processes in exercise and sport. *Journal of Sport and Exercise Psychology, 14,* 339-351.

Leitenberg, H. (1990). *Handbook of social and evaluation anxiety.* New York: Plenum Press

¥Lindwall, M., and Lindgren, E. (2005). The effects of a 6-month exercise intervention programme on physical self-perceptions and social physique anxiety in non-physically active adolescent Swedish girls. *Psychology of Sport and Exercise, 6,* 643-658.

Mack, D. E., Strong, H. A., Kowalski, K. C., and Crocker, P. R. E. (2007a). Does friendship matter? An examination of social physique anxiety in adolescence. *Journal of Applied Social Psychology, 37,* 1248-1264.

Mack, D. E., Strong, H. A., Kowalski, K. C., and Crocker, P. R. E (2007b). Self-presentational motives in eating disordered behavior: A known groups differences approach. *Eating Behaviors. 8,* 98-105.

Martin Ginis, K. A., Lindwall, M., and Prapavessis, H. (2007). Who cares what other people think? Self-presentation in sport and exercise. In G. Tenenbaum and R. Eklund (Eds.) *Handbook of Sport Psychology*, (3rd ed., pp. 136–157). New York: Wiley.

¥Martin Ginis, K. A., Eng, J. J., Arbour, K. P., Hartman, J. W., and Phillips, S. M. (2005). Mind over muscle? Sex differences in the relationship between body image change and subjective and objective physical changes following a 12-week strength-training program. *Body Image, 2,* 363-372.

Martin, K. A., and Leary, M. R. (2001). Self-presentational determinants of health risk behavior among college freshmen. *Psychology and Health, 16*, 17 –27

Martin, K. A., Rejeski, W. J., Leary, M. R., McAuley, E., and Bane, S. (1997). Is the social physique anxiety scale really multidimensional? Conceptual and statistical arguments for a unidimensional model. *Journal of Sport and Exercise Psychology, 19,* 360-368.

Motl, R. W. and Conroy, D. E. (2001). The social physique anxiety scale: Cross validation, factorial invariance, and latent mean structure. *Measurement in Physical Education and Exercise Science, 5*, 81-95.

Orwin, R. G. (1983). A fail-safe *N* for an effect size in meta-analysis. *Journal of Educational Statistics, 8,* 157-159.

Pedhazur, E. J., and Pedhauzer Schmelkin, L. P. (1991). *Measurement, design, and analysis: An integrated approach.* Hillsdale, NJ: Lawrence Erlbaum.

Pendleton, V. R., Goodrick, G. K., Poston, W. S. C., Reeves, R. S., and Foreyt, J. P. (2002).Exercise augments the effects of cognitive-behavioral therapy in the treatment of binge eating. *International Journal of Eating Disorders, 31*, 172-184.

Prentice, D. A. and Miller, D. T. (1992). When small effects are impressive. *Psychological Bulletin, 112*, 160-164.

¥Russell, W. D. (2002). Comparison of self-esteem, body satisfaction, and social physique anxiety across males of different exercise frequency and racial background. *Journal of Sport Behavior, 25*, 74-91.

Russell, W. D., and Cox, R. H. (2003). Social physique anxiety, body dissatisfaction and self-esteem in college females of differing exercise frequency, perceived weight discrepancy, and race. *Journal of Sport Behavior, 26*, 298-319.

Sabiston, C., Sedgwick, W. A., Crocker, P. R. E., Kowalski, K. C., and Mack, D. E. (2007). Social physique anxiety in adolescence: An exploration of influences, coping strategies, and health behaviors. *Journal of Adolescence, 22*, 78-101.

¥Sabiston, C. M., Crocker, P. R. E., and Munroe-Chandler, K. J. (2005). Examining current-ideal discrepancy scores and exercise motivations as predictors of social physique anxiety in exercising females. *Journal of Sport Behavior, 28*, 668-686.

¥Schwerin, M. J., Corcoran, K. J., Fisher, L., Patterson, D., Askew, W., Olrich, T., and Shanks,S. 1996). Social physique anxiety, body esteem, and social anxiety in bodybuilders and self-reported anabolic steroid users. *Addictive Behaviors, 21*, 1-8.

Schlenker, B. R., and Leary, M. R. (1982). Social anxiety and self-presentation: A conceptualization and model. *Psychological Bulletin, 92*, 641-669.

Shroff, H., L. Thornton, R. L., Tozzi, F., Klump, K. L., Berrettini, W. H., Brandt, H., Crawford, S., Crow, S., Fichter, M. M., Goldman, D., Halmi, K. A., Johnson, C., Kaplan, A. S., Keel, P., LaVia, M., Mitchell, J., Rotonda, A., Strober, M., Treasure, J., Woodside, D. B., Kaye, W. H., and Bulik, C. M. (2006). Features associated with excessive exercise in women with eating disorders. *International Journal of Eating Disorders, 39*, 454-461.

Striegel-Moore, R., and Bulik, C. (2007). Risk factors for eating disorders. *American Psychologist, 62*, 181-198.

Sundgot-Borgen, J., Rosenvinge, J. H., Bahr, R., and Schneider, L. S. (2002). The effect of exercise, cognitive therapy and nutritional counselling in treating bulimia nervosa. *Medicine and Science in Sports and Exercise, 34*, 190-195.

Swinbourne, J. M., and Touyz, S. W. (2007). The co-morbidity of eating disorders and anxietydisorders: A review. *European Eating Disorders Review, 15*, 253-274.

Thompson, A. M., and Chad, K. E. (2002). The relationship of social physique anxiety to risk for develop an eating disorder in young females. *Journal of Adolescent Health, 91*, 207-211.

Thornton, B., and Maurice, J. (1997). Physique contrast effect: Adverse impact of idealized body images for women. *Sex Roles, 37*, 433-439.

Trochim, W. M. K. (2001). *The research methods knowledge base* (2nd ed). Atomic Dog Publishing.

Welk, G. J. (2002). *Physical activity assessments for health related research.* Human Kinetics; Champaign, IL.

Whitener, E. M. (1990). Confusion of confidence intervals and credibility intervals in meta-analysis. *Journal of Applied Psychology, 75*, 315-321.

¥Williams, P. A., and Cash, T. F. (2001). Effects of a circuit weight training program on the body images of college students. *International Journal of Eating Disorders, 30*, 75-82.

Yanovski, S. Z. (1993). Binge eating disorder: Current knowledge and future directions. *Obesity Research*, *1*, 306-318.

¥indicates articles that were included in the meta-analysis

In: Eating Disorders in Adult Women
Editor: Julian N. Fuchs

ISBN 978-1-60456-673-4

Chapter 10

EATING ATTITUDES AND MENTAL HEALTH AMONG CANADIAN WOMEN CONCERNED ABOUT THEIR WEIGHT

Jungwee Park* and Marie P. Beaudet
Statistics Canada, Ottawa, Ontario, K1A 0T6, Canada

ABSTRACT

Objectives: This article aimed to explore the associations between four attitudinal dimensions of the EAT-26 and selected mental health measures among women aged 15 or older concerned about their weight. The dimensions studied were food and body weight preoccupation, self-imposed dieting and external pressure to eat. The mental health measures selected were self-perceived mental health, having experienced a depressive episode in the last year and a diagnosis of an eating disorder.

Methods: The analyses were based on a sub-sample of women who were classified as concerned about their weight and who were surveyed as part of a national representative sample of the Canadian population in 2002. Weighted cross-tabulations were used to describe the characteristics of weight-concerned women. Logistic regression models were constructed to examine the associations between eating attitudes and mental health measures when selected confounders were controlled.

Results: Women preoccupied with food were more likely to rate their mental health negatively, to have experienced a depressive episode in the last year and to report having received a diagnosis of an eating disorder. Body image preoccupation was associated with depression and an eating disorder while external pressure to eat was related to a diagnosed eating disorder. Self-imposed dieting was not associated with the mental health indicators studied.

Conclusion: The findings presented are based on a national representative sample and are generally consistent with those obtained with smaller communities or clinical samples that have used the EAT-26. Thus, they are more generalizable. Moreover,

* Corresponding author (responsible for correspondence and reprints) Jungwee Park Statistics Canada D-6 9th Floor, Jean Talon Building 170 Tunney's Pasture Driveway, Ottawa, Ontario, K1A 0T6 Tel: (613)951-4598 Fax: (613)951-4179 jungwee.park@statcan.ca.

significant associations between specific dimensions of eating attitudes and mental health indicators were revealed.

Key words: *Eating attitudes, Eating disorder, Mental health, EAT-26*

INTRODUCTION

Unhealthy eating attitudes tend to be associated with psychological problems.[1,2] They have been shown to be related to self-perceived mental health and well-being.[3,4] Previous studies indicate that disordered eating attitudes often coexist with other mental disorders, such as mood, personality and anxiety disorders.[5-13] It has been reported that unhealthy eating attitudes are suggestive of an eating disorder. Some researchers have argued that abnormal eating attitudes are positively associated with the severity of an eating disorder.[14-17] Also, people with poor eating attitudes may be at risk for developing a full eating disorder syndrome over time.[15, 18-21]

Up to now, most research has examined the association of a global measure of eating attitudes on mental health by relying on the overall score of the Eating Attitudes Test (EAT).[2,6,12,22-24] Studies have documented the distinct dimensions of eating attitudes with factorial analyses of the EAT.[25-31] This research has been concentrated on identifying the dimensions of the EAT or on demonstrating relationships between factors identified and an eating disorder.[25,26,29]

It is expected that different dimensions of eating attitudes may have distinct associations with various measures of mental health. However, associations between specific dimensions of eating attitudes and mental health indicators are less well known. The main purpose of this article is to fill this information gap by examining the relationship between four dimensions of the EAT-26 (food and body image preoccupation, self-imposed dieting and external pressure to eat) and selected measures of mental health. Mental health measures studied are self-perceived mental health, a major depressive episode in the last year and a self-reported diagnosis of an eating disorder.

METHODS

Data Source

The analyses are based on data from the Canadian Community Health Survey (CCHS), cycle 1.2 conducted in 2002. One person aged 15 or older was randomly selected from a sample of households selected in a multi-stage stratified cluster sample from an area frame. The overall response rate was 77%.

The CCHS 1.2 contained questions on a wide range of mental disorders and problems, including the EAT, a measure originally developed by Garner et al.[26] to identify people at risk of an eating disorder. In the CCHS 1.2, the EAT questionnaire was administered to 5,116 respondents (1,324 men and 3,792 women), who answered positively two screening questions on concerns about their weight. This article is based on the 3,792 women who answered the

EAT component of the survey. These women represent 18.5% (approximately 2.4 million) of the population of community residing women 15 or older in Canada and are referred to, from now on, as weight-concerned women. Their characteristics are presented in Appendix A.

Compared to women who were classified as not concerned about their weight, weight-concerned women were younger, average age of 46 and 39 years respectively (Table I). Controlling for age, they were more likely to be overweight or obese as measured by their BMI and to perceive themselves as overweight.

MEASURES

The EAT was originally developed as an objective and valid index of symptoms frequently observed in anorexia nervosa. Since then, it has been employed as a screening tool for eating disorders in both clinical and non-clinical samples. The EAT has been utilized extensively as a research tool for identifying abnormal eating attitudes and behaviours and how these relate to eating disorders.[26,32] As a screening tool for identifying eating disorders, the EAT is usually administered to individuals who have displayed symptoms or expressed concerns about their weight. In the CCHS 1.2, it was administered to persons who answered "yes" to two screening questions.

The dimensions of the EAT retained for this analysis are based on the results of a factor analysis which have been published elsewhere.[30] Four factors were identified and were labelled food preoccupation, body image preoccupation, self-imposed dieting, and perceived external pressure to eat.

The four dimensions of the EAT-26 as well as other health-related variables considered in this analysis are described in Appendix B.

Analytical Techniques

Multiple logistic regressions were used to model the relationship between the four EAT dimensions and the three selected mental health indicators. Socio-demographic characteristics such as age, household income, educational attainment, employment, marital status were included in the models as control variables. Body mass index and perceived weight, which have been identified as important correlates of eating attitudes and which were available in the CCHS 1.2 were also included.

To account for survey design effects, the variance used in the calculation of coefficients of variation and confidence intervals was estimated with the bootstrap technique.[33,34] Additional details about the sample, the interviews, the variable definitions, and the derivation of the sampling weights can be found in published reports and on the Statistics Canada Web site @ www.statcan.ca.[35]

Table I. Selected characteristics of weight-concerned and non weight-concerned women, household population, aged 15 or older, Canada excluding territories, 2002

	Weight-concerned	Non weight-concerned
Average age	38.6†	46.0
Obesity rate*	36.5†	12.1
Overweight rate*	33.2†	24.2
Perceived overweight rate*	77.3†	37.2

Data source: 2002 Canadian Community Health Survey, cycle 1.2
*adjusted for age
†significantly different from non weight-concerned women

Results

Self-Perceived Mental Health

In the CCHS, self-perceived mental health was based on a respondent's self-evaluation of her psychological health and well-being. Among women concerned about their weight, women preoccupied with food were more likely to perceive their mental health as poor (Table II, Appendix C). None of the other dimensions of the EAT were associated with this indicator of mental health. Perceiving oneself as overweight, a diagnosis of a chronic condition, a diagnosis of a mental disorder, being previously married, unemployed, having a secondary education and living in a comparatively low-income household were positively associated with low ratings of one's perceived mental health. In contrast, women in the 65 or older age group were less likely to rate their mental health as fair or poor compared to middle age women, those in the 45 to 64 age group. BMI was the only dimension not associated with self-perceived mental health.

Depression

Many of the factors associated with self-perceived mental health were also associated with depression. Food and body image preoccupation were positively related to a major depressive episode in the last year when mental illnesses other than depression, chronic condition, and socio-demographic variables were controlled (Table II, Appendix C). According to this analysis, self-imposed dieting and a perception of external pressures to eat were not statistically associated with depression.

Women concerned about their weight who lived in household classified as middle, lower-middle or low income were more likely to have experienced a depressive episode in the last year compared to women living in households in the upper-middle or high income adequacy group. Women who reported being previously married, who perceived themselves as underweight, who were diagnosed with a physical chronic condition or a mental disorder other than depression, also had higher odds of having experienced a depressive episode in the previous 12 months. Women's highest level of educational attainment, employment and BMI were not associated with a greater likelihood of having experienced a depressive episode in the last year.

Diagnosed Eating Disorder

Weight-concerned women who were classified as preoccupied with food, preoccupied with their body image and as reporting external pressure to eat were more likely to have been diagnosed with an eating disorder (Table II, Appendix C). Self-imposed dieting was the only dimension of the EAT-26 studied which did not show a higher likelihood of reporting a diagnosis of an eating disorder.

Not surprisingly, underweight women had a greater likelihood of having been diagnosed with an eating disorder compared to women with a BMI in the acceptable range. In contrast, women classified as overweight were less likely to have been diagnosed with an eating disorder while self-perceived weight was not associated with a diagnosis of an eating disorder. Women living in households with an income adequacy in the low, lower-middle and middle ranges were less likely to have been diagnosed with an eating disorder compared to women in the upper middle and highest income adequacy quintiles. Being unemployed, having never married and a diagnosis of another mental disorder increased the odds of having been diagnosed with an eating disorder. A diagnosis of a chronic condition, age and education were not associated with a diagnosis of an eating disorder.

DISCUSSION

According to this analysis, almost one in five women (19% or an estimated 2.4 million) was concerned about her weight in Canada in 2002. In recent years, it has been reported that more people, young women in particular, suffer from serious eating disorders in Canada and that approximately 3 percent of women are affected by an eating disorder during their lifetime.[36] In 2002, based on the CCHS, when a number of factors including eating attitudes were controlled, being young was not an independent risk factor for mental health problems among Canadian women who were classified as concerned about their weight.

Women who were preoccupied with food and those preoccupied with their body image had higher odds of being depressed in the last 12 months and were more likely to have been diagnosed with an eating disorder. The former group was also more likely to view their mental health negatively. Not surprisingly, women who report external pressure to eat were more likely to have received a diagnosis of an eating disorder.

Previous research has documented that the EAT scores have an accuracy of at least 90% when used to identify persons who have been diagnosed with an eating disorder based on the DSM-IV criteria in clinical samples.[37]

Findings of this article are generally consistent with the literature that suggests an association between poor eating attitudes and depression.[5,10,24,38] They also are consistent with research findings that have reported that eating problems and depression are often co-morbid conditions [9,14,39] and the findings that document the association between unhealthy eating attitudes and mental well-being.[3,4] Like findings of a number of previous studies,[14-21] results of this article also support significant association between poor eating attitudes and eating disorder.

Table II. Adjusted odds ratios relating mental health outcomes to the dimensions of eating attitudes, weight-concerned women aged 15 or older, Canada excluding territories, 2002

	Self-rated mental health				Depression				Diagnosed eating disorder			
Eating attitudes dimensions	adjusted OR		95% CI		adjusted OR		95% CI		adjusted OR		95% CI	
Food preoccupation	1.79	*	1.25	2.58	1.77	*	1.23	2.54	3.05	*	1.38	6.74
Body image preoccupation	1.08		0.75	1.55	1.56	*	1.09	2.23	2.88	*	1.28	6.45
Self-imposed dieting	0.70		0.47	1.06	1.24		0.84	1.82	0.67		0.30	1.51
Perceived external pressure to eat	1.17		0.77	1.77	1.17		0.75	1.83	3.88	*	2.02	7.47

Data source: 2002 Canadian Community Health Survey, cycle 1.2

Notes: Each model included age, household income, education, employment, marital status, BMI, perceived weight, physical chronic conditions and mental disorders (Appendix B).

"Missing" categories for household income, employment, BMI, and perceived weight were included in the model to maximize sample size, but their odds ratios are not shown.

* p<0.05

... Not applicable

Contrary to the other dimensions of the EAT-26 studied, self-imposed dieting was not associated with mental health measures included in this analysis. This dimension may be measuring a cognitive or a behavioural predisposition while the other dimensions studied have a stronger component of affectivity.

A number of limitations are associated with the present analysis. All the information in the CCHS 1.2 is based on self-report. It is therefore not possible to separate from the results the part played by social desirability, poor recall, denial, or unwillingness to disclose personal information.

The risk of an eating disorder is only available for women who answered positively two screening questions. Thus, results from this study cannot be generalized to the eating attitudes of all women, but only to those who voiced concerns about their weight.

Since the CCHS is a cross-sectional survey, the causal direction between the dimensions of eating attitudes and other variables cannot be inferred. For example, it is not possible to determine if the higher odds of having a major depressive episode found among women who were preoccupied with food is because food preoccupation leads to depressive symptoms [9] or because depression will result in a strong preoccupation with food.[12,38] Also, since the CCHS does not include longitudinal information, it is not possible to adjust the findings for time of onset of the attitudes or the mental health outcomes nor is it possible to examine the long-term health effects of the respondents' eating attitudes.

Despite the limitations of this study, the findings presented are based on a national representative sample and are generally consistent with those obtained with smaller communities or clinical samples that have used the EAT-26. Thus, it is believed that they are more generalizable results. Moreover, significant associations between specific dimensions of eating attitudes and mental health indicators were revealed.

REFERENCES

[1] Ball K, Lee C, Brown W. Psychological stress and disordered eating: An exploratory study with young Australian women. *Women and Health* 1999; 29 (2): 1-15.

[2] Button EJ, Sonuga-Barke EJ, Davies J, Thompson M. A prospective study of self-esteem in the prediction of eating problems in adolescent schoolgirls: questionnaire findings. *British Journal of Clinical Psychology* 1996; 35(Pt.2): 193-203.

[3] Blaase H, Elklit A. Psychological characteristics of women with eating disorders: Permanent or transient features? *Scandinavian Journal of Psychology,* 2001; 42(5): 467-478.

[4] Hay P. Quality of life and bulimic eating disorder behaviors: Findings from a community-based sample. *International Journal of Eating Disorders* 2003; 33(4): 434-442.

[5] Abrams KK, Allen LR, Gray JJ. Disordered eating attitudes and behaviors, psychological adjustment, and ethnic identity: A comparison of black and white female college students. *International Journal of Eating Disorders* 1993; 14(1): 49-57.

[6] Buddeberg-Fischer B, Bernet R, Schmid J, Buddeberg C. Relationship between disturbed eating behavior and other psychosomatic symptoms in adolescents. *Psychotherapy and Psychosomatics* 1996; 65 (6): 319-326.

[7] Horner TN Jr, Utermohlen V. A multivariate analysis of psychological factors related to body mass index and eating preoccupation in female college students. *Journal of the American College of Nutrition* 1993; 12(4): 459-465.

[8] Lane A. Relationships between attitudes towards eating disorders and mood. *Journal of Science and Medicine in Sport* 2003; 6(2): 144-154.

[9] Lewinsohn PM, Striegel-Moore RH, Seeley JR. Epidemiology and natural course of eating disorders in young women from adolescence to young adulthood. *Journal of the American Academy of Child and Adolescent Psychiatry* 2000; 39(10): 1284-1292.

[10] Oates-Johnson T, DeCourville N. Weight preoccupation, personality, and depression in university students: An interactionist perspective. *Journal of Clinical Psychology* 1999; 55(9): 1157-1166.

[11] Siegel JM, Yancey AK, Aneshensel CS, Schuler R. Body image, perceived pubertal timing, and adolescent mental health. *Journal of Adolescent Health* 1999; 25(2): 155-165.

[12] Wichstrøm L. Psychological and behavioral factors unpredictive of disordered eating: A prospective study of the general adolescent population in Norway. *International Journal of Eating Disorders* 2000; 28(1): 33-42.

[13] Williamson DA, Kelley ML, Davis CJ, Ruggiero L, Blouin DC. Psychopathology of eating disorders: A controlled comparison of bulimic, obese, and normal subjects. *Journal of Consulting and Clinical Psychology* 1985; 53(2): 161-166.

[14] Dancyger IF, Garfinkel PE. The relationship of partial syndrome eating disorders to anorexia nervosa and bulimia nervosa. *Psychological Medicine* 1995; 25(5): 1019-1025.

[15] Drewnowski A, Yee DK, Kurth CL, Krahn DD. Eating pathology and DSM-III-R bulimia nervosa: A continuum of behavior. *American Journal of Psychiatry* 1994; 151(8): 1217-1219.

[16] Franko DL, Omori M. Subclinical eating disorders in adolescent women: A test of the continuity hypothesis and its psychological correlates. *Journal of Adolescence* 1999; 22(3);389-396.

[17] Stice E, Killen JD, Hayward C, Taylor CB. Support for the continuity hypothesis of bulimic pathology. *Journal of Consulting and Clinical Psychology* 1998; 66(5): 784-790.

[18] Attie I, Brooks-Gunn J. Development of eating problems in adolescent girls: A longitudinal study. *Developmental Psychology* 1989; 25(1): 70-79.

[19] King MB. Eating disorders in a general practice population: Prevalence, characteristics and follow-up at 12 to 18 months. *Psychological Medicine, Monograph Supplement* 1989; 14: 1-34.

[20] King MB. The natural history of eating pathology in attenders to primary medical care. *International Journal of Eating Disorders* 1991; 10(4): 379-387.

[21] National Eating Disorders Screening Program. *Eating disorders: Frequently asked questions.* Retrieved March 1, 2006 from http://www.mentalhealthscreening. org/eat /eat-faq.htm. 2004.

[22] Button EJ, Loan P, Davies J, Sonuga-Barke EJ. Self-esteem, eating problems, and psychological well-being in a cohort of schoolgirls aged 15-16: A questionnaire and interview study. *International Journal of Eating Disorders* 1997; 21(1): 39-47.

[23] Button EJ, Reveley C, Palmer R. An ethnic comparison of eating attitudes and associated psychological problems in young British women. *International Journal of Eating Disorders* 1998; 23(3):317-323.

[24] Wichstrøm L. Social, psychological and physical correlates of eating problems: A study of the general adolescent population in Norway. *Psychological Medicine* 1995; 25(3): 567-579.

[25] Dotti A, Lazzari R. Validation and reliability of the Italian EAT-26. *Eating and Weight Disorders* 1998; 3(4): 188-194.

[26] Garner DM, Olmsted MP, Bohr Y, Garfinkel PE. The eating attitudes test: Psychometric features and clinical correlates. *Psychological Medicine* 1982; 12(4):871-878.

[27] Johnson CS, Bedford J. Eating attitudes across age and gender groups: A Canadian study. *Eating and Weight Disorders* 2004; 9(1): 16-23.

[28] Koslowsky M, Scheinberg Z, Bleich A, Mark M, Apter A, Danon Y, et al. The factor structure and criterion validity of the short form of the Eating Attitudes Test. *Journal of Personality Assessment* 1992; 58(1): 27-35.

[29] Nasser M. The psychometric properties of the Eating Attitude Test in a non-Western population. *Social Psychiatry and Psychiatric Epidemiology* 1994; 29(2): 88-94.

[30] Park J, Beaudet MP Eating attitudes and their correlates among Canadian women concerned about their weight. *European Review of Eating Disorders* 2007; 15(4):311-320.

[31] Wells JE, Coope PA, Gabb DC, Pears RK. The factor structure of the Eating Attitudes Test with adolescent schoolgirls. *Psychological Medicine* 1985; 15(1): 141-146.

[32] Button EJ, Whitehouse A. Subclinical anorexia nervosa. *Psychological Medicine* 1981; 11(3): 509-516.

[33] Rao JNK, Wu CFJ, Yue K. Some recent work on resampling methods for complex surveys. *Survey Methodology (Statistics Canada, Catalogue 12-001)* 1992; 18(2): 209-217.

[34] Rust KF, Rao JN. Variance estimation for complex surveys using replication techniques. *Statistical Methods in Medical Research* 1996; 5(3): 283-310.

[35] Statistics Canada. *Canadian Community Health Survey -- Mental Health and Well-being.* Catalogue 82-617-XIE. Ottawa, ON: Industry Canada, 2004

[36] Health Canada. *A Report on Mental Illnesses in Canada.* Ottawa, ON: Author, 2002.

[37] Mintz LB, O'Halloran MS. The Eating Attitudes Test: Validation with DSM-IV eating disorder criteria. *Journal of Personality Assessment* 2000; 74(3): 489-503.

[38] Lee AM, Lee S. Disordered eating and its psychosocial correlates among Chinese adolescent females in Hong Kong. *International Journal of Eating Disorders* 1996; 20(2): 177-183.

[39] Viesselman JO, Roig M. Depression and suicidality in eating disorders. *Journal of Clinical Psychiatry* 1985; 46(4): 118-124.

[40] Garner DM. Psychoeducational principles in treatment. In: Garner DM, Garfinkel PE (Eds.), *Handbook of Treatment for Eating Disorders*. New York: Guilford Press, 1997.

[41] American Psychiatric Association. *Diagnostic and Statistical Manual of Mental Disorders. 4th rev. ed. DSM-IV-TR.* Washington, DC: Author, 2000.

[42] Health Canada. *Canadian Guidelines for Body Weight Classification in Adults.* Ottawa, ON: Author, 2003.

[43] Cole TJ, Bellizzi MC, Flegal KM, Dietz WH. Establishing a standard definition for child overweight and obesity worldwide: International survey. *British Medical Journal* 2000; 320(7244): 1240-1243.

Appendix A. Distribution of Selected Characteristics, Weight-Concerned Women Aged 15 or Older, Canada Excluding Territories, 2002

	Sample size	Estimated population	
		000	%
Total	3792	2351	100.0
Age groups			
15-24	804	525	22.3
25-44	1669	1036	44.0
45-64	1000	636	27.0
65 or older	319	155	6.6
Household income adequacy			
Low/lower-middle	617	262	11.1
Middle	809	454	19.3
Upper-middle/high	2050	1411	60.0
Missing	316	224	9.5
Educational attainment			
Less than secondary graduation	932	566	24.1
Secondary graduation	713	482	20.5
Some postsecondary	393	247	10.5
Postsecondary graduation	1738	1026	43.6
Missing	16	30	1.3
Employment status			
Yes	2757	1756	74.7
No	943	559	23.8
Missing	92	36	1.5
Marital status			
Never married	1208	722	30.7
Previously married	495	215	9.1
Married	2085	1410	60.0
Missing	4	4	0.2
Food preoccupation			
Yes	637	376	16.0
No	3139	1966	83.6
Missing	16	9	0.4
Body image preoccupation			
Yes	613	375	16.0
No	3163	1970	83.8
Missing	16	7	0.3
Self-imposed dieting			
Yes	675	434	18.4
No	3097	1900	80.8
Missing	20	17	0.7
Perceived external pressure to eat			
Yes	455	271	11.5
No	3315	2067	87.9
Missing	22	13	0.6

Data source: 2002 Canadian Community Health Survey, cycle 1.2

Notes: Because of rounding, detail may not add to totals.

APPENDIX B: SURVEY QUESTIONS OR VARIABLE DEFINITIONS

i) The EAT-26 and its Sub-scales

In the CCHS 1.2, the EAT-26 was administered to persons who answered “yes” to two screening questions:

(1) “Was there ever a time in your life when you had a strong fear or a great deal of concern about being too fat or overweight? “ and

“During the past 12 months, did you have a strong fear or a great deal of concern about being too fat or overweight?”

The EAT-26 consists of twenty-six questions answered on a 6-point scale labelled “always” (scored 3), “usually” (scored 2), “often” (scored 1), and “sometimes” “rarely,” and “never” (all scored 0). The rationale for the restriction of range from 1 to 6 to 0 to 3 rests on the theoretical assumption that item scaling on the EAT-26 is continuous only for the responses weighted 1 to 3.[40] Thus, a higher score on the index indicates a greater risk of an eating disorder.

The scores on the dimensions were calculated by summing the responses to the items. The cut-off point selected to convert each subscale into a dichotomous variable corresponded approximately to the 17th highest percentile of its distribution. This percentile was chosen because it represents the proportion of weight-concerned women who scored 20 or higher on the distribution of the overall EAT-26 score, and a score of 20 was the cut-off point chosen by Garner et al.[26] to indicate the risk of having an eating disorder.

The food preoccupation dimension has a potential range of 0 to 18. It is based on 6 items: “find oneself preoccupied with food”, “go on eating binges”, “feel extremely guilty after eating”, “feel that food controls your life”, “give too much time and thought to food”, and “feel uncomfortable after eating sweets”. Women identified as concerned with their weight who scored 4 or more on the food preoccupation dimension were considered to be preoccupied with food.

For body image preoccupation, the cut-off was 8 out of a potential range of 0 to 12. The dimension is based on 4 items: “terrified about being overweight”, “preoccupied with a desire to be thinner”, “think about burning up calories when exercising”, and “preoccupied with the thought of having fat on your body”.

To be regarded as positive on the self-imposed dieting dimension, a respondent had to score 7 or more out of a total score of 18. Scores are based on 6 questions: “aware of calorie content of the foods”, “avoid food with a high carbohydrate”, “avoid foods with sugar”, “eat diet foods”, “display self-control around food”, and “engage in dieting behaviour”.

If a respondent had at least 1 point on the last dimension, she was considered as perceiving external pressure to eat. The dimension of perceived external pressure to eat is based on 3 question items: “feel that others prefer you to eat more”, “others think that you are too thin”, and “feel that others pressure you to eat”.

ii) Health variables

	Survey questions/definitions
Self-perceived mental health	"In general, would you say your mental health is: excellent? very good? good? fair? poor?" For this article, respondents who answered excellent, very good or good were considered to have positive mental health and those who answered fair or poor were classified as having negative mental health.
Depression	Depression was measured with the World Mental Health version of the Composite International Diagnostic Interview (WMH-CIDI).[41] It is characterised by a loss of interest in most activities or a depressed mood most of the day on most days for at least a two-week period and is accompanied by other symptoms such as change in weight or appetite, insomnia, fatigue or loss of energy, feelings of worthlessness, inability to concentrate and suicide ideation.
Mental disorder	Respondents were classified as having a *mental disorder* if they met the WHO-CIDI criteria for at least one of four mental disorders (major depression, mania, panic episode, social phobia and agoraphobia)* or the criteria for alcohol or drug dependence.
Eating disorder	Respondents were also asked if they had an *eating disorder* such as anorexia or bulimia which was expected to last or had lasted 6 months or more and had been diagnosed by a health professional.
Chronic condition	Respondents were asked about long-term conditions that had lasted or were expected to last six months or longer and that had been diagnosed by a health care professional. The eighteen conditions considered in this analysis were asthma, fibromyalgia, arthritis or rheumatism, back problems, high blood pressure, migraine, chronic bronchitis, emphysema, diabetes, epilepsy, heart disease, cancer, ulcers, the effects of a stroke, bowel disorder, thyroid disorder, chronic fatigue syndrome and multiple chemical sensitivities.
Body mass index (BMI)	*Body mass index* (BMI) is the result of dividing self-reported weight in kilograms by the square of self-reported height in metres. Cut-offs of the International BMI guidelines for women aged 19 or older were used to classify respondents into four groups: underweight (BMI less than 18.5), acceptable weight (BMI ranging from 18.5 to less than 25), overweight (a BMI value between 25 and 29.9) and obese, 30 or over.[42] The age and sex specific cut-offs defined by Cole et al.[43] were used to classify the BMI's of women under age 19. Pregnant women were excluded from the analysis because BMI is not an appropriate measure for them.
Self-perceived body weight	To measure *self-perceived body weight*, respondents were asked, "Do you consider yourself, overweight, underweight, or just about right?" Women were assigned to one of three groups (perceived overweight, perceived underweight, and perceived acceptable weight) based on the option they selected.

* Depression is excluded from this count when it is used as a dependent variable.

Appendix C. Adjusted odds ratios of selected mental health measures weight-concerned women aged 15 or older, Canada excluding territories, 2002

	Poor/fair self-perceived mental health				Depression				Diagnosis of an eating disorder			
Characteristics	adjusted OR		95% CI		adjusted OR		95% CI		adjusted OR		95% CI	
Age groups												
15-24	0.96		0.55	1.69	1.52		0.85	2.72	0.85		0.16	4.43
25-44	1.27		0.89	1.82	1.13		0.76	1.69	2.29		0.68	7.76
45-64 †	1.00		...	...	1.00		...	...	1.00		...	...
65 or older	0.44	*	0.23	0.85	0.24	*	0.09	0.63	0.48		0.05	4.61
Household income adequacy												
Low/lower-middle	1.71	*	1.15	2.56	1.66	*	1.06	2.60	0.41	*	0.17	0.98
Middle	1.65	*	1.51	2.38	1.75	*	1.22	2.50	0.37	*	0.16	0.87
Upper-middle/high †	1.00		...	...	1.00		...	...	1.00		...	...
Educational attainment												
Less than secondary graduation	1.39		0.95	2.05	0.80		0.54	1.20	0.71		0.28	1.82
Secondary graduation	1.43	*	1.01	2.02	0.98		0.64	1.48	0.81		0.27	2.43
Some post-secondary	0.85		0.51	1.43	0.61		0.36	1.02	0.64		0.26	1.57
Post-secondary graduation †	1.00		...	...	1.00		...	...	1.00		...	...
Employment												
Unemployed	2.00	*	1.43	2.80	1.48		0.98	2.25	5.05	*	2.08	12.26
Employed†	1.00		...	...	1.00		...	...	1.00		...	...
Marital status												
Never married	1.45		0.97	2.17	1.35		0.92	1.98	3.98	*	1.66	9.56
Previously married	2.12	*	1.49	3.03	2.82	*	1.78	4.47	1.94		0.58	6.50
Married †	1.00		...	...	1.00		...	...	1.00		...	...
Eating attitudes												
Food preoccupation	1.79	*	1.25	2.58	1.77	*	1.23	2.54	3.05	*	1.38	6.74
Body image preoccupation	1.08		0.75	1.55	1.56	*	1.09	2.23	2.88	*	1.28	6.45
Self-imposed dieting	0.70		0.47	1.06	1.24		0.84	1.82	0.67		0.30	1.51
Perceived external pressure to eat	1.17		0.77	1.77	1.17		0.75	1.83	3.88	*	2.02	7.47
BMI												
Obese	0.99		0.69	1.42	0.77		0.50	1.19	0.75		0.32	1.73
Overweight	0.96		0.64	1.45	0.92		0.62	1.34	0.27	*	0.11	0.67
Underweight	0.77		0.21	2.87	1.07		0.29	3.99	4.15	*	1.16	14.88
Acceptable weight †	1.00		...	...	1.00		...	...	1.00		...	...
Perceived weight												
Perceived overweight	1.83	*	1.18	2.82	1.58		0.97	2.58	0.80		0.37	1.73
Perceived underweight	2.22		0.66	7.50	4.31	*	1.26	14.81	3.40		0.61	18.93
Perceived acceptable weight †	1.00		...	...	1.00		...	...	1.00		...	...
At least one chronic condition	1.61	*	1.16	2.23	1.93	*	1.34	2.76	1.04		0.48	2.26
At least one mental disorder	5.59	*	4.20	7.45	3.59	*	2.65	4.86	5.91	*	2.76	12.66
Model information												
Sample size	3617				3595				3618			
Records dropped because of missing values	175				197				174			

Data source: 2002 Canadian Community Health Survey, cycle 1.2
Notes: "Missing" categories for household income, employment, BMI, and perceived weight were included in the model to maximize sample size, but their odds ratios are not shown.
* p<0.05
... Not applicable

In: Eating Disorders in Adult Women
Editor: Julian N. Fuchs

ISBN 978-1-60456-673-4

Chapter 11

IS RESTRAINED EATING A RISK FACTOR IN WOMEN EXECUTIVES?

Lotte Habermann-Horstmeier*
STZ Companies and Managers, Klosterring 5.
D 78050 Villingen-Schwenningen
Germany

ABSTRACT

Aim: It is not easy for overweight women to participate in professional life. They are often considered less efficient. If you think about a ′typical businesswoman`, you expect her to be a slim and attractive person. But is that true? Are women executives slimmer than other women? If yes, how do they achieve this goal?

Method: We wanted to find out the answers to these questions through a questionnaire we sent out by e-mail in 2006 to 300 women in leading positions (top and middle management) in Germany. The questionnaire contained a mix of open- and closed-ended questions. The subject of eight of the 50 questions was nutrition and health.

Results: We found an average body mass index in the low to normal range. The group of underweight women was nearly twice as large as it is in the average German female population. Additional questions showed that many of these female executives achieve this goal of staying slim through restrained eating.

Conclusion: A slim and well-styled body shows, "I am successful, I am perfect. I am managing my life as successfully as my career." In order to keep such a slim body in our affluent society over a long period of time, one's eating behavior must permanently be geared to loose weight or avoid weight gain. In this context, cognitive control of eating behavior is of prime importance. Ignoring physiological hunger signals and psychological appetence signals are important as well. However, such kind of eating behavior may lead to impaired eating, which is a risk factor for developing an eating disorder.

Keywords: *Women executives, nutrition, body-mass-index (BMI), restrained eating.*

---

* Contact: Dr. med. Lotte Habermann-Horstmeier, Deputy Director of STZ Companies and Managers, Klosterring 5. D 78050 Villingen-Schwenningen. Germany. Telephone: 0049/7721/2069970; Fax: 0049/7721/2069971. Email: stz952@stw.de

Introduction

In German society, in which nearly every second person is overweight (Statistisches Bundesamt, 2005), being slim is a synonym for success and power. We know how important it is today, especially for young girls and women, to be slim. A slim body stands for youth, beauty and attractiveness. Being slim also means competence and acknowledgement. Perpetuating this stereotype, women's magazines regularly publish new dietary plans and pharmaceutical companies offer appetite suppressants. In addition, liposuction and other surgical measures have become a completely natural way for many people to achieve an ideal, slim body. Studies done in the US show that overweight women are recognizably handicapped throughout their working life. They often have trouble getting a job and if they get one, they earn less money than slim women with similar qualifications or positions (Frieze et al, 1991; Cawley, 2000). In our society, overweight persons are often seen as less efficient and emotionally and physically less resilient. It is not surprising, that overweight people are often more self-conscious and therefore less successful in their jobs.

Is it absolutely necessary as a woman to be slim in order to get a particular working position? If you look at a ′typical businesswoman`, you naturally expect her to be slim and attractive. U. Renz (2006) believes that this is connected with the Protestant ethos of performance. A slim and well-styled body shows "I am successful, I am perfect." "I do not enjoy life, I am working to improve my abilities - I am eating with self-control. I am managing my life as successful as my career." In order to keep such a slim body in our affluent society over a long period of time, one's eating behavior must permanently be geared to loose weight or avoid weight gain. It is in this context that Herman first used the term "restrained eating" in scientific literature in the 1970s. He used this word to denote all efforts made to consciously cut down on the amount one eats (Herman and Mack, 1975). Later Westenhöfer und Pudel (1991) expanded this definition. They understand "restrained eating" to be a long-term pattern of the intake of food, which is characterized by cognitive surveillance and the ignoring of physiological hunger and psychological appetence signals. The aim of this pattern is to supply only a small amount of calories to help in reducing weight and/or staying the same weight (Westenhöfer, 1991).

But is it not true that diets and restrained eating are a part of everyday life in our modern society? In addition, aren't such patterns of behavior common in all sectors of society? In this context, what are the distinctive/special features of the nutrition behavior of female executives? Lastly, what is the real problem here? With all the negative health consequences of being overweight, isn't it more desirable to be slim? In our society, it is more likely that slim people are admired and envied. Health risks are mainly seen in overweight people and not in the slim ones. To find out the answers to some of these questions we not only asked German female executives about their height and weight, but also about their nutrition behavior.

Subjects and Methods

Our empirical study "Career obstacles for women in leading positions", planned and delivered in 2006 by STZ Companies and Managers in cooperation with the International

Business Faculty of Furtwangen University, included one section that is about the connection of nutrition and health on the one hand and job and career on the other hand. Following the Gabler Wirtschaftslexikon (2005), the survey defines women in leading positions as those working in the areas of senior management and middle management. The female executives were contacted mainly via e-mail, the survey having been sent to networks of women, companies, administrative institutions, clinics and universities. Altogether, more than 300 women agreed to complete the e-mail questionnaires consisting of 50 questions. Three hundred women returned the completed questionnaires. As expected only 15 percent of the women were between 25 and 35 years old, more than 50 percent were between 36 and 45 years old and about one third of the women were older than 46 years (Table 1).

Table 1. Age of participants

	Number of participants	Percentage
25 to 35 years	44	14.7 %
36 to 45 years	161	53.7 %
46 to 55 years	76	25.3 %
56 to 65 years	19	6.3 %
Sum	300	100 %

RESULTS

In the last section of our questionnaire the participating women were asked about their height and their weight, about their nutrition behavior in the occupational and private sector and about possible weight problems and the possible connections they saw between their "career" and "nutrition and health".

Height, Weight and Body-Mass-Index

The Height of the Participants

Two hundred and sixty nine of the 300 participating women reported their height (Figure 1). According to this, they were 168.94 centimeters (66.56 inches) tall on average [standard deviation 5.95 cm, median 169 cm]. Fifty percent of the women asked were between 165 cm [first quartile (Q_1): 65.01 inches) and 172 cm (third quartile (Q_3): 67.77 inches] tall and 80 percent were between 160 cm (63.04 inches; that means only 10 percent were shorter) and 177 cm (69.74 inches; that means 10 percent were taller) tall. The calculated mean value was almost three centimeters (1.18 inches) more than the average height of all German women aged between 25 and 65 years, which is 166 cm (65.40 inches; data according to the micro census survey of the Statistisches Bundesamt Deutschland, 2005). Comparing the average height in the four determined age groups, it is evident that the average height of the women that participated in our survey is almost three centimeters greater in all the age groups when compared to the average height of German women as a whole (Table 2).

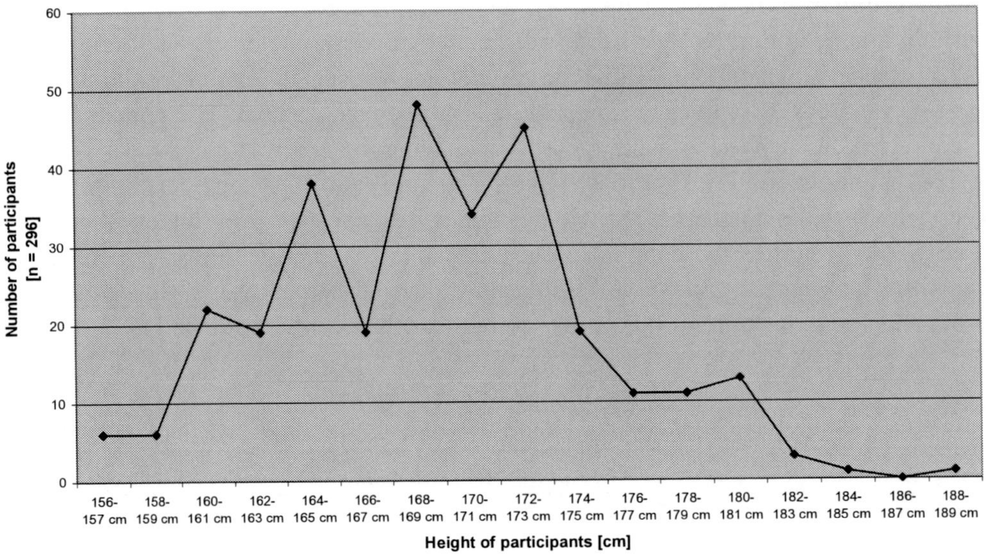

Figure 1. Height of participants [n = 296].

Table 2. Average height of participants compared with the average height of all German women

Age groups	Average height of participants	Average height of all German women (according to the German micro census 2005)
25 to 35 years	170.2 cm	167.5 cm
36 to 45 years	169.6 cm	166.5 cm
46 to 55 years	167.0 cm	165.5 cm
56 to 65 years	167.3 cm	164.5 cm

Weight of Participants

Two hundred and ninety five of the 300 participants did name their present weight (figure 2). The average weight of the women was 64.79 kg (standard deviation 9.86 kg, median 63 kg), or 142.86 pounds (standard deviation 21.74 lb, median 138.92 lb). Fifty percent of the women asked weighed between 58 kg (127.89 lb; first quartile) and 70 kg (154.35 lb; third quartile). Eighty percent weighed between 54 kg (119.07 lb) and 77 kg (169.79 lb). From this data it is clear that the calculated mean value is almost 3 kg (6.62 lb) less than the average weight of all German women in the age groups falling between 25 and 65 years.

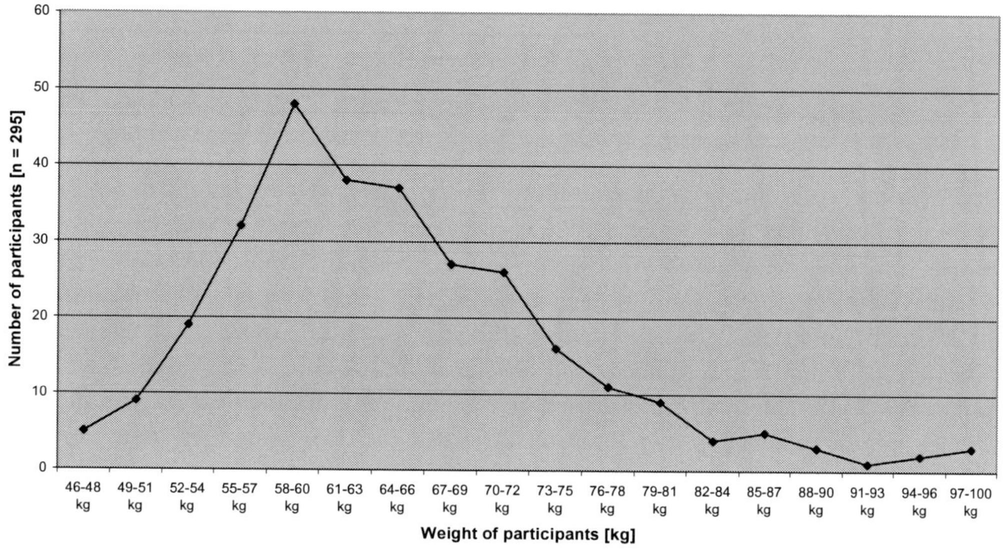

Figure 2. Weight of participants.

The average weight data was established by the German Statistisches Bundesamt within the bounds of the micro census survey in 2005 (Mikrozensus, 2005). According to Aubele (2006), earlier statistical surveys have shown that both women and men systematically underestimate their body weight around 2 kg (4.41 lb) and overestimate their height around 0.3 to three cm (0.12 in to 1.18 in). As all the values of this study are not empirical but ones obtained from the subjects, it is legitimate to compare both average values.

Body Mass Index of the Subjects

More expressive than only giving the height and weight of the subjects is including the body mass index (BMI). The BMI is defined as a quotient of body weight and the square of the body height. Usually the BMI is important in recognizing being underweight and overweight, respectively. Based on its correlation to the proportion of body fat, the BMI makes it possible to roughly estimate the body composition, especially in extreme cases. It also allows the estimating of the weight associated with health risks. However, the BMI gives no exact information about the body composition respective to the proportion of body fat, especially in older people with their different age related body changes and their common changes in water balance (Volkert, 2006).

Calculating of the body mass index (BMI):

$$\frac{\text{Body weight [kg]}}{\text{Body height}^2\ [m^2]} = \text{BMI } [kg/m^2]$$

In 1998, the world health organization (WHO) arranged weight classifications for adults based on the body mass index. These weight classifications consist of underweight (BMI < 18.5 kg/m^2), normal weight (18.5 – 24.9 kg/m^2) and overweight (BMI ≥ 25 kg/m^2, containing pre-obense [BMI 25 – 29.9 kg/m^2], obese class I [BMI 30 – 34.9 kg/m^2], obese class II [BMI 35 – 39.9 kg/m^2] and obese class III [BMI ≥ 40 kg/m^2]). It is important to recognize that this classification does not consider the age and gender of the subjects, but is based on an average physique. The BMI values can only be used on a limited basis for men with a high proportion of muscles and for small and very tall persons. Usually, the BMI categories are used to assess whether one is underweight. According to the WHO, being underweight is defined as having a BMI < 18.5 kg/m^2. One of the WHO's diagnosis criteria for anorexia nervosa (taken from the ICD-10 classification of mental and behavioural disorders) is a BMI ≤ 17.5 kg/m^2.

In our study, we calculated the body mass index of all the women that provided their height and weight. The average BMI of the subjects was 22.2 kg/m^2 [standard deviation 3.4 kg/m^2, median 22 kg/m^2]. Fifty percent of the women executives had a BMI between 20 kg/m^2 (first quartile) und 23 kg/m^2 (third quartile). Eighty percent had a BMI between 19 kg/m^2 and 26 kg/m^2. Figure 5 shows the BMI values of the subjects with a steep peak at 20.0 to 21.5 kg/m^2 and a little peak at 23.0 to 24.5 kg/m^2. The majority of the subjects' BMI values (73.2 percent) are within the limits of what the WHO has defined as normal weight; however, many fall within the lower part of the normal weight range (figure 3).

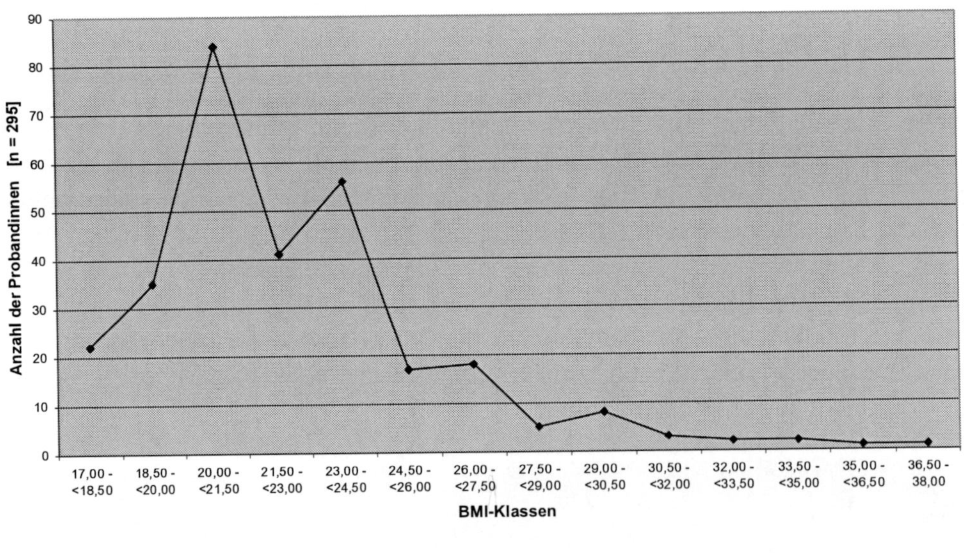

Figure 3. Participant Body Mass Index (BMI).

Seven point five percent of the women executives surveyed had a BMI in the underweight range. When distinguishing between moderately underweight (BMI <18.5 kg/m^2) and severely underweight (BMI ≤ 17.5 kg/m^2, see diagnosis criteria of anorexia nervosa), 5.1 percent of the women executives surveyed are moderately underweight and 2.4 percent are severely underweight (table 3).

Table 3. Participant BMI, scaled to the WHO weight classes including a discrimination between moderately and severely underweight [n = 295 subjects]

weight classes, BMI in kg/m^2	number of subjects	percentage
17.00 to <17.50	7	2.4%
17.50 to <18.50	15	5.1%
18.50 to <25.00	216	73.2%
25.00 to <30.00	44	14.9%
30.00 to <35.00	11	3.7%
35.00 to <40.00	2	0.7%

When we compared the BMI values of our subjects to the average BMI values of the German female population between the ages of 25 to 65 years (Auberle, 2006), according to the WHO criteria, nearly two thirds of the women executives surveyed are in the normal weight range. In contrast, only 56 percent of the German female population falls within this range. Seven point five percent of the women executives were classified as underweight. This percentage was much higher than what was found in the German female population (4 percent). Considerable differences were also found in the overweight category. The percentage of overweight women executives was considerably lower than the percentage of overweight females in the German population (figure 4).

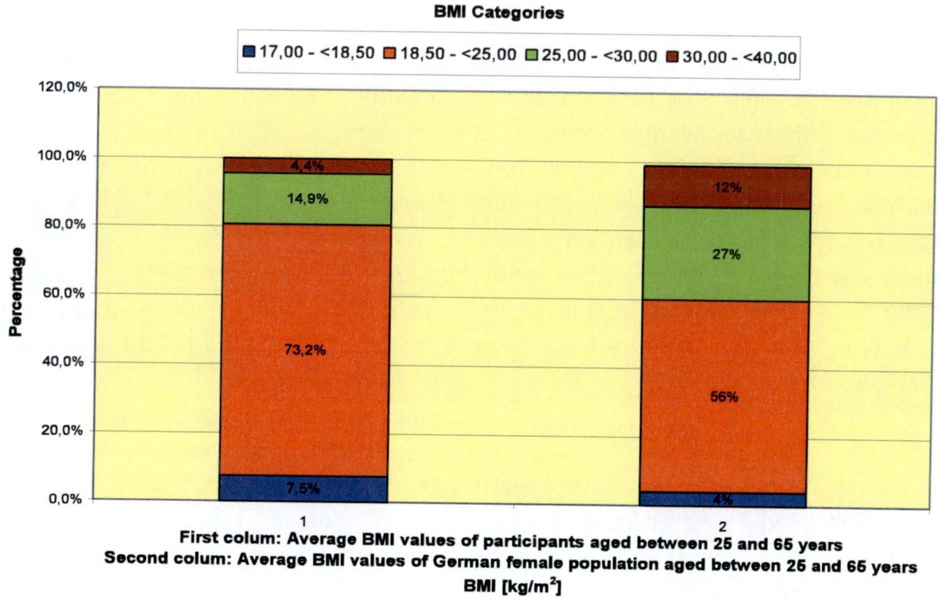

Figure 4. Participant BMI compared to average BMI of German women [based on Mikrozensus 2005].

Unexpectedly, the number of underweight women in all age groups was more than twice as high in the group of women executives than in the average German female population. A comparison of the overweight women showed that the women executives surveyed were on average less overweight than the average German female population. None of the women executives were classified as overweight grade III. Also, it was observed that the BMI of the women executives hardly rose with age, in contrast to the German female population where it rose considerably. Only in the 56 to 65 years old age group, are an above average percentage of the women executives classified as pre-obese (table 4).

Table 4. Participant BMI compared to average BMI of German women (calculated on the German micro census survey 2005), scaled in age classes

BMI categories	subjects 25 to 35 years	German women: 25 to 35 years	subjects 36 to 45 years	German women: 36 to 45 years	subjects 46 to 55 years	German women: 46 to 55 years	subjects 56 to 65 years	German women: 56 to 65 years
17.00 - <18.50	11.4%	6.0%	7.6%	3.5%	5.3%	2.5%	5.3%	2.0%
18.50 - <25.00	77.3%	69.0%	75.2%	64.0%	74.7%	53.5%	42.1%	44.5%
25.00 - <30.00	11.4%	18.0%	14.0%	22.5%	10.7%	29.5%	47.4%	36.5%
30.00 - >40.00	0.0%	7.0%	3.2%	9.5%	9.3%	14.5%	5.3%	18.0%

Career, Nutrition Habits and Weight

Additionally, we asked our subjects about their nutrition habits. One question inquired about there being a connection between working situations and eating too much or too little. More than one fifth of the women surveyed (20.7 percent) said that in some situations they eat too much and more than one quarter (26.0 percent) said that in some situations they eat too little. Many subjects said that both situations were relevant and pertained to them at times. Altogether one third of the women surveyed (31.3 percent) admitted to paying attention to their nutrition during work hours, while more than half of the women (54.7 percent) did so during their time off. Twenty eight point seven percent of the women surveyed said they did not pay attention to their nutrition while at work. Only 15.3 percent did not do so during their time off (figure 5).

More than half of the women asked (54.3 percent) said their weight did not change until they began their work as an executive. Thirty-one percent gained weight (until 5 kg: 14.3 percent; 5 to 10 kg: 10.7 percent; more than 10 kg: 6.0 percent) and 5.4 percent (until 5 kg: 3.0 percent; 5 to 10 kg: 1.7 percent; more than 10 kg: 0.7 percent) lost weight. Eight percent of the women indicated that their weight varied greatly; they gained and lost a large amount of weight. Surprisingly, most of these women (nearly 80 percent) had a normal BMI between 18.5 and 24.5 kg/m^2. Approximately half of these were in the lower part of the normal weight range (BMI 18.5 to 21.5 kg/m^2). It is also surprising that 90 percent of the underweight women (BMI < 18.5 kg/m^2) maintained a constant weight. In this group, only two women actually lost weight (until 5 kg respectively 5 to 10 kg).

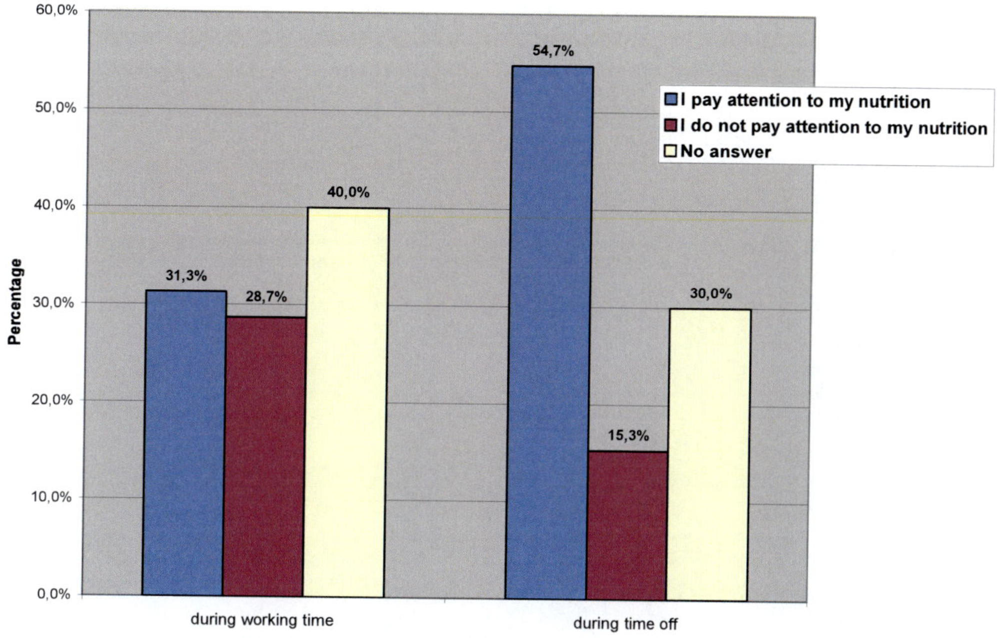

Figure 5. Did our subjects pay attention to nutrition during working time/time off?

According to these values, it was very astonishing that only 41.7 percent of the women surveyed said that it was not a problem for them to stay at the same weight when asked about the reasons for their weight changes. Many women did name numerous reasons why their weight changed. Many of these women (40 percent) said they have no time or energy for sports or exercise because of their jobs. About 18.3 percent of the women maintained that they did not have enough time for well-planned out and nutritious eating during work hours. Twenty-two percent thought the reason for this was strain and stress from the job. Another 15 percent said that their weight problems were a result of the stress caused by the multiple roles they had to play. When comparing the percentage of subjects whose weight stayed constant and the percentage of women who said they did not have any problem staying at the same weight, a discrepancy is noticed. Up to 80 percent of the women in leading positions were only able to stay at a normal weight with a supreme effort (figure 6).

Most of these women (70.3 %) did not stay on a diet to reduce their weight until after taking on a leading position. Only 2.7 percent permanently lived on a diet. Nearly all of the women who had been on a diet one or more times had a normal BMI (18% of the women with a BMI between 18.5 to < 20 kg/m^2 and 33 % of the women with a BMI between 23 to < 24.5 kg/m^2).

The last question wanted to know what kind of connection the subjects saw between "career" and "nutrition and health". It is of interest that 8 percent of the women surveyed thought a good balance between the body, mind, requirements of the job and family were important in order to have successful career. Many women used the sentence: "Mens sana in corpore sano." These women often connect this sentence with the view that one has to learn to establish priorities. Six percent of the women said that it was all a question of organization; when organized, they could handle their job and manage their nutrition and health. This is similar to the view held by 6 percent of the women surveyed who preferred a disciplined and controlled form of eating. For at least 12 percent of the women executives, nutrition is connected with organization, discipline and oversight.

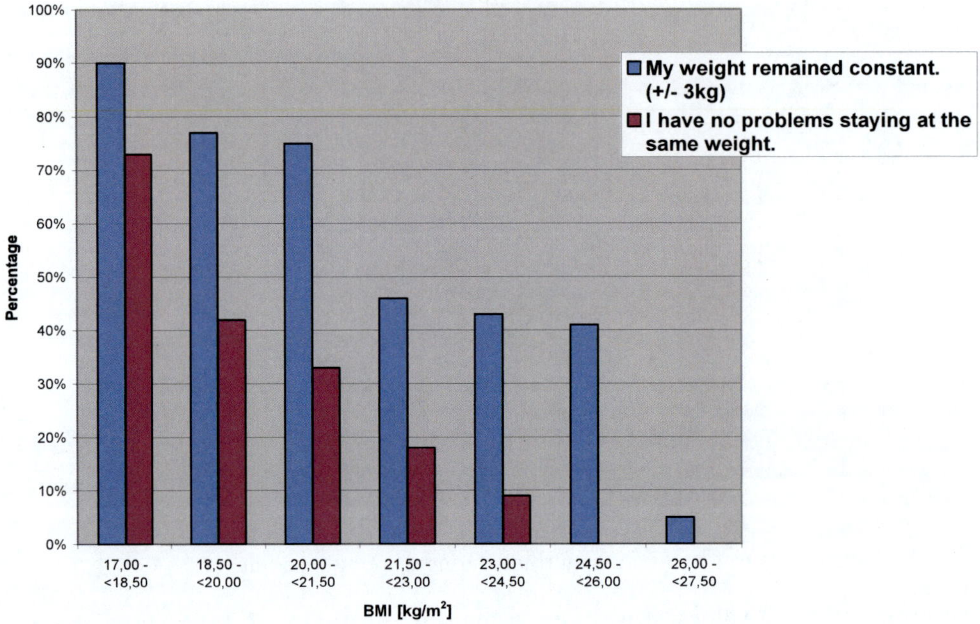

Figure 6. Percentage of participants who declared that their weight remained constant compared to the percentage of participants who said that they have no problem staying at the same weight (related to BMI groups).

DISCUSSION

Attractive – and that usually means, slim – women usually have a better chance of quickly advancing up the corporate ladder (Frieze et al. 1991). One of the women surveyed expressed this sentiment in the following way: "A sporty body suggests vitality, capability and success. This leads people to suppose that one is also full of life and capable of high-performance and success on the job." People believe slim and beautiful women more than they believe other women. It has been shown that slim women have more self-confidence and better communicative skills than other women, which they can use to their advantage in salary negotiations e.g. (Hamermesh and Biddle, 1994; Mobius and Rosenblat, 2006).

We found out that the average BMI of the women executives surveyed, fell in the lower part of normal weight range. In all age groups, the percentage of underweight women was close to more than twice as high as in the average German female population. Similar results were found in Vienna in 2001. The mean BMI value of women executives in the Vienna study was 22.4 kg/m^2 and that is nearly identical to our value (22.2 kg/m^2). Many more women in non-management jobs were found to be overweight than women in executive functions [Stadt Wien, 2001 and 2003].

EATING DISORDERS, THE OTHER SIDE OF OBSESSION WITH SLIMNESS

As written in the DGE-special, journal of the German Nutrition Society (04/2000), "in our slim and beautiful society, being underweight is not seen as a problem. On the contrary, people envy those that are slim. However, the other side of the obsession with slimness is eating disorders." In the headlines of media, you mainly find references to the so-called XXL generation, overweight kids and young persons that do not exercise enough, have poor nutrition habits and in many cases have already been diagnosed with typical subsequent illnesses at a young age. Being overweight and binge eating disorders are one extreme, while being underweight and anorectic eating disorders are on the other extreme.

The Diagnostic and Statistical Manual of Mental Disorders, 4th ed. (DSM IV) differentiates between three groups of eating disorders: anorexia nervosa, bulimia nervosa and other eating disorders not otherwise specified. Such subsyndromal, not otherwise specified eating disorders do not fulfil all criteria of anorexia or bulimia, but are of clinical relevance. This includes a kind of eating behaviour Herman and Mack (1975) called *restrained eating*. Well aware of today's 'slim' obsessed society, even children are beginning to watch and control their weight (Brunner and Franke, 1997). This can be achieved by diets, which, meanwhile, has become a common part of every day life. As reported by Pudel and Westenhöfer (2003), every second women in Germany has dieted at least one time. At first glance, this contradicts our results whereby 70 percent of the women asked said that they had never been on a diet since operating in an executive capacity. Although 60 percent of our subjects told us that their weight remained constant since beginning their jobs as executives, only approximately 42 percent said they had no problem staying at the same weight. The other 58 percent named many reasons why it is not easy for them to maintain their weight. It is evident that many of the women that have been able to maintain a constant weight have only been able to do so with difficulty. In addition, it is interesting to note that eight percent of the subjects said their weight varied greatly; they had lost and gained a large amount of weight. Even most of the BMI values of this eight percent were in the normal area.

′Businesswomen‵ Strive for a BMI in the Lower Part of the Normal Weight Range

"On the one hand, being successful in one's career requires physical resilience and good health. On the other hand, being in a leading position involves long working hours and frequent business trips and dinners that often do not allow for time to exercise or nutritious eating. Striking a balance between professional obligations and staying healthy is often a challenge – but, like other challenges managers and executives face, it is one they should be able to and do overcome." Many of our subjects see themselves in this dilemma and try to solve it in their own way. Many women executives also feel the pressure of living up to the idea that a ′businesswoman‵ has to be slim. Her body is supposed to show that she is managing her body as successfully as her career. She is striving for perfection in any situation in life. The women executives surveyed know that, "Slim women have better career chances, because they are seen as more attractive and healthier…" For most 'business women' being slim means having a BMI in the lower part of the normal weight range. As early as 1987, a study done by Westenhöfer et al. showed that 35000 female readers of a German women's magazine wanted to have an ideal figure with a BMI in the lower part of normal weight range. This shows that overweight women are not the only ones dissatisfied with their weight.

Cognitive Control of Nutrition Habits

In reaching this ideal, most of the women surveyed did not prefer weight reduction diets, which are likely to fail. They prefer a form of diet that they do not consider to be a diet at all; they consciously reduce their intake of food on a long-term basis. Such a long-term pattern of intake of food is characterized by cognitive control and ignoring physiological hunger signals and psychological appetence signals, the result of which is a lower calorie supply that helps to reduce weight and/or stay at the same weight (definition of restrained eating according to Pudel and Westenhöfer, 1989). Typical patterns of behaviour according to the scale of ´Cognitive control of nutrition habits` are to leave out meals, consciously eat smaller portions to avoid weight gain or to classify food according to its calorie content, e.g. For example, some of the women surveyed told us they never eat anything at night. It is typical for these women to say, "I do not have any problems with being overweight because I am not able to have lunch due to time constraints and I am working every weekend." They compensate by eating less or nothing at all in the next few days after business dinners. At least 12 percent of the women executives surveyed said nutrition is a question of self-discipline. They used words like ´control`, ´discipline`, ´will`, and ´staying power`. However, these are the only subjects that explicitly named this aspect in our question asking for a possible connection between career and nutrition. It is likely that a much larger percentage of the women try to maintain their weight through restrained eating - as the difference between the number of women who say they have no problems staying at the same weight and the number of women who say their weight remained constant. Not everyone who skips a meal is considered a ´restrained eater`. However, from a medical perspective, it becomes alarming if this behaviour requires a high behaviour control (Herman and Mack, 1975; Woody et al, 1981; Pudel and Westenhöfer, 1989).

Physiological Mechanism to Regulate Hunger and Fullness Are Disturbed

In cases of restrained eating, physiological mechanisms of appetite, hunger and fullness no longer play any role. Normally appetite and the intake of food are regulated by a complex network of different signals that work together. Such signals are hormones and neurotransmitters. There is scientific data that suggests our brain is programmed to make us feel ´hungry` (Klaus, 2006). This state does not change until the brain records signals of fullness. It takes a considerable amount of psychological work to have hunger signals under cognitive control. The hypothalamus, limbic system and cortex play a crucial role in this process. New studies show that especially brain areas, which are important areas in the reward system, are also important here (Roth, 2006). Neurotransmitters like dopamine and serotonin as well as endogenous opioids and cannabinoids play an important role here.

Disturbances of Eating Behaviour - Inhibition of Cognitive Control

Restrained eating affects the somatic area, resulting in neuroendocrine disturbances and changes in energy metabolism. The effect on the HPA axis caused by restrained eating due to anorexia nervosa is a typical example of this. This condition leads to amenorrhoea and a general form of defeminisation, e.g., an aspect that some ′businesswomen‵ may perhaps unconsciously feel positive about because feminine women have fewer chances to get a leading position (von Rennenkampf, 2004).

There are also consequences of restrained eating in psychical area including cognitive disturbances, affective instability and poor satisfaction of hedonistic needs (de Zwaan, 2006). Due to the disturbance of body image, the persons affected feel too fat even after they permanently loose weight. The absence of hunger and satiety feeling increases the fear of losing control when eating. In some ′restrained eaters‵ this leads to the inhibition of cognitive control and spontaneous attacks of ravenous hunger and eating fits. One distinguishes between different grades of cognitive control. Particularly in case of rigid control intensified hunger for sweets, ravenous hunger, stress forced hunger and/or hunger in case of boredom will appear. In a management environment, ravenous hunger is encouraged by the typical working situation, which is described like this by one of our subjects: "Because of time pressure one is not able to eat calmly. One does not have a normal feeling of satiety. Sometimes there is no ability to have lunch at all, so that when you get home you are totally ravenous and scarf down all the food you can find."

Emotions and Their Influence on the Disturbances of Eating Behaviour

The statistics show that many ′restrained eaters‵ are not successful in controlling their eating behaviour. ′Restrained eaters‵ have a disposition to eat more if they are dysphoric, while unrestrained eaters eat less in this mood (Baucom and Aiken, 1981; Ruderman, 1985). According to Westenhöfer et al. (1987), body weight correlates best with the variable ′Disturbances of eating behaviour‵. Women that practice less restrained eating, but have high disturbances, have the highest body weight. In a survey conducted on the webpage belonging to DEBInet (Gellen, 2003), more than 1000 visitors reported information about their nutrition behaviour. This survey showed that women have values at least twice as high as men on scales for ′cognitive control‵ and ′disturbances‵. People that are underweight only sporadically show a high disturbances level combined with less cognitive control. They probably use other measures, including vomiting or using laxative drugs, to keep their weight low. Most underweight women only have a low disturbances level. It is typical for this group to show severe forms of restrained eating.

Perfectionism and Restrained Eating – A Tool To Make One's Career or a Risk Factor for Developing an Eating Disorder?

Striving for perfectionism, being highly self-motivated and putting forth maximum effort are all beneficial when making one's career, but they can also be relevant risk factors for developing an eating disorder. It is no wonder that the Eating Disorder Inventory-2 (Paul and Thiel, 2004) includes the dimension "perfectionism". Typical characteristics of persons suffering from a restrained form of anorexia nervosa are ambition, discipline, consistency, toughness, intentness of purpose and diligence (Diaz-Marsa et al, 2000; Karwautz et al, 2003). Effort and discipline are very important in order to be successful on the job and to finally reach a leading position. Therefore, it does not surprise us that there are more persons with the characteristic perfectionism in leading positions than on the average in society. It is not uncommon to see a persistent drive towards superior performance and recognition, especially in women that have managed to break the glass ceiling and obtained a leading position (Women in Leadership, 2002). Even the expressions our subjects mentioned above in reference to nutrition, ´control`, ´discipline`, ´will`, and ´staying power`, indicate that perfectionism plays a role in the lives of many of the women executives surveyed.

Probable Health and Psychosocial Consequences of Restrained Eating

Although physical deficiency symptoms may be caused by restrained eating, there are no grounds for assuming that older women have a higher rate of somatic illnesses when they eat in a restrained way, e.g. (Hays et al, 2002). Ford et al. (2001), who analyzed the age and gender corrected data of more than 100000 Americans in 1996, showed an impairment of quality of life only at BMI values of $< 18{,}5$ and ≥ 30 kg/m^2. For Pudel and Westenhöfer (2003) restrained eating is a risk factor for a disturbed eating behaviour. Nevertheless, this does not mean that all the women surveyed who practice restrained eating, have a clinical eating disorder. However, their risk to develop such an eating disorder is greater than in the average population. It has been determined that in underweight women, extreme restrained eating is linked to substantial psycho-mental demands and emotional disturbances as well as to sleep disturbances with exhaustion, poor psychosexual interest, and problems within a partnership. These conditions can lead to impaired physical and mental ability, a decrease in the ability to concentrate and learn, and interaction problems. All of these factors can negatively influence one`s professional and personal life. In practice, it is of bigger importance to note that restrained eating is connected with considerable psycho-mental strain and emotional dysfunction, which may lead to a lower physical and mental ability to cope with pressure and a decline of the ability to concentrate, the ability to learn and the ability to interact socially. Beyond all of this, it may lead to augmented impulse breakthroughs. All these factors may impair the working and social life of a person in the management field.

RESULTS

A result of restrained eating may be mental disturbances. The considerable demands faced by managers every day, are frequently overwhelming. Therefore, it is important to inform all women executives about the bio-psychosocial aspect of working and of having a career if possible. Most women do not realize the central meaning of nutrition in this context. Besides getting a basic nutrition consultation, talking about stress prevention is also an important part of such a consultation. This may take place within circles and forums made up of and for women executives. Company doctors also play an important role in contacting the women in leading positions within their firms. It is important that they offer individual health consultations and advancement opportunities to current and future women executives. In Germany there are enough offers of help and assistance to women with existing eating disorders, however it is feared that these women will not accept help because of their mental state. Company doctors also need to keep an eye on this problem and should offer support if necessary. Up until now, scientific studies on the ′eating behaviour of women executives` hardly existed. The information presented here only gives a small glimpse into this complex field and is meant to serve as a catalyst for further research in this area.

REFERENCES

Alisch K, Winter E, Arentzen U (Hrsg.). *Gabler Wirtschaftslexikon*. Gabler Verlag, Wiesbaden, 16. Aufl. 2005.

Aubele U. Body-Mass-Index – Ergebnisse aus der Mikrozensusbefragung. In: Ernährung in Bayern. Bayerisches Staatsministerium für Umwelt, Gesundheit und Verbraucherschutz; Bayerisches Landesamt für Gesundheit und Lebensmittelsicherheit; Stand Nov 2006: http://www.visernaehrung.bayern.de/de/left/fachinformationen/ernaehrung/uebergewicht/bmi.htm.

Baucom DH, Aiken PA. Effect of depressed mood in eating among obese and nonobese dieting and nondieting persons. *J. Pers. Soc. Psychol.* 1981, 41(3): 577-585.

Brunner E, Franke A. Ess-Störungen. Eine Information für Ärztinnen und Ärzte. Informationsschrift der Deutschen Hauptstelle gegen die Suchtgefahren. Bergisch Gladbach: Media Print, 1997.

Cawley J. Body weight and women`s labor market outcomes. *National Bureau of Economic Research*; NBER Working Papers No. 7841, August 2000.

de Zwaan M. Essstörungen. Folien zur Vorlesung am 29./30.11.2006, Institut für Psychosomatische Medizin und Psychotherapie des Universitätsklinikums Erlangen; Stand Nov. 2006: www.psychosomatik.klinikum.uni-erlangen.de/e1848/e423/inhalt432/EssstoerungenWS06_07.pdf.

DGE (Deutsche Gesellschaft für Ernährung e.V.). Ess-Störungen – die Kehrseite des Schlankheitswahns. DGE spezial 04/2000 vom 06.09.2000; http://www.dge.de/modules.php?name=Newsandfile=printandsid=131 (Stand: Nov. 2006).

Diaz-Marsa M, Carrasco JL, Saiz J. A study of temperament and personality in anorexia and bulimia nervosa. *J. Personal. Disord.* 2000, 14(4): 352-359.

Ford ES, Moriarty DG, Zack MM, Mokdad AH, Chapman DP. Self-reported body mass index and health-related quality of life: findings from the behavioral risk factor surveillance system. *Obesity Research* 2001, 9: 21-31.

Frieze IH, Olson JE, Russell J. Attractiveness and income for men and women in Management. *J. Appl. Social. Psychol.* 1991, 21(13): 1039-1057.

Gellen D. Praxissemesterarbeit über eine Umfrage zum Essverhalten der Besucher der Homepage des Deutschen Ernährungsberatungs- und –informationsnetzes (DEBInet) am Institut für Ernährungsinformation. Hochschule Niederrheim, 2003; Stand Nov. 2006: http://www.ernaehrung.de/aktuell/archiv/ErgebnisUmfrage.htm.

Hamermesh DS, Biddle JE. Beauty and the labor market. *American Economic Review* 1994, 84: 1174-1194.

Hays NP, Bathalon GP, McCrory MA, Roubenoff R, Lipman R, Roberts SB. Eating behavior correlates of adult weight gain and obesity in healthy women aged 55-65 y. The American Journal of Clinical Nutrition 2002, 75(3): 476-483.

Herman CP, Mack D. Restrained and unrestrained eating. *Journal of Personality* 1975; 43(4): 647-660.

Karwautz A, Troop NA, Rabe-Hesketh S, Collier DA, Treasure JL. Personality disorders and personality dimensions in anorexia nervosa. *J. Personal. Disord.* 2003, 17(1): 73-85.

Klaus S. Regulation von Hunger und Sättigung. *Ärztemagazin Phoenix* 4/06, 2006, 4: 4-5.

Mobius MM, Rosenblat TS. Why beauty matters. *American Economic review* 2006, 96(1), 222-235.

Paul T, Thiel A. Eating Disorder Inventory-2. *Deutsche Version*. Hogrefe Verlag, Göttingen, 2004.

Pudel V, Westenhöfer J. Ernährungspsychologie. *Eine Einführung*, Hofgrefe, Göttingen, 3. Aufl., 2003.

Pudel V, Westenhöfer J. Fragebogen zum Eßverhalten (FEV). *Handanweisung*. Hogrefe Verlag, Göttingen, 1989.

Renz U. Schönheit. *Eine Wissenschaft für sich*. Berlin Verlag, Berlin 2006.

Roth G. Fühlen, Denken, Handeln. Wie das Gehirn unser Verhalten steuert. Neue, vollständig überarbeitete Ausgabe. Suhrkamp Verlag, Frankfurt 2003.

Ruderman AJ. Dysphoric mood and overeating: a test of restraint theory`s disinhibition hypothesis. *J. Abnorm. Psychol.* 1985, 94(1): 78-85.

Stadt Wien (Hrsg.), Gesundheit in Wien (Health in Vienna). Wiener Gesundheits- und Sozialsurvey (Vienna Health and Social Survey) AutorInnen: Freidl W, Stronegger W-J, Neuhold Ch, Wien, 2001; www.wien.gv.at/who/survey/ (Stand: Nov. 2006).

Stadt Wien (Hrsg.), Lebensstile in Wien (Lifestyles in Vienna). AutorInnen: Freidl W, Stronegger W-J, Neuhold Ch, Wien, 2003; www.wien.gv.at/who/lebensstile/ (Stand: Nov 2006).

Statistisches Bundesamt Deutschland. Leben in Deutschland – Haushalte, Familien und Gesundheit – Mikrozensus 2005. Körpermaße der Bevölkerung nach Altersgruppen. Ergebnisse der Mikrozensus-Befragung im Jahr 2005; http://www.destatis.de/basis/d/gesu/gesutab8.php (Stand: Nov. 2006).

Volkert D. Der Body-Mass-Index (BMI) – ein wichtiger Parameter zur Beurteilung des Ernährungszustands. *Akt Ernähr Med.* 2006; 31: 126-132.

von Rennenkampf A. Aktivierung und Auswirkungen geschlechtsstereotyper Wahrnehmung von Führungskompetenz im Bewerbungskontext. Dissertation an der Universität Mannheim, Fakultät für Sozialwissenschaften, 2004.

Westenhöfer J, Pudel V, Maus N, Schlaf G. Das kollektive Diätverhalten deutscher Frauen als Risikofaktor für Essstörungen. *Aktuelle Ernährungsmedizin*. 1987, 12: 154-159.

Westenhöfer, J. Dietary restraint and disinhibition: is restraint a homogeneous construct? *Appetite* 1991, 16: 45 – 55.

Westenhöfer, J., Pudel, V. Cognitive control of eating behavior, disinhibition of control, and successful weight reduction [Abstract]. *International Journal of Obesity* 1991, 15(1): 91.

WHO (World Health Organization). Obesity: preventing and managing the global epidemic. *Report of a WHO consultation on obesity*. Geneva: World Health Organisation, 1998.

Women in Leadership: A European Business Imperative. The Catalyst, New York and The Conference Board. Brussels; 2002, www.catalystwomen.org/bookstore/files./exe/WICLEUexesum.pdf.

Woody EZ, Costanzo PR, Liefer H, Conger J. The effect of taste and caloric perceptions on the eating behavior of restrained and unrestrained subjects. *Cognitive Therapy and Research* 1981, 5(4): 381-390.

In: Eating Disorders in Adult Women
Editor: Julian N. Fuchs

ISBN 978-1-60456-673-4

Chapter 12

ACTUAL - DESIRED BMI DISCREPANCY, BODY DISSATISFACTION AND SELF CONCEPT IN WOMEN WITH BULIMIA NERVOSA AND BINGE EATING DISORDER

Giorgio A. Tasca[1,2,3], Louise Balfour[1,2], Kanchan Kurichh[2], Monique Potvin-Kent[2] and Hany Bissada[1,2]
[1]Ottawa Hospital, [2]University of Ottawa, [3]Carleton University

ABSTRACT

It was hypothesized that higher levels of actual-desired BMI discrepency (ADBD) would be associated with higher binge eating symptoms, lower self concept, and higher body dissatisfaction for a clinical sample of women with Bulimia Nervosa (BN) and Binge Eating Disorder (BED). A theoretical frame for ADBD was put forward based on self discrepancy theory. Also hypothesized was that women with BN would have greater eating and self related pathology than those with BED. Fifty-one participants diagnosed with BN and 41 with BED drawn from a clinical sample completed questionnaires assessing eating disorder and general psychopathology. Greater ADBD was related to greater body dissatisfaction for the BN and BED groups, and lower self concept for the BN group. Those with BN had more self-related pathology. ADBD can be easily assessed by clinicians and may be used as an index of body dissatisfaction and overall self concept. ADBD may be a vulnerability factor for developing an eating disorder for women.

Researchers have identified actual-desired body weight discrepancy (ADBD) among those with eating disorders as an important variable in the clinical assessment of eating disorder symptoms (Crowther and Sherwood, 1997), and ADBD has been implicated in the clinical literature in the etiology of Bulimia Nervosa (BN; Casper, 1983). Similarly, Thompson (1996) argued that discrepancies between actual body size and desired body size is an index of body dissatisfaction (Thompson, 1996). Within these clinical conceptualizations of ADBD, there is little theoretical formulation for why this particular discrepancy may have an impact on psychological functioning, well being, and/or eating disorder symptoms. A notable exception is McKinley (1998) who suggested that the negative impact of ADBD on the body esteem of college women is a result of internalized cultural standards encouraging negative body experiences. In general however, the impact of ADBD on eating disorder symptomatology has received little empirical attention.

Tiggeman, Winefield, Winefield and Goldney (1994) looked at the relationship between ADBD and psychological well being among young adults. They found that greater ADBD, defined as Aperceived overweight was related to low self evaluation and to lower levels of psychological well being. In a sample of undergraduate women, McKinley (1998) found that ADBD was related to body esteem and high body shame. She also reported higher ADBD among women than among men. Snyder (1997) found a significant correlation between perceived overweight and the Body Dissatisfaction, Drive for Thinness and Interoceptive Awareness scales of the Eating Disorders Inventory –2 (EDI-2; Garner, 1991). These studies of general population college women were all suggestive of the role of ADBD for a clinical sample of women with eating disorders.

Some studies have looked at ADBD among an eating disordered population. A recent study by Doll and Fairburn (1998) found that women with BN had a greater ADBD than normal controls. Similarly, studies have found that adolescent girls with BN and severe binge eating reported greater ADBD than those with mild binge eating and normal controls (Crowther and Chernyk, 1986; Post and Crowther, 1985). Few studies have looked at the relationship between ADBD and severity of eating disorder symptoms and psychological variables. Heffernen (1996), studied a sample of lesbians with BN, and found a significant correlation between ADBD and body dissatisfaction. Heffernen's (1996) study looked at ADBD as a variable of secondary interest, and did not conceptualize ADBD within a broaden psychological context in order to increase our understanding of ADBD's role in eating disorder pathology.

The current study looked at the importance of assessing for ADBD in a clinical context and developed a conceptual understanding of this variable as a potential risk factor for eating disorders (Casper, 1973). ADBD was seen as important in women with eating disorder symptoms when desired body weight was lower than actual body weight. ADBD was defined as a different but related construct to body dissatisfaction. Body dissatisfaction is specifically related to body shape and size but not necessarily to a self discrepancy. Because ADBD was defined in terms of a discrepancy between one=s weight and one=s personal ideal or what is proscribed as an ideal, then ADBD likely taps into core issues of ideal self image based on personal or cultural standards, and self evaluation (Tiggeman et al., 1994). In this study, ADBD's relationship with eating disorder symptoms and psychological sequelae of eating disorders in a clinical sample of women diagnosed with BN or with BED was studied. First, a theoretical formulation of how ADBD may be an important predictor of eating disorder symptoms and psychological problems in women with BN or BED is proposed. To do so Higgins= (1987) self discrepancy theory is used as a framework.

SELF DISCREPANCY THEORY

There is an increasing consensus in the literature that Western sociocultural values emphasize thinness and appearance for young women (Heffernan, 1996). Striegel-Moore

(1993) argued that the internalization of these values as ideals among women constitute a risk factor for the development of an eating disorder. This may be due to the discrepancy between cultural standards of unrealistic thinness that may be internalized, and actual BMI and body shape that generally do not meet these standards. This discrepancy likely leads to a sense of not living up to a social standard among some women, resulting in further attempts to attain this ideal. With repeated failures at reaching this goal, some women may experience a sense of personal failure, low self esteem, and dissatisfaction with their self and body.

Higgins (1987) proposed similar notions of discrepancy with regard to the self in his self discrepancy theory. Higgins (1987) suggested that there are several domains of self including the actual self, ideal self and ought self. Actual self refers to aspects and attributes of the self that one actually possesses. Ideal self refers to aspect or attributes that one would like to possess. Ought self refers to aspects or attributes that one believes one should possess. Ideal self and ought self are self guides that are personal standards that people set up. These standards may be those established as important by others, or may be internally held standards, or both. For the purposes of this study, a culturally sanctioned ideal of thinness is seen as a self guide (i.e. ought self), especially if it has been internalized by women (i.e. ideal self).

Moretti and Higgins (1990) found that discrepancies between self guides and actual self can lead to emotional distress and potential emotional problems; the greater the discrepancy, the greater the distress and problems. In a study looking at self discrepancy among college women, Strauman, Vookles, Berenstein, Chaiken, and Higgins (1991) found that self discrepencies were related to body dissatisfaction and maladaptive eating in female college students. Snyder (1997) found significant correlations between actual - ideal self discrepancies and body dissatisfaction even after actual BMI was controlled.

Body weight and weight related self perceptions are integral parts of the experience of the self for women with eating disorders. The emphasis and importance placed on actual weight is a pivotal part of the disorder. Just as the discrepancy between actual self and self guides is related to psychological distress, problems with self concept, and eating disorder related psychopathology (Snyder, 1997; Strauman et al, 1991), we hypothesized that the discrepancy between actual and desired BMI for women with BN and BED will be related to eating disorder symptoms, body dissatisfaction, and low self concept. ADBD represents a tangible parallel to actual-desired self discrepancies that is particularly salient to women who are vulnerable to eating disorders. Because of the parallel, ADBD could represent a core self related construct for those with eating disorders. Although one could argue that body dissatisfaction may imply some discrepancy from an ideal or standard, ADBD is a more direct measure of such a discrepancy.

Bulimia Nervosa and Binge Eating Disorder

BED has recently been included as a diagnosis requiring further research in the Diagnostic and Statistical Manual for Mental Disorders (DSM-IV; APA, 1994). Research has indicated that in a community sample (Hay and Fairburn, 1998) and in a clinical sample (Tasca, Wood, Demidenko, Bissada, 2002) those with BED had lower levels of psychopathology than those with BN. Other researchers have found those with BED to be distinct from obese controls, and to be a homogeneous group on a number of variables. For example, obese people who binge eat compared to obese people who do not binge eat show greater psychopathology (Marcus, Wing, Ewing, Kern, Gooding and McDermott, 1990), greater eating pathology (Yanovski, Nelson, Dubbert, and Spitzer, 1993), lower self esteem and greater discrepancy between their current and ideal body size (Striegel-Moore, Wilson, Wilfley, Elder, and Brownell, 1998). Although Striegel-Moore et al, (1998) found greater body dissatisfaction among binge eaters than controls, other studies have not found the same result (de Zwaan et al, 1994; Antoniou, Tasca, Bissada, and Balfour, 2002). Binge eating is a symptom held in common between BN and BED and often the criteria for evaluating binge eating is similar for both disorders (Walsh and Garner, 1997). Problems with self esteem and self concept are also shared among these disorders (Striegel-Moore, et al., 1998). Body image disturbance and dissatisfaction is a hallmark symptom of BN (Kearney-Cook and Striegel-Moore, 1997).

Hypotheses

The first hypothesis for this study was that a greater ADBD, where actual body weight is greater than desired body weight, will be associated with greater binge eating symptoms, lower self concept, and greater body dissatisfaction for women in the BN and BED groups. Second, women with BN will exhibit more eating disorder and self related problems than women with BED on the measures used in this study. We predict that those with BN will have greater ADBD, more binge eating symptoms, lower self concept and greater body dissatisfaction than women with BED.

Method

Participants

A total of 92 women were assessed as part of this study. These were patients referred by family physicians to a consultation service of a center for the treatment of eating disorders in a medium sized urban setting. Of the 92, 51 patients met diagnostic criteria for BN and 41 met diagnostic criteria for BED. Table 1 presents diagnostic and demographic data of these patients. Results of univariate comparisons of these variables will be discussed below.

Procedure

Patients were assessed by a psychiatrist or a psychologist. Just prior to the consultation, patients completed a battery of tests including the Eating Disorders Inventory-2 (EDI-2; Garner, 1991), the Personality Assessment Inventory (PAI; Morey, 1991), and the Diagnostic Survey of Eating Disorders (DSED; adapted from Johnson and Connors, 1987). They were then given a DSM-IV multiaxial diagnosis by the psychiatrist or psychologist (APA, 1994). A referral to one of several treatment options offered by the Center or in the community was often suggested. As a validation check on the diagnosis, 10% of all initial consultations (N = 210) referred to the Center were randomly selected and re-evaluated by an independent clinician blind to the diagnosis. Identifying information and diagnostic conclusions were removed from the re-evaluated reports. Agreement between the independent clinician and the original diagnosis was 86% suggesting a high level of agreement.

Table 1. Demographic and Clinical Data for Women With Bulimia Nervosa (BN) and Binge Eating Disorder (BED), With Univariate Comparisons and Effect Size (d).

	BN (*n*=51)		BED (*n*=41)				
	M	*sd*	*M*	*sd*	*F*	*p*	*d*
Age	30.81	8.85	40.88	9.92	27.33	<.001	.95
Actual BMI	28.59	7.28	41.74	9.41	58.84	<.001	1.24
Desired BMI	22.76	3.21	27.20	5.37	31.63	<.001	.91
ADBD	17.69	13.02	33.15	12.07	35.47	<.001	1.04
Binge Episodes in 28 days	16.96	15.94	16.98	20.31	.00	.997	.00
Binge Days in 28 days	14.95	9.52	14.37	9.64	.07	.786	.06
Body Dissatisfaction	21.02	6.90	22.57	5.40	1.41	.238	- .25
Self Concept Factor	2.86	.93	3.34	1.01	5.69	.019	.48
High Self Esteem (Man-G)	45.51	11.02	46.58	12.09	0.18	.714	- .09
Low Self Efficacy (DEP-C)	73.79	17.24	65.93	16.91	4.96	.028	.45
Identity Instability (BOR-I)	70.89	11.75	61.81	13.50	12.26	.001	.68

Note: Effect sizes (*d*) are small (>.20), medium (>.50) or large (>.80) effects (Cohen, 1988).

MEASURES

Actual-Desired BMI Discrepancy (ADBD).

Actual height and body weight were measured at the time of assessment and Body Mass Index (BMI; k/m^2) was calculated from these. As part of the DSED, patients were asked what their desired weight was. Based on this and their actual height, a desired BMI was calculated, and then desired BMI was subtracted from actual BMI. To control for the effect of actual body weight, the difference between actual and desired BMI was divided by actual BMI. The result was multiplied by 100 so that ADBD was expressed as a percent deviation from actual BMI ([actual BMI - desired BMI / actual BMI] x 100).

Binge Eating Symptoms

Objective binges were assessed using the criteria outlined in the Eating Disorder Examination (EDE; Fairburn and Cooper, 1993). Consistent with DSM-IV (APA, 1994), frequency of binges were used for the BN group and days binged was used for the BED group. The number of symptoms over the past 28 days were counted using a calendar recall method.

Body Dissatisfaction

The Body Dissatisfaction Scale of the EDI-2 (Garner, 1991) is a 9-item scale that measures dissatisfaction with overall shape and size. Internal consistency was reported at alpha = .92 (Garner, 1991).

Self Concept

Morey (1996) described self concept to encompass domains of self esteem, stability of identity, and self efficacy. Self Concept was measured by using three scales from the Personality Assessment Inventory (PAI; Morey, 1991). The Mania - Grandiosity (MAN-G) scale was used to assess self esteem, as an evaluative component of self perception. The Depression - Cognitive (DEP-C) scale measured personal competence and perceived control, and is considered a measure of self efficacy (Morey, 1991). Stability of identity was measured by the Borderline - Identity Problems (BOR-I) scale and represents vulnerability to environmental stressors. Morey (1996) looked at the configuration of scores on these three scales to assess self concept. High self concept is suggested by high scores on MAN-G and low scores on DEP-C and BOR-I. Low self concept is suggested by low scores on MAN-G, and high scores on DEP-C and BOR-I. Tasca, et al. (2002) report adequate psychometric properties of PAI scales and subscales for eating disordered populations.

RESULTS

Initial Inspection of the Data

There were no univariate or multivariate outliers in the data, all variables had acceptable distributions, and there was no multicolinearity among dependent variables. Table 2 shows the zero order Pearson Product Moment correlations among the variables for each diagnostic group.

SELF CONCEPT FACTOR

As stated, Morey (1996) suggested an analysis of the configuration of three PAI scales in order to assess self concept. However, this approach does not easily lend itself to using self concept as a continuous variable in a data analysis. Therefore, a self concept factor was created by conducting a principal components factor analysis with no rotation of the MAN-G, DEP-C and BOR-I scales of the PAI (Morey, 1991) for both the BN group and the BED group. As expected, and consistent with Morey's (1996) conceptualization, one factor emerged for the BN and BED groups separately accounting for 59.15% and 65.26% of the variance respectively. Also as expected, the component matrix had the MAN-G load negatively (-.65 and -.60 respectively), the DEP-C scale load positively (.93 and .94 respectively), and the BOR-I scale load positively, (.70 and .84 respectively). These findings are consistent with Morey's (1996) configural approach but allows for a single score representing self concept for each participant. Scores on the self concept factor were reversed so that low scores on this factor represents low self concept and high scores represent high self concept.

Table 2. Correlations among variables for women with Bulimia Nervosa (BN) and Binge Eating Disorder (BED) groups.

	ADBD		Binge Symptoms[1]		Body Dissatisfaction	
	BN (n=51)	BED (n=41)	BN	BED	BN	BED
Binge Symptoms[1]	-.093	.261				
Body Dissatisfaction	.465* *	.427**	.175	-.062		
Self Concept	-.284*	-.298	-.100	-.223	-.263	-.309*

[1]Binge symptoms for BN are binge episodes in 28 days, and for BED are binge days in 28 days.
*$\underline{p}$<.05, **$\underline{p}$<.01The SPSS General Linear Model (GLM) program was used to perform an overall multivariate analysis among ADBD and all the other variables for each diagnotic group. Individual Pearson correlations were calculated to assess for the relationship between ADBD and the number of binge episodes in the past 28 days (for the BN group), days binged in the past 28 days (for the BED group), the EDI-2 Body Dissatisfaction Scale, and the PAI Self Concept Factor for the BN and BED groups separately.

Actual-Desired BMI Difference

Bulimia Nervosa Group

Using the Wilks' criterion, the combined variables (binge episodes, body dissatisfaction and self concept) were significantly related to the parameter ADBD for the BN group, approximate $F(3, 47) = 5.395$, $\underline{p} < .003$. There was a strong association between ADBD and the combined dependent variables ($\eta^2 = .26$) (Cohen, 1988). Table 2 shows the correlations between ADBD and individual variables for the BN group. Higher ADBD was significantly related to higher scores on the Body Dissatisfaction Scale and lower scores on the Self Concept Factor. ADBD was not significantly associated with binge episodes for the BN group.

Binge Eating Disorder Group

The Wilks' criterion suggested that the combined variables (binge days, body dissatisfaction, and self concept) were significantly related to ADBD for the BED group, approximate $F(3, 37) = 3.791$, $\underline{p} < .018$. There was a strong association between ADBD and the combined dependent variables ($\eta^2 = .26$) (Cohen, 1988). Table 2 shows the individual bivariate correlations between ADBD and each of the other variables. Higher ADBD was significantly associated with higher scores on the Body Dissatisfaction Scale. The correlation approached significance for the relationship between ADBD and the Self Concept Factor. ADBD was not significantly associated with days binged for the BED group.

Comparing Bulimia Nervosa to Binge Eating Disorder

As indicated in Table 1, those with BN were significantly younger, had a lower actual BMI and lower desired BMI than those with BED. Because older patients may weigh more, age was covaried when the groups were compared on actual BMI. The difference in actual BMI remained significant even when age was covaried in an ANCOVA ($F(3,88) = 55.50$, $p < .001$). Those with BED had a significantly higher ADBD than those with BN (Table 1). In this study, ADBD was calculated as the percent discrepancy from actual BMI, so it is possible that the higher BMI of those with BED may account for this difference. To test this, an ANCOVA covarying actual BMI was conducted. When the variance accounted for by actual BMI was covaried, there was no significant difference on ADBD between those with BN and those with BED ($F(3,88) = .083$, $p > .05$). That is, any difference in ADBD is likely due to those with BED weighing significantly more than those with BN, and so the percent discrepancy can be accounted for by the initial difference in weight between the two groups. There were no differences between the BN and BED groups on measures of binge episodes or binge days. There was also no significant difference between the two groups on the Body Dissatisfaction scale.

On the overall Self Concept Factor derived from the PAI, those with BN had significantly lower self concept than the BED group. When the individual scales making up that factor were considered (Table 1), it was apparent that the BN group had lower self efficacy (DEP-C), and greater identity instability (BOR-I). There were no differences in level of self esteem (MAN-G) between the two groups.

Discussion

This study looked at ADBD among women with BN and BED, and conceptualized the impact of ADBD on eating disordered women within the framework of self discrepancy theory (Higgins, 1987). Despite clinical references to the importance of ADBD (Crowther and Sherwood, 1997), this is the first known attempt to look directly at the relationship between ADBD and eating disorder related psychopathology in a clinical sample. The hypothesis that ADBD would be related to higher eating disorder symptoms, higher body dissatisfaction and lower self concept in women with BN and BED was partially supported. It was clear that for the BN group, greater ADBD was significantly related to body dissatisfaction and low self concept. For the BED group, greater ADBD was associated with greater body dissatisfaction, and there was a trend toward a correlation with low self concept.

In self discrepancy theory (Higgins, 1987) greater actual self vs ideal self dicrepancies predict more emotional discomfort and distress (Moretti and Higgins, 1990). This appears to be paralleled in the ADBD of our eating disordered samples. ADBD likely results in a number of vulnerabilities such as a sense of personal shortcomings and personal dissatisfaction, especially for eating disordered women for whom body weight and shape are so crucial to self evaluation. In light of internalized social ideals of thinness for women with eating disorders (Striegel-Moore, 1993), and given the results of this study, ADBD may be viewed as a potential vulnerability factor for women in developing BN and BED. Prospective studies among adolescent girls using ADBD would provide a stronger test of this hypothesis.

ADBD was not related to binge eating symptoms for either the BN or BED groups, and so no support was found for this hypothesis. It is possible that while ADBD is related to self related experiences, such as body dissatisfaction and self concept, it may not be directly related to symptoms of binge eating.

Comparing Bulimia Nervosa and Binge Eating Disorder

The clearest difference between the two diagnostic groups in this study was on self concept, with women with BN having lower self concept as measured by the PAI (Morey, 1991; Morey, 1996). Specifically, those with BN had greater identity instability (BOR-I) and lower self efficacy (DEP-C). This suggested greater self related problems and pathology among those with BN as compared to women with BED. This is consistent with reports in the literature indicating that BN is a more severe disorder than BED (Hay and Fairburn, 1998; Tasca, et al., 2002), and that there is a high comorbid diagnosis of self related pathology, such as borderline personality disorder, among those with BN (Dennis and Sansone, 1991; Rossiter, Agras, Telch and Schneider, 1993). Had this study focused on self esteem (e.g. MAN-G) only, differences between groups would not have emerged. This is consistent with a study finding no differences between eating disorder diagnostic groups on two measures of self esteem (Griffiths, et al., 1999). The Self Concept Factor, allowed for differences to emerge among the diagnostic groups by defining self related problems in broader terms that includes self esteem, identity stability and self efficacy. This broader self construct may be more meaningful to the understanding of an eating disordered population than self esteem alone.

There were no differences between the BN and BED groups on the number of binge episodes or days binged over the previous 28-day period. This is consistent with previous research that found no difference in the number of objective binges between BN and BED samples (Hay and Fairburn, 1998). The means for these two groups in this study were almost identical (Table 1). This result does not support the notion that BED is a less severe than BN when it comes to objective binge eating symptoms.

Our study did not find differences in body dissatisfaction between those with BED and BN. In addition, both diagnostic groups had mean Body Dissatisfaction Scale scores above the clinical cutoff for the EDI-2 (Garner, 1991), suggesting severe problems in this area for the majority of women in both groups. This result is consistent with the work of Striegel-Moore, et al (1998) who found greater body dissatisfaction among obese binge eaters than controls. The results of this study also indicated that body dissatisfaction among these eating disordered samples were related to ADBD and their associated self discrepancies.

Self Concept Factor

To our knowledge this is the first report in the literature using self concept as defined by the PAI (Morey, 1991) with an eating disordered population. As stated, our results suggested that this broader construct may be more meaningful to the study of an eating disordered population that self esteem alone. Furthermore, this is the first report to create a self concept factor based on the configural analysis of self concept from the PAI as suggested by Morey (1996). The prinicpal components analysis produced a factor with loadings from the component scales (MAN-G, DEP-C, and BOR-I) that parallel Morey=s (1996) configural interpretation of those scales. The advantage of using this approach is that it allows for the creation of a single continuous variable measuring self concept that lends itself to multifactorial analysis. The disadvantage is that unique information provided by the individual component scales gets diluted within the overall factor score.

Clinical Implications of ADBD

Using 95% confidence intervals, cutoffs for the percent deviation from individuals= actual BMI were calculated. In our sample, if an individual with BN had a desired BMI that was less than 21% of their actual BMI, then it would be considered clinically significant. For example, the mean actual BMI in our sample of women with BN was 28.59. A clinical cutoff could be established so that a patient with BN who had a BMI of 28.59 and a desired BMI of 22.59 (21% below actual BMI for the BN group) or less would have a 95% probability of having problems with body dissatisfaction and low self concept. Interestingly, in our BN sample, the mean desired BMI was 22.76, which is almost exactly 21% below the mean BMI for the BN group. Clinicians could easily calculate the percent deviation from actual BMI, use the clinical cutoffs suggested by our sample, and have an index of how problematic body dissatisfaction and self concept are for those with BN. Similar calculations could be made for the BED group for whom a desired BMI of less than 37% of actual BMI would be considered clinically significant.

Limitations and Future Research

The small sample size of the BED group may have reduced the power of some of the analyses. This is particularly apparent in Table 2 where correlations between binge symptoms for the BN group is significantly correlated with Self Concept (r = -.284), but a slightly higher correlation within the BED groups for the same variables(r = -.298) was not statistically significant.

Given that ADBD was related to eating disorder related variables in these clinical samples, it would be interesting to see if this discrepancy predicted problems with self concept, body dissatisfaction, mood, and other psychological variables in a female sample in the general population. One would expect a similar pattern of results in a general population as well. However, the relationship between ADBD likely will be more salient within the clinical and subclinical range of that population. Longitudinal research starting with an adolescent sample and then following that sample could be done to see if ADBD is a risk factor for developing an eating disorder. We do not expect ADBD to be as important an issue for men since cultural standards of unrealistic thinness is more likely to occur with women (Striegel-Moore, 1993), and McKinley (1998) found higher ADBD among women. If, as our theory suggests, ADBD is a core self discrepancy that leads to negative mood and eating disorder symptoms, then we would expect ADBD to be a risk factor for developing an eating disorder for young women but not necessarily for men. For men, issues related to ideal body shape (e.g. muscle and low body fat percentage) and not body weight per se may be a more important variable predicting self concept and eating disorder related symptoms.

Conclusion

A theory of ADBD as a self discrepancy is presented that may represent a risk factor for eating disorders among women. Self discrepancy theory suggests that a greater discrepancy between actual self and ideal self leads to greater distress and emotional problems (Moretti and Higgins, 1990). Similarly, the results of this study indicated that ADBD is associated with lower self concept and greater body dissatisfaction. ADBD could be an issue targeted in the assessment and treatment of women with BN, and also for those with BED. Its assessment is relatively straight forward, and the 95% confidence intervals presented here could be used as cutoffs for clinical samples. Targeting ADBD in treatment by focusing on its relevance to eating disordered individuals, its impact on feelings about their body, and its impact on self concept may allow women with eating disorders to begin to moderate the effects of these discrepancies. The impact of ADBD found in this study continue to lend importance to the notion that the internalization of culturally sanctioned ideals of thinness (Striegel-Moore, et al., 1998) are corrosive to women=s body and self esteem (McKinley, 1998).

References

American Psychiatric Association (1994). *Diagnostic and statistical manual of mental disorders* (4th ed.). Washington, DC: Author.

Antoniou, M., Tasca, G.A., Wood, J., Bissada, H. (2003). Binge Eating Disorder versus overeating: A failure to replicate and common factors in severely obese treatment seeking women. *Eating and Weight Disorders, 8,* 145-149.

Brownell, K.D., and Rodin, J. (1994). The dieting maelstrom. *American Psychologist, 49,* 781-791.

Casper, R.A. (1983). On the emergence of Bulmia Nervosa as a syndrome: A historical view. *International Journal of Eating Disorders, 2,* 3-16.

Cohen, J. (1988). *Statistical power analysis for the behavioral sciences.* (2nd ed.). Hillsdale, NJ: Earlbaum.

Crowther, J.H. and Chernyk, B. (1986). Bulimia and binge eating in adolescent females: A comparison. *Addictive Behaviors, 11,* 415-424.

Crowther, J.H and Sherwood, N.E. (1997). Assessment. In D.M. Garner and P.E. Garfinkel (Eds.) *Handbook of treatment for eating disorders*. New York: Guilford.

Dennis, A.B. and Sansone, R.A. (1991). The clinical stages of treatment for the eating disorder patient with borderline personality disorder. In C. Johnson (Ed.) *Psychodynamic treatment of anorexia nervosa and bulimia*. New York: Guilford.

de Zwaan, M., Mitchell, J.E., Seim, H.C., Specker, S.M.., Pyle, R.L., Raymond, N.C. and Crosby, R.B. (1994). Eating related and general psychopathology in obese women with binge eating disorder. *International Journal of Eating Disorders, 15*, 43-52.

Doll, H.A. and Fairburn, C.G. (1998). Heightened accuracy of self-reported weight in bulimia nervosa: A useful cognitive Adistortion. *International Journal of Eating Disorders, 24*, 267-273.

Fairburn, C.G. and Cooper, Z. (1993). The Eating Disorder Examination (12th Ed.). In C.G. Fairburn, and G.T. Wilson (Eds.) *Binge eating: Nature, assessment, and treatment*. New York: Guilford.

Garner, D. (1991). *Eating Disorders Inventory-2 Professional Manual*. Odessa, FL: Psychological Assessment Resources.

Griffiths, R.A., Beumont, P.J., Giannakopoulos, E., Russell, J., Schotte, D., Thornton, C., Touyz, S.W., Varano, P. (1999). Measuring self-esteem in dieting disordered patients: The validity of the Rosenberg and Coopersmith contrasted. *International Journal of Eating Disorders, 25*, 227-231.

Hay, P. and Fairburn, C.G. (1998). The validity of the DSM-IV scheme for classifying bulimic eating disorders. *International Journal of Eating Disorders, 23*, 7-15.

Heffernen, K. (1996). Eating disorders and weight concern among lesbians. *International Journal of Eating Disorders, 19*, 127-138.

Higgins, E.T. (1987). Self-discrepancy: A theory relating self and affect. *Psychological Review, 94*, 319-340.

Johnson, C. and Connors, M.E. (1987). *The etiology and treatment of bulimia nervosa: A biopsychosocial approach*. New York: Basic.

Kearney-Cook, A., and Striegel-Moore, R. (1997). The etiology and treatment of body image disturbance. In D.M. Garner and P.E. Garfinkel (Eds.) *Handbook of treatment for eating disorders*. New York: Guilford.

McKinley, N.M. (1998). Gender differences in undergraduates= body esteem: The mediating effect of objectified body consciousness and actual/ideal weight discrepancy. *Sex Roles, 39*, 113-123.

Marcus, M.D., Wing, R.R., Ewing, L., Kern, E., Gooding, W., and McDermott, M. (1990). Psychiatric disorders among obese binge eaters and non-binge eaters. *International Journal of Eating Disorders, 9*, 69-77.

Moretti, M.M., and Higgins, E.T. (1990). Relating self-discrepancy to self-esteem: The contribution of discrepancy beyond actual-self ratings. *Journal of Experimental Social Psychology, 26*, 108-123.

Morey, L.C. (1991). *Personality assessment inventory*. Odessa, FL: Psychological Assessment Resources.

Morey, L.C. (1996). *An interpretive guide to the personality assessment inventory (PAI)*. Odessa, FL: Psychological Assessment Resources.

Post, G., and Crowther, J.H. (1985). Variables that discriminate bulimic from nonbulimic adolescent females. *Journal of Youth and Adolescence, 14*, 85-98.

Rossiter, E.M., Agras, W.S., Telch, C.F., and Schneider, J.A. (1993). Cluster B personality disorder characteristics predict outcome in treatment of bulimia nervosa. *International Journal of Eating Disorders, 13*, 267-274.

Snyder, R. (1997). Self discrepancy theory, standards for body evaluation, and eating disorder symptomatology among college women. *Women and Health, 26*, 69-84.

Strauman, T.J., Vookles, J., Berenstein, V., Chaiken, S., and Higgins, E.T. (1991). Self-discrepancies and vulnerability to body dissatisfaction and disordered eating. *Journal of Personality and Social Psychology, 61*, 946-956.

Striegel-Moore, R.H. (1993). Etiology of binge eating disorder: A developmental perspective. In C.G. Fairburn and G.T. Wilson (Eds.) *Binge eating: Nature, assessment, and treatment*. New York: Guilford.

Striegel-Moore, R.H., Wilson, G.T., Wilfley, D.E., Elder, K.A., and Brownell, K.D. (1998). Binge eating in an obese community sample. *International Journal of Eating Disorders, 23,* 27-37.

Tasca, G.A., Wood, J., Demidenko, N., and Bissada, H. (2002). Using the PAI in an eating disordered population: Scale characteristics and differences among diagnostic groups. *Journal of Personality Assessment, 79*, 337-356.

Thompson, J.K. (1996). Assessing body image disturbance: Measures, methodology and implementation. In J.K. Thompson (Ed.) *Body image, eating disorders and obesity: An integrative guide for assessment and treatment.* Washington, DC: American Psychological Association.

Tiggeman, M.., Winefield, H.R., Winefield, A.H., and Goldney, R.D. (1994). Gender differences in the psychological correlates of body-weight in young adults. *Psychology and Health, 9*, 345-351.

Walsh, B.T., and Garner, D.M. (1997). Diagnostic issues. In D.M. Garner and P.E. Garfinkel (Eds.) *Handbook of treatment for eating disorders*. New York: Guilford.

Yanovski, S.Z., Nelson, J.E., Dubbert, B.K., and Spitzer, R.L. (1993). Association of binge eating disorder and psychiatric comorbidity in obese subjects. *American Journal of Psychiatry, 150*, 1472-1479.

INDEX

A

B

C

D

E

H

I

J

K

L

M

N

S

T

U